Color Atlas of Uveitis

(Second Edition)

Joseph B. Michelson, MD, FACS
Director, Retina-Uveitis Service
Head, Division of Ophthalmology
SCRIPPS CLINIC and RESEARCH FOUNDATION
La Jolla, California, USA

Consultant in Retina
U.S. Naval Regional Medical Center, San Diego

Mosby Year Book

St. Louis   Baltimore   Boston   Chicago   London   Philadelphia   Sydney   Toronto

Mosby–Year Book, Inc.
11830 Westline Drive
St. Louis, MO 63146

Copyright © Wolfe Publishing Ltd, 1992
All rights reserved.
Published in 1992 with rights in the USA, Canada and Puerto Rico by Mosby–Year Book, Inc.

ISBN 0-8151-5872-6

First published in 1980 by Wolfe Publishing Ltd,
2–16 Torrington Place, London WC1E 7LT, UK.

All rights reserved. No part of this publication may be reproduced, stored in a retrieval system, or transmitted, in any form or by any means, electronic, mechanical, photocopying, recording, or otherwise, without written permission from the publisher.

Permission to photocopy or reproduce solely for internal or personal use is permitted for libraries or other users registered with the Copyright Clearance Center, provided that the base fee of $4.00 per chapter plus $.10 per page is paid directly to the Copyright Clearance Center, 21 Congress Street, Salem, MA 01970. This consent does not extend to other kinds of copying, such as copying for general distribution, for advertising or promotional purposes, for creating new collected works, or for resale.

Library of Congress Cataloging-in-Publication Data has been applied for.

Contents

The Classification of Uveitis	5
Signs of Uveitis	6
Rheumatoid Arthritis	37
Juvenile Rheumatoid Arthritis	41
Ankylosing Spondylitis	45
Reiter's Disease	47
Sarcoidosis	49
Acquired Immune Deficiency Syndrome (AIDS)	55
Lyme Disease	59
Syphilis	63
Collagen Vascular diseases (*Connective Tissue Inflammation*)	65
Vogt–Koyanagi–Harada Syndrome	69
Uveal Effusion	75
Presumed Ocular Histoplasmosis	77
Coccidioidomycosis	83
Ocular Toxocariasis	85
Toxoplasmosis	91
Behçet's Disease	97
Reticulum Cell Sarcoma	103
Mycobacteria	109
Herpes Virus	115
Cytomegalic Virus Inclusion Disease (CID)	119
Serpiginous Choroidopathy (*Geographic Choroiditis, Helicoid Choroiditis*)	121
Subacute Sclerosing Panencephalitis (SSPE)	124
Pars Planitis (*Peripheral Uveitis, Chronic Cyclitis*)	125
Acute Multifocal Placoid Pigment Epitheliopathy (AMPPE)	127
Multiple Evanescent White Dot Syndrome (MEWDS)	129
Bilateral Acute Retinal Necrosis (*BARN Syndrome or ARN Syndrome*)	131
Birdshot Choroidopathy	133
Fuchs' Heterochromic Iridocyclitis	135
Relapsing Polychondritis	137
Drug Abuse	139
Natural and Intraocular Lenses	145
References	147
Index	153

To Karen, Kerith, Seth, and Matthew, as always.

The content and spirit of this volume are also dedicated to Michael A. Bedford, Jerry A. Shields, and G. Richard O'Connor and Robert A. Nozik to whom I owe so much.

The Classification of Uveitis

The accurate diagnosis of uveitis is important because treatments for different types of uveitis can vary considerably. For example, the typical iridocyclitis of juvenile rheumatoid arthritis is chronic and would require the judicious application of steroids. Steroid overdose would lead to cataract and glaucoma. Certain other arthritic uveitides, however, like ankylosing spondylitis or Reiter's disease are acute and intermittent in their nature and may require aggressive, short-term application of steroids. Reticulum cell sarcoma and other pseudoinflammations that present as uveitis and represent the masquerade syndrome of a malignant infiltrate necessitate irradiation and chemotherapy. Other of the uveitides, such as pars planitis, may require no treatment at all; or as in the case of a toxoplasmic retinochoroiditis, which is quite peripheral to the macula and disc, the physician may choose no treatment as the course of best judgement.

Several steps must be taken to properly classify a case of uveitis. The proper naming of the inflammation's anatomic distribution as an iritis, 'cyclitis,' vitreitis, pars planitis, intermediate uveitis, retinitis, choroiditis, chorioretinitis, retinal-choroiditis, choroiditis or panuveitis is the all-important first step in assessing the type of uveitis present. The second step is to describe the disorder as acute, chronic, acute and intermittent, etc., and to determine the pertinent characteristics of it. The next step is to look for specific details that may be idiosyncratic to a certain type of inflammation.

All of the diagnostic considerations can be included in the patient's physical description. An example of this would be a chronic iridocyclitis in a child with arthritis in the hand. This description indicates chronic for the chronicity, iridocyclitis for the location, and a child with arthritis for the pertinence. This description would easily lead to a diagnosis of juvenile rheumatoid arthritis type of inflammation. Similarly, a chronic bilateral diffuse granulomatous uveitis with retinal vasculitis (predominantly a phlebitis) in a black woman might specifically implicate sarcoidosis, and very few other entities need be considered. Another example might be a chronic unilateral iridocyclitis with secondary cataract, open angle glaucoma, and heterochromia in a 34-year-old white man. All of these clinical signs would indicate a Fuch's heterochromic cyclitis. An even more dramatic description is a chronic bilateral diffuse granulomatous recurrent uveitis with serious macular detachment in a 32-year-old Japanese with alopecia areata, tinnitis, and dizziness. Such a description suggests a Vogt–Koyanagi–Harada disease. These considerations, based on the specific location of inflammation, the chronicity, and the other pertinent characteristics gleaned from the history yield a simple naming and meshing technique for the firsthand suggestive diagnosis of uveitis as promulgated by Nozik, *et al.* The diagnostic considerations lead to a proper categorization of uveitis.

It is the goal of this atlas to demonstrate those uveitic signs that will familiarize the reader with specific common uveitis disease entities so he can diagnose accurately and treat these very complicated ophthalmologic disorders. The meshing of clinical signs base upon the history and a considered differential diagnostic list used to evaluate special laboratory tests and consultations should determine the ultimate and accurate diagnosis.

CLASSIFICATION OF UVEITIS

	granulomatous/nongran	unilat/bilateral
Rheumatoid arthritis: acute iridocyclitis,	ng,	b
Juvenile rheum. arth: chronic iridocyclitis	ng,	b
Ankylosing spondylitis: acute, recurrent i-c	ng	b
Reiter's disease: acute iridocyclitis	ng	b
Sarcoidosis: any pattern inflammation (predominant retinal phlebitis)	g,	b
AIDs: retinitis (CMV, pneumocystis, lues)	g,	b
Lyme disease: vasculitis, papillitis	ng,	b
Syphilis: any pattern inflammation	g,	b
Collagen vascular disease: vasculitis, i-c	ng,	b
Vogt–Koyanagi–Harada disease: pan-uveitis (exudative retinal detachment)	g,	b
Uveal effusion: exudative ret. detachment	ng,	b
Presumed Ocular Histoplasmosis: choroiditis (sub retinal neovascularization)	g,	b

	granulomatous/ nongran	unilat/ bilateral		granulomatous/ nongran	unilat/ bilateral
Coccidioidomycosis: acute choroiditis	g,	b	choroiditis	ng,	b
Ocular Toxocariasis: retinal abscess	g,	u	Subacute Sclerosing Panencephalitis: acute choroiditis/retinitis	g,	u or b
Toxoplasmosis: pure retinitis first, acute	g,	u or b	Intermediate uveitis (pars plantis): recurrent vitritis, cystoid macular edema	ng,	u or b
Behçet's disease: i-c, retinitis, vasculitis	ng,	b	AMPPE: acute ret. pigment epitheliitis	ng,	b
Reticulum cell sarcoma: vitritis, choroidal infiltrate	ng,	b	MEWDS: acute ret. pigment epitheliitis	ng,	b
Mycobacteria: leprosy-iridocyclitis tuberculosis: choroiditis, vasculitis	g, g,	b b	ARN: acute retinal necrosis Birdshot choroidopathy: acute choroiditis	g, ng,	b b
Herpes virus: HSV 1-keratitis, iritis H zoster-i-c, papillitis, retinitis CMV-retinitis Epstein–Barr-i-c, choroiditis, keratitis	ng, ng, ng, ng,	u u or b b u or b	Fuch's heterochromic: acute/chronic iridocyclitis, chronic glaucoma Relapsing polychondritis: keratitis, i-c Drug abuse: acute endophthalmitis, vitritis, retinal emboli	ng, ng, g,	u or b b u or b
Serpiginous choroiditis: chronic					

Signs of Uveitis

SIGNS OF UVEITIS

Skin:
- Vesicles (herpetic disease) 1
- Erythema nodosum (Behçet's, Tbc, ulcerative colitis, strep) 208
- Erythema migrans 'concentric' (Lyme disease) 136
- Vitiligo (Vogt–Koyanagi–Harada) 149, 151
- Lepromata (Hansen's Disease) 5
- Lupus pernio (Sarcoidosis) 3, 116, 117
- Mucous membranes/aphthous ulcers (Behçet's; Reiter's) 4, 7

Conjunctiva:
- Nodules 2, 3, 118
- Infiltrates 2, 3
- Papillae (Reiter's) 111
- Scleral nodules 97, 236
- Episcleritis 13, 99
- Scleritis 97, 99

Cornea:
- Keratic precipitates–fine
  –mutton-fat 19, 22
  –stellate (stellactite–Fuch's 20
  –pigmented 14
- Pattern of k.p.: outside of lower 1/3–Fuch's 20
- Vessels, neovascularization
- Phlyctenules (Tbc, allergy, etc)
- Band keratopathy (JRA, chronic glaucoma, chronic inflammation) 16
- Dendrites (herpetic disease) 10, 247, 249

Iris:
- Nodules: Koeppe 28
  Bussacca 32
  Berlin
  stromal-sarcoid; lepromata on surface 31
- Synechiae: peripheral anterior
  posterior 33
  ring on anterior lens capsule 21
- Infiltrates
- Loss of iris pigment epithelium: transillumination (H. Zoster, Fuch's) 11

Lens:
- Cataract nuclear sclerosis 25
  posterior subcapsular 43
  zonular
  iatrogenic
  intraocular lens

Vitreous:
- Cells: diffuse, focal (inflammatory vs masquerade) 37

                    intermediate uveitis (pars planitis) 35
                    snowballs 36
- Syneresis
- Cholesterol crystals

Retina/choroid:
- Level and pattern–focal infiltrate
                    diffuse infiltrate
- Vasculitis–diffuse 48, 49
                    focal 50, 51, 52

- Pars plana infiltrates 36
- Pattern of exudates 72, 129, 130, 269, 273
                    hemorrhages
                    scar tissue (i.e. toxocara 60, 61, 62;
                    toxoplasmosis 56, 57; histo 65, 67)
- Infarction-central (Behçet's, H. Zoster, etc) 50
                    peripheral (ARN) 274, 275

1 Excoriated vesicular lesion adjacent to the lateral canthus. Primary herpes simplex infection of the skin spread to the eye causing keratitis and secondary uveitis.

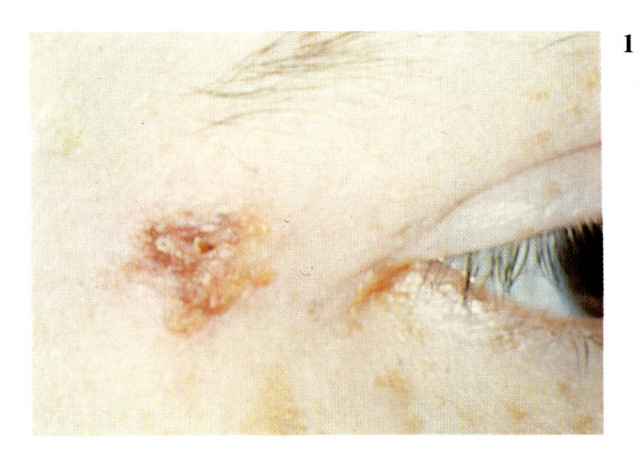

2 Conjunctival biopsy candidate. Eversion of the lower lid demonstrates pinkish-yellow lesion. It is all-important to search the conjunctiva for biopsy material to establish a diagnosis of sarcoid in a patient with a granulomatous uveitis. This specific lesion turned out to be a subconjunctival lymphoma; however, when such lesions are noted in the conjunctiva, the yield is quite high in order to establish a histologic diagnosis of sarcoidosis. All such patients should have double eversion of the eyelid in order to search for conjunctival lesions for quick and easy biopsy in the office. Blind biopsy of the conjunctiva is considered by many to be fruitless.

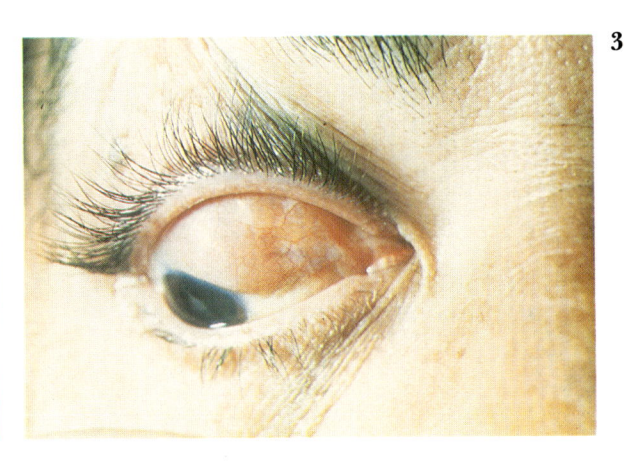

3 Biopsy lesion. Another patient who demonstrates a subconjunctival lymphoma infiltrate has double eversion of the lids achieved in order to search for a conjunctival lesion consistent with sarcoidosis for biopsy.

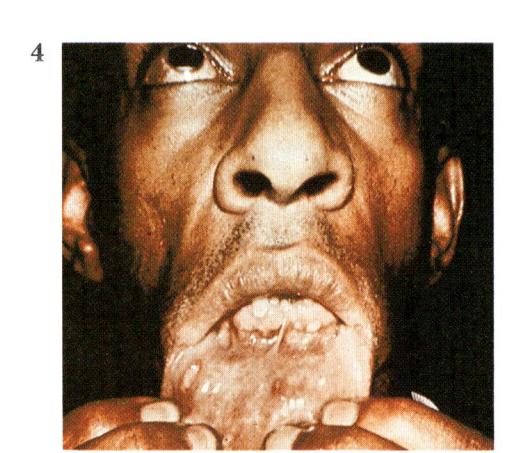

4 Behçet's disease. The patient demonstrates a painful, red, injected right eye with classical hypopyon, everting the lower lip to demonstrate aphthous ulceration of the buccal mucosa. This patient has classical findings of Behçet's disease, which remains a clinical diagnosis. (*Courtesy of the Wills Eye Hospital Residents' Teaching Collection.*)

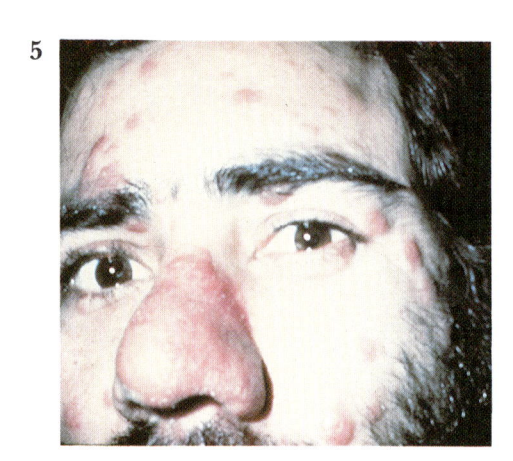

5 Lepromatous iridocyclitis. Patient with lepromatous iridocyclitis of a chronic serous nature in the left eye who demonstrates facial nodular lepromata, which when biopsied histologically yield the diagnosis.

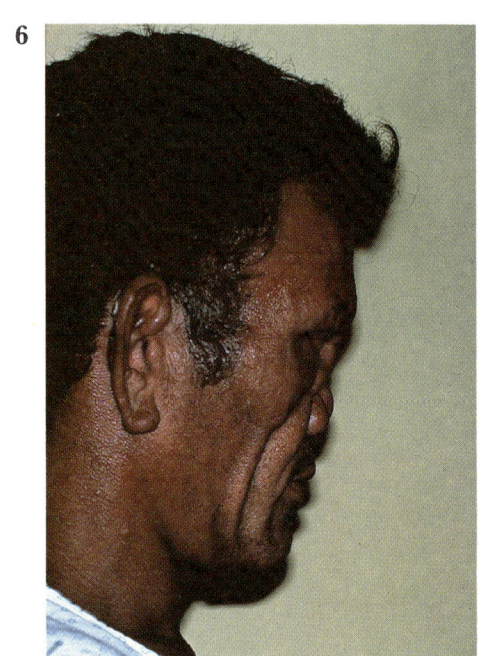

6 Resorbed nasal cartilage. Patient with lepromatous leprosy and lepromatous uveitis whose striking facial profile demonstrates the resorption of the nasal cartilage.

7 Aphthous ulceration on the tongue of a patient with granulomatous iridocyclitis secondary to Behçet's disease.

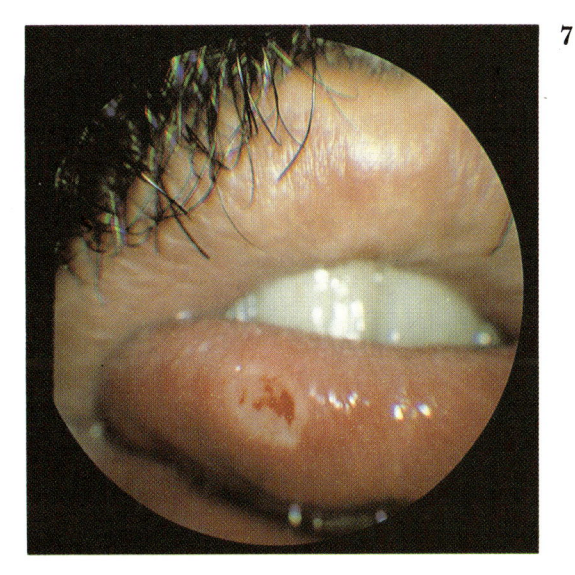

8 Iris heterochromia. Patient with anterior segment ischemia who is demonstrating unilateral iris heterochromia due to early rubeosis iridis at the pupillary margin, a moderate cell and flare in the anterior chamber. This is caused by large vessel obstruction.

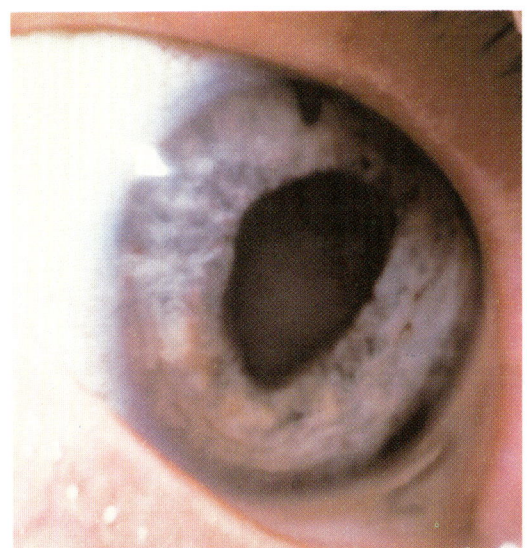

9 Anterior segment ischemia. Patient demonstrates a marked subconjunctival hemorrhage secondary to a scleral buckling procedure for retinal detachment. Of note is the corneal haze, the moderate cell and flare in the anterior chamber, and the marked rubeosis iridis that is hemorrhaging at the pupillary margin interiorly due to anterior segment ischemia from a very tight scleral buckling procedure. The anterior segment ischemia was manifest first by an intense iridocyclitis.

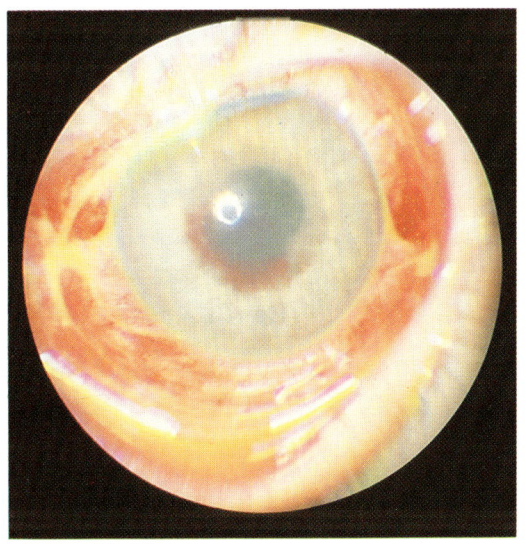

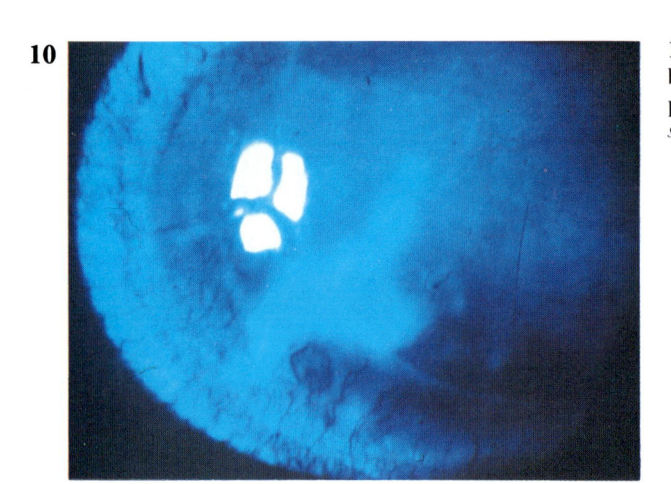

10 Herpes dendrite. Active keratitis manifested by bright fluorescein-stained dendrite in a patient with herpetic keratouveitis. (*Courtesy of the Wills Eye Hospital Residents' Teaching Collection.*)

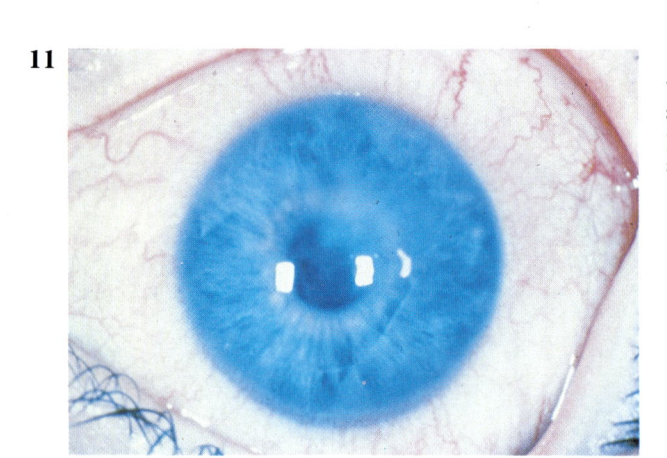

11 Herpetic iridocyclitis with iris atrophy. Patient with herpes simplex keratouveitis manifesting a stromal scar. Evidence in the iris of areas of atrophy in the iris pigment epithelium give rise to an uneven pigment intensity.

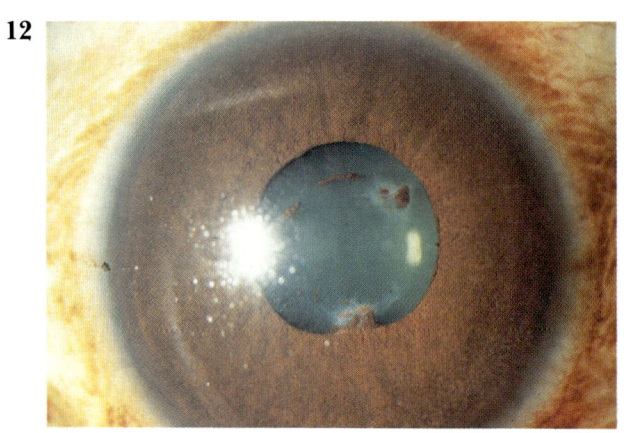

12 Sarcoid uveitis. Patient with sarcoid uveitis demonstrating synechiae and iris pigment deposition on the anterior lens capsule where previous synechiae had been broken by dilatation of the pupil.

13 Sturge–Weber telangiectasia mistaken for episcleritis. Patient thought to have mild episcleritis and rheumatoid arthritis. A larger feeder vessel coming off inferotemporally from the limbus is actually a Sturge–Weber syndrome of telangiectasia of the conjunctiva and upper lid with hemangioma of the choroid. This patient was treated with drops by a referring ophthalmologist for episcleritis that was recalcitrant.

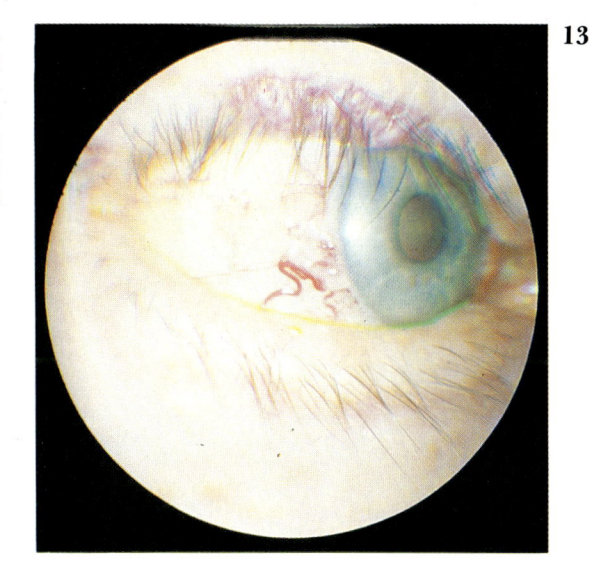

14 Pigmented keratic precipitates (KP). Note all KP are white, as evidenced by the corneal endothelial deposits in this patient suffering from anterior chamber intraocular lens-induced itiris.

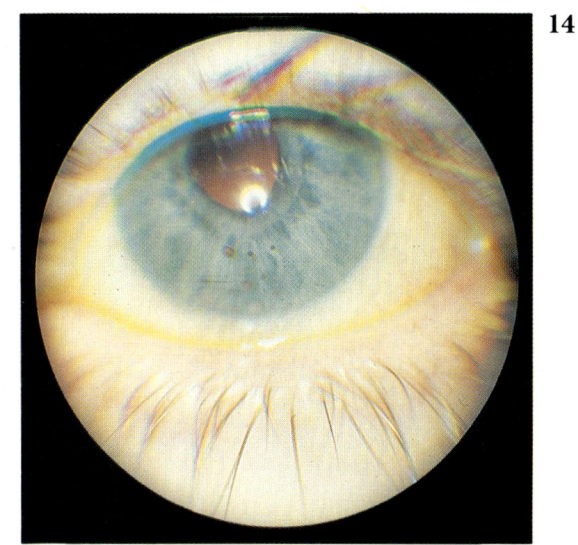

15 Cyclitic membrane. A child with juvenile rheumatoid arthritis, chronic iridocyclitis, and status post-intracapsular cataract extraction done many years previously with cyclitic membrane and development of phthisis bulbi. The patient's cornea now demonstrates invasion by limbal vessels as one other manifestation of the eventual demise of this eye due to its involutional changes and phthisis secondary to ciliary body detachment by the cyclitic membrane.

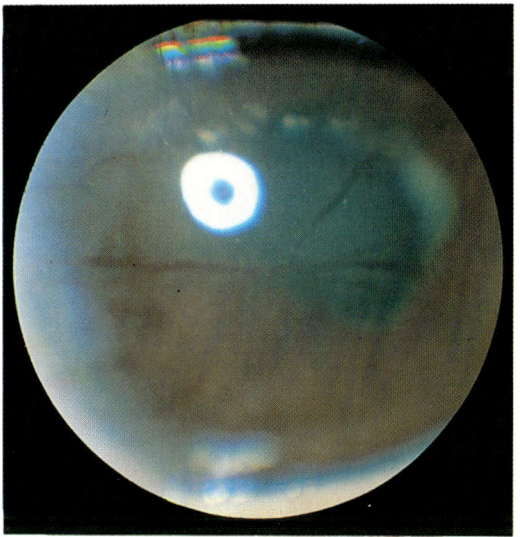

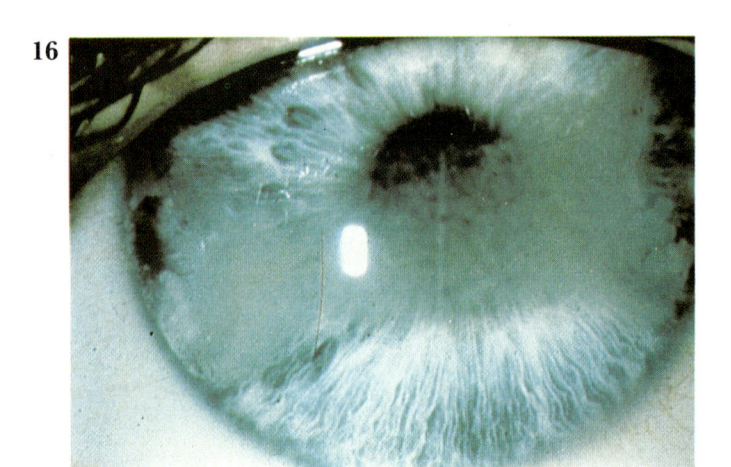

16 Band keratopathy. Typical calcific band keratopathy in the otherwise seemingly quiet white eye of a 9-year-old child. The patient has juvenile rheumatoid arthritis with chronic, unremitting iridocyclitis.

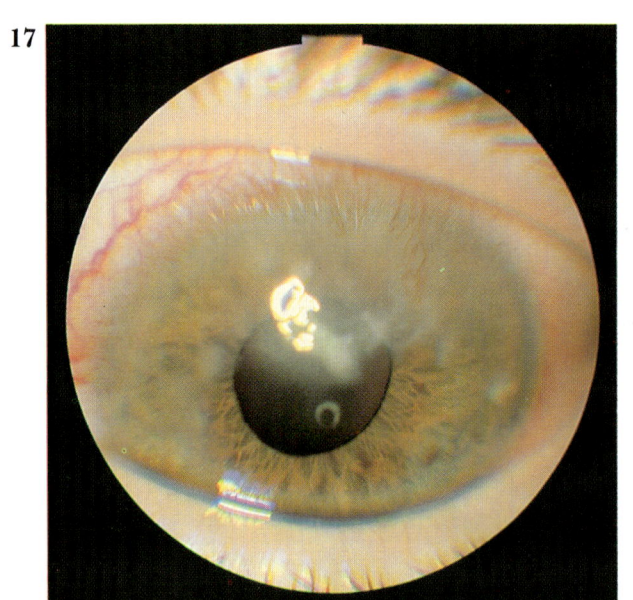

17 Chronic relapsing polychondritis. A 24-year-old woman with scleritis, epithelial and anterior stromal infiltrate in the superior cornea secondary to chronic relapsing polychondritis.

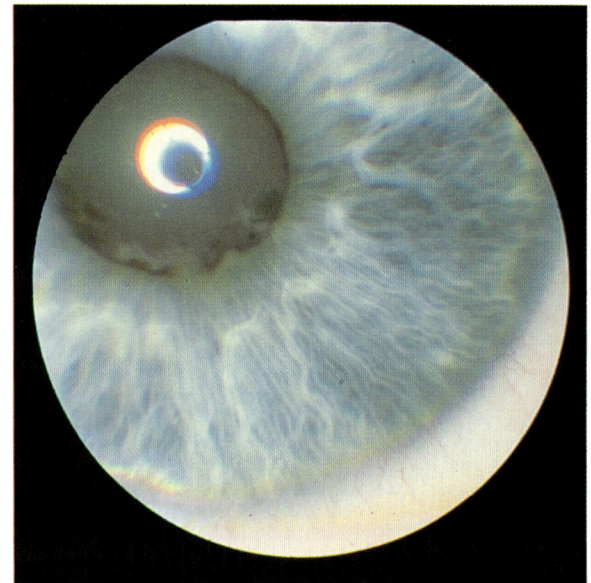

18 Reiter's disease. Patient with fibrous synechiae unresponsive to pupillary dilatation as a sequela of acute, intermittent iridocyclitis of a profound nature caused by Reiter's disease.

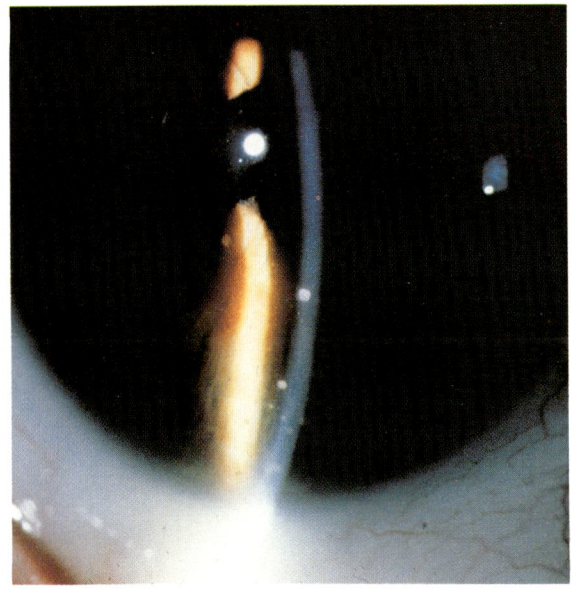

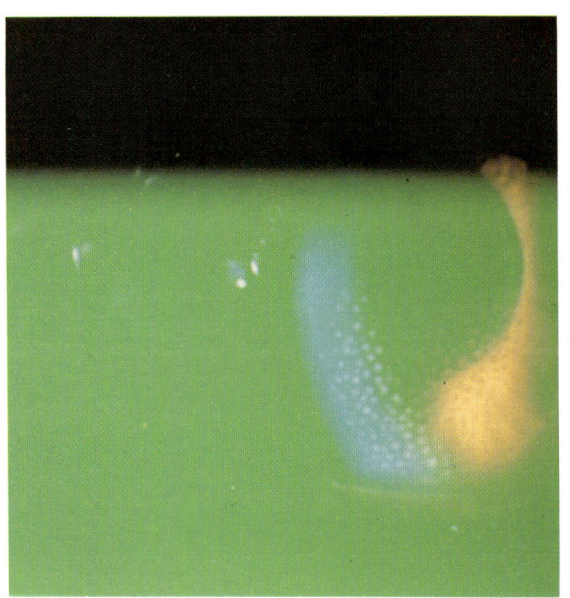

19 Granulomatous KP. Typical large white mutton-fat granulomatous type KP in a patient with sarcoid uveitis. Granulomatous type KP are usually found in those uveitides that are granulomatous on histologic demonstration, such as sarcoidosis, syphilis, and tuberculosis. However, a profound iridocyclitis that results from a nongranulomatous type inflammation such as ankylosing spondylitis or Reiter's disease may be so severe in its presentation as to show the same type of precipitates on the corneal endothelium. Therefore, the designation of granulomatous precipitates for this large mutton-fat type is misleading when it only implies the histologically granulomatous type disease.

20 Fuchs' heterochromic cyclitis. Very diffuse broad band of white mutton-fat type KP on the corneal endothelium extending in a uniform pattern up over the whole bottom half of the cornea in patients with a Fuchs' heterochromic cyclitis. The KP are not concentrated in the inferior triangle of the cornea as they usually are in other diseases but are rather evenly distributed throughout the back of the endothelium as depicted here. Often these precipitates are not pigmented, disappear and reappear sporadically, are seen with retroillumination or transillumination, and may have stellate and/or crystalline projections extending posteriorly from the precipitates themselves.

21 Vogt–Koyanagi–Harada disease. Patient with diffuse anterior segment haze from a moderate iridocyclitis secondary to Vogt–Koyanagi–Haradi disease. Pigmented KP are present on the corneal endothelium in back of which is a Voissus' ring where the iris had previously been stuck down on the anterior lens capsule.

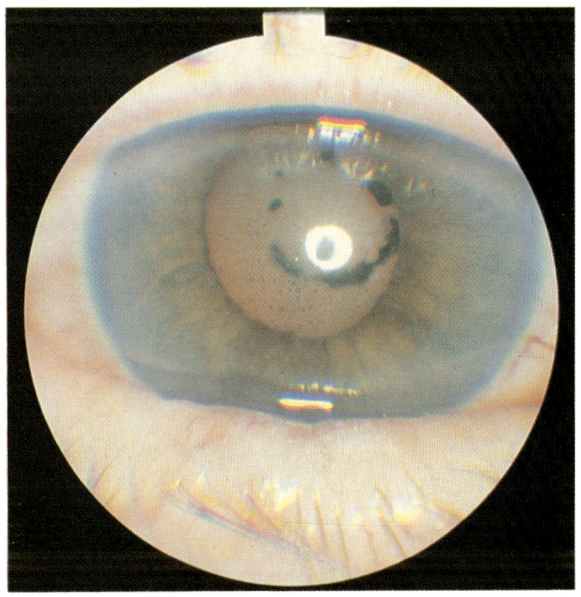

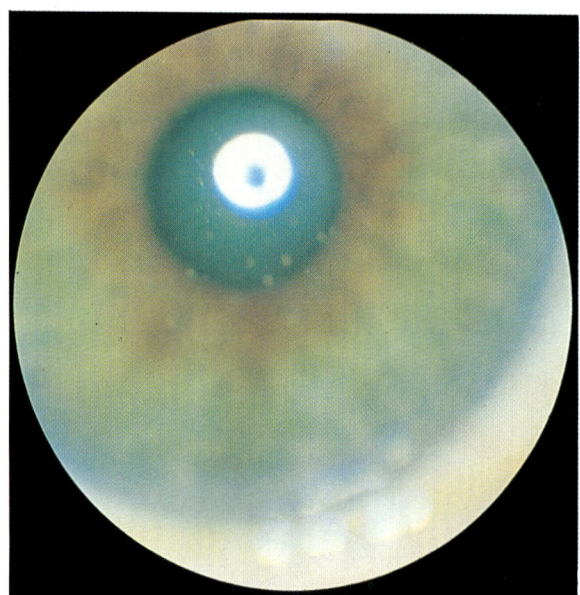

22 Large mutton-fat KP. Large white mutton-fat KP seen typically on the lower one third of the corneal triangle in a patient with a granulomatous iridocyclitis. Synechia formation has not yet occurred at the pupillary margin.

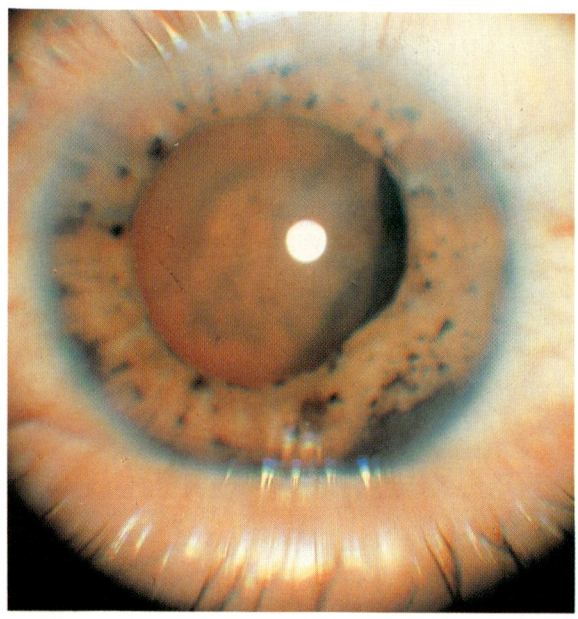

23 Masquerade syndrome of iritis. A 54-year-old white woman with a profound anterior segment inflammation has a dense cell and flare in the anterior chamber and the anterior vitreous. The iris surface is speckled with small punctate black pigmented lesions, but note the rather coalescent lesion at the 5 o'clock position and the large coalescent black pigment on the iris pupillary margin, extending from the 2 to the 4:30 o'clock position. This pseudo-uveitis was actually due to malignant melanoma infiltration of the ciliary body, iris, and anterior chamber in a patient with metastatic melanoma from the skin of her back.

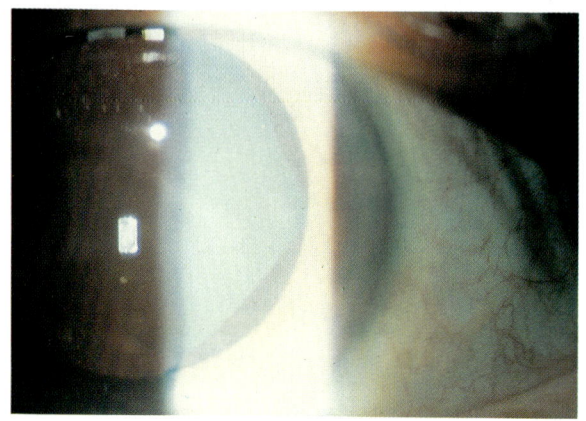

24 Cysts of iris pigment epithelium. A 53-year-old white woman in whom iris nodules thought to be Busacca nodules of a uveitic nature were actually cysts of the iris pigment epithelium. When the iris is dilated to full extent as seen here, these cysts peek around the corner of the iris pupillary margin and can transilluminate on retroillumination on the slit-lamp beam. Such cysts in the iris pigment epithelium are normal and may be confused with iris stromal nodules that are often seen as typical manifestations of uveitis in patients with granulomatous diseases, such as sarcoidosis and tuberculosis.

25 Juvenile rheumatoid arthritis. Typical quiet-appearing white eye from an external view which, when looked at in the slit-lamp, would demonstrate a mild to moderate chronic iridocyclitis caused by juvenile rheumatoid arthritis. This eye demonstrates a very prominent, dense, white cataract as a manifestation of the ongoing, long-standing, chronic iridocyclitis of this disease. Such children with juvenile rheumatoid arthritis should be examined often to look for the complicated sequelae of their chronic iridocyclitis that might be otherwise missed. Many of these eyes don't manifest the angry red appearance of the other uveitides. Such a quiet white external appearance often belies the fact that either juvenile rheumatoid arthritis, pars planitis or reticulum cell sarcoma might actually be manifesting a profound degree of inflammation inside one of the eyes of a patient who might not have any type of external inflammatory signs.

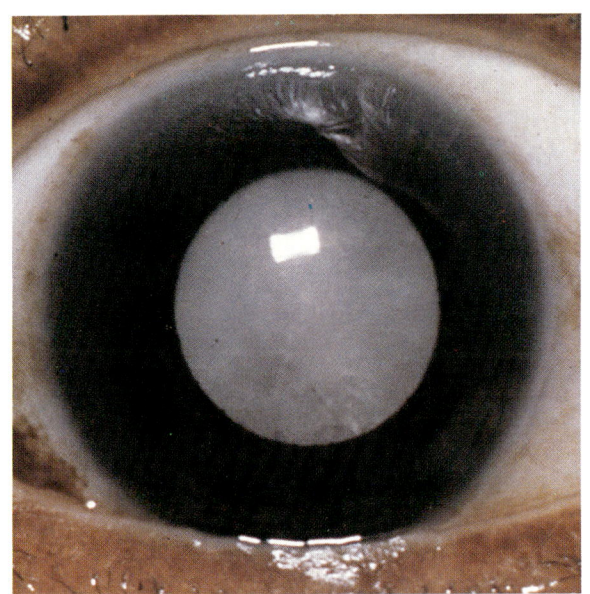

26 Endophthalmitis. A 52-year-old man with intense, conjunctival injection, corneal epithelial sloughing, hypopyon, and intense iridocyclitis suggestive of endophthalmitis; however, this patient actually has geographic herpetic ulceration of the cornea with secondary uveitis of such a profound nature that it simulates a true endophthalmitis of bacterial origin.

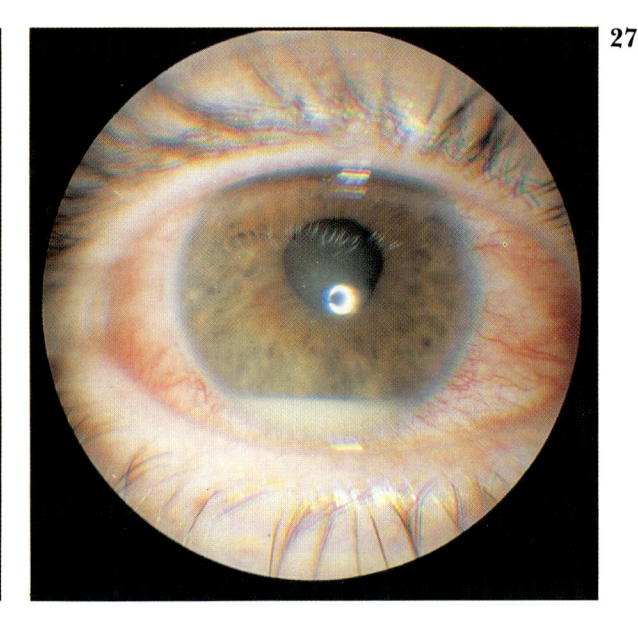

27 Behçet's disease. A 23-year-old patient with diffuse scleral injection and hypopyon with a moderate cell and flare in the anterior chamber suggestive of endophthalmitis. The patient actually has a classic presentation of hypopyon, aphthous ulceration of the mouth, erythema nodosum, and arthropathy of Behçet's disease. This hypopyon cleared rapidly with corticosteroid treatment.

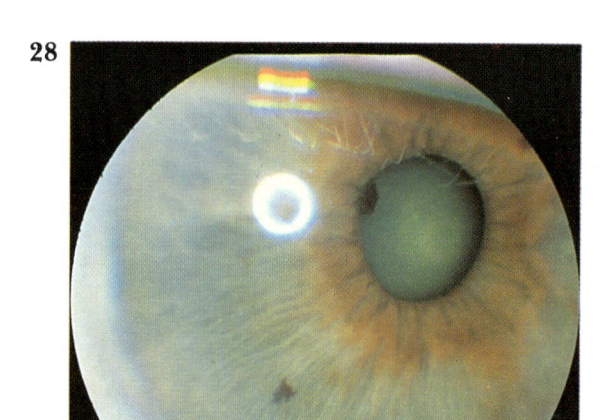

28 Koeppe nodule. Patient with isolated Koeppe nodule at the 10 o'clock position at the pupillary margin secondary to acute intermittent iridocyclitis caused by long-standing ankylosing spondylitis.

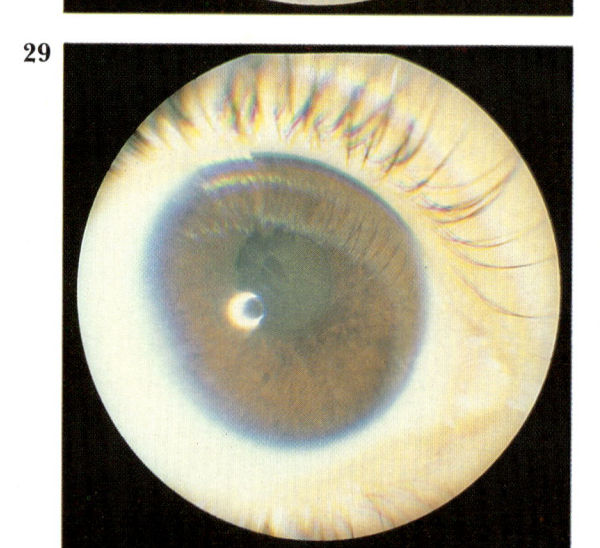

29 Juvenile rheumatoid arthritis. A 15-year-old patient with the typical external appearance of a quiet white eye caused by juvenile rheumatoid arthritis. The arthritis along with chronic iridocyclitis is manifested by a moderate cell and flare and a cyclitic membrane as an overgrowth from old intracapsular cataract surgery. Originally, these eyes were thought to have a poor surgical prognosis after cataract surgery because of the development of a phthisis bulbi caused by detachment of the ciliary body from cyclitic membrane such as this. With the development of pars plana surgical techniques via the vitrectomy instruments, such cyclitic membranes can be removed in toto, preventing the ultimate demise of this eye from phthisis bulbi.

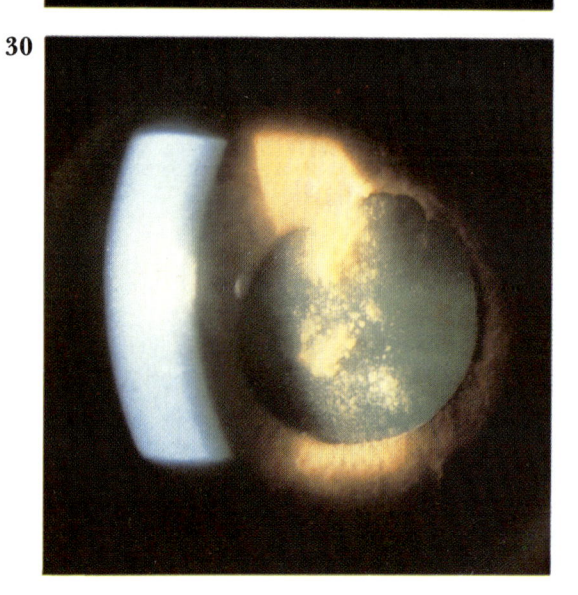

30 Leprosy. A 30-year-old man with a chronic serous iridocyclitis secondary to lepromatous leprosy demonstrating nodular lepromata or cheesy iris deposits that are also forming synechiae and pigmentary changes over the anterior lens capsule.

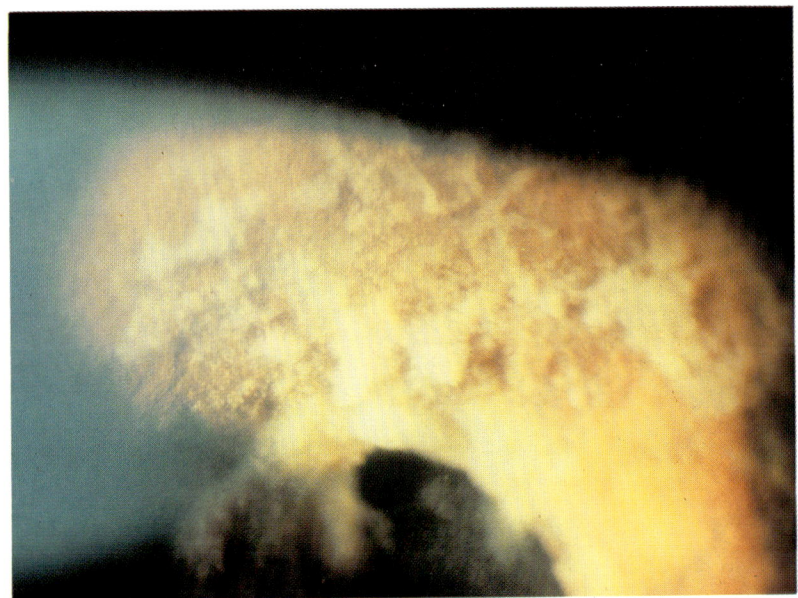

31 Nodular lepromata from lepromatous iridocyclitis forming on the surface of the iris. This typically cheesy infiltration exquisitely powdered over the iris surface is easily differentiated from Busacca nodules that are in the iris stroma itself in chronic uveitis. This classic presentation of these lepromatous lesions should suggest the diagnosis of lepromatous iridocyclitis.

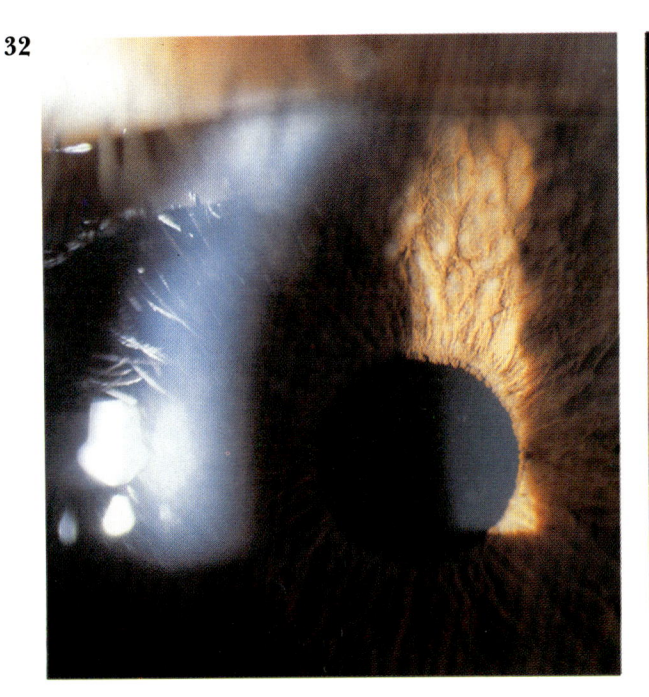

32 Busacca nodules are seen as superficial white excrescences on the surface of the superior iris in this patient with Vogt–Koyanagi–Harada disease. The nodules melted away with corticosteroids.

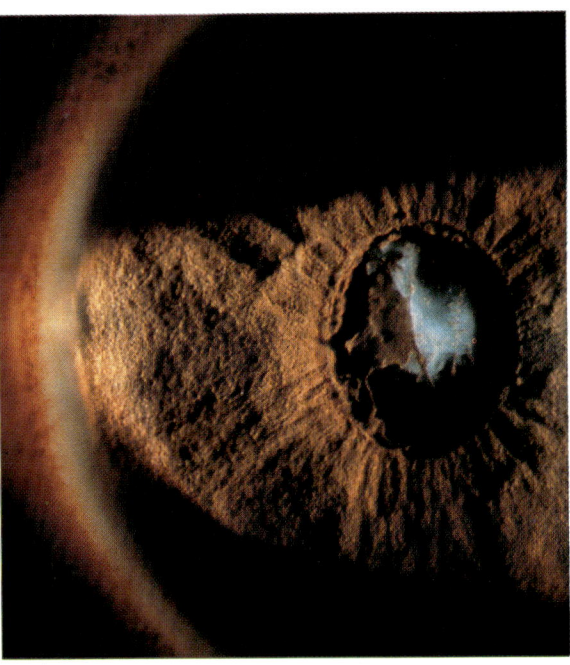

33 Vogt–Koyanagi iridocyclitis. Prominent fibrotic synechiae and pigment deposition on the anterior lens capsule in a patient with Vogt–Koyanagi–Harada uveitis. Side illumination at the slit-lamp shows an almost obscured pupil.

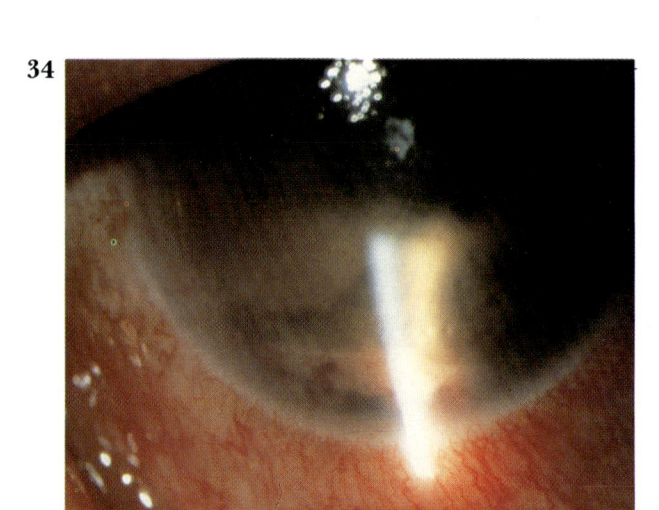

34 Hypopyon speckled with petechiae at the inferior cornea and chamber angle. Endophthalmitis and Berlin's nodule must be differentiated from this collection of white cells in this patient who actually suffers from lepromatous iridocyclitis.

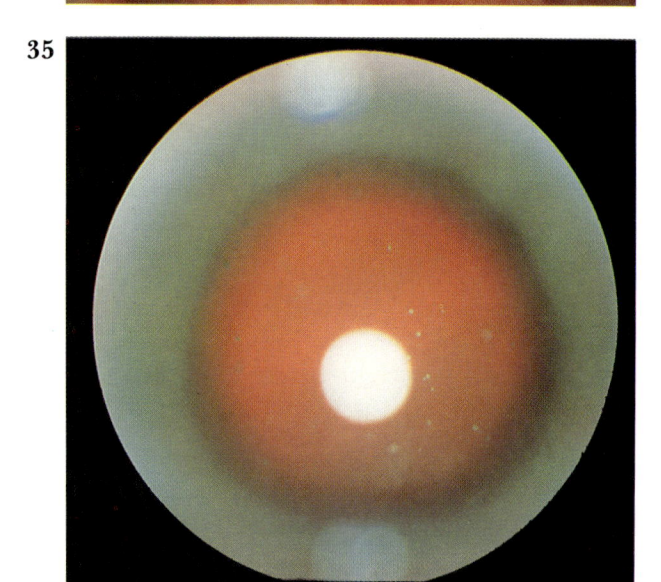

35 Pars planitis. Anterior vitreous showing diffuse clumps of white infiltration in a patient with pars planitis or chronic cyclitis. The external appearance of the eye is quiet and white and the iris demonstrates no synechiae as its usual presentation. Often, these vitreous infiltrates are more inferior in their location, but this patient has a diffuse vitreitis of equal intensity anteriorly and posteriorly and superiorly and inferiorly.

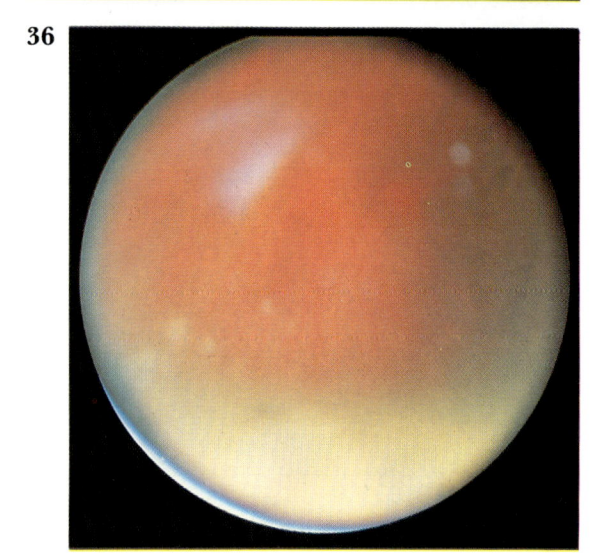

36 Pars plana infiltrate. A 21-year-old patient with pars planitis or chronic cyclitis demonstrating white snowballs of vitreous infiltrate overlying the dense white snowbanking of the pars plana. The pars plana is elevated by external scleral depression.

37 Reticulum cell sarcoma. A patient with dense vitreous infiltrate with some prominent snowballs in the vitreous; however, this is a case of reticulum cell sarcoma in an older patient in which there is also a quiet, white external appearance commonly seen in the pars planitis picture. Profound anterior segment inflammation may be present, including thick synechiae, even in the face of a quiet external picture.

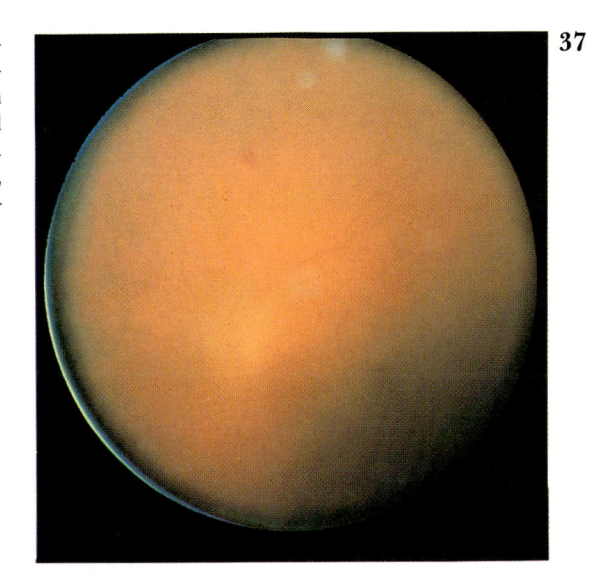

38 Toxoplasmosis. A 26-year-old man with acute toxoplasmosis in the macula as viewed through a fairly dense vitreitis. This might be interpreted as a mild 'lighthouse in the fog' clinical picture.

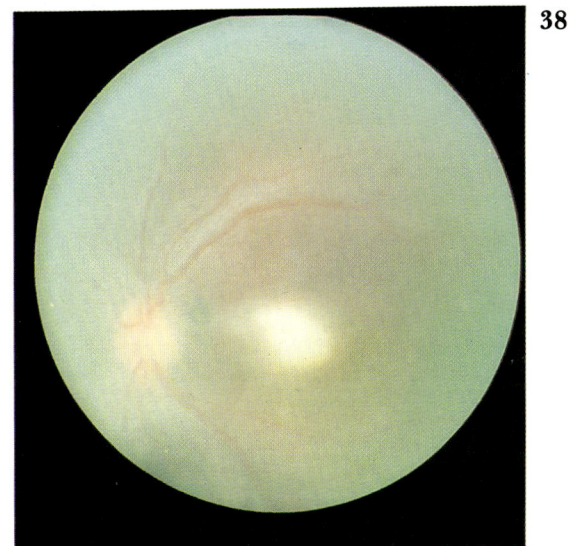

39 Toxoplasmosis reactivation. A prominent but peripheral satellite reactivation of toxoplasmosis in a patient with a dense vitreitis surrounded by snowballs. Note a localized necrotizing vasculitis in the area of this acute reactivating lesion next to its old original lesion that now has scarring of the retinal pigment epithelium and appears inactive.

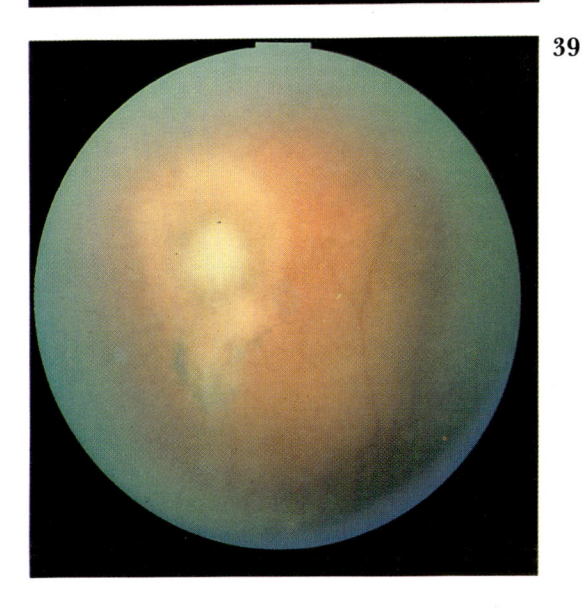

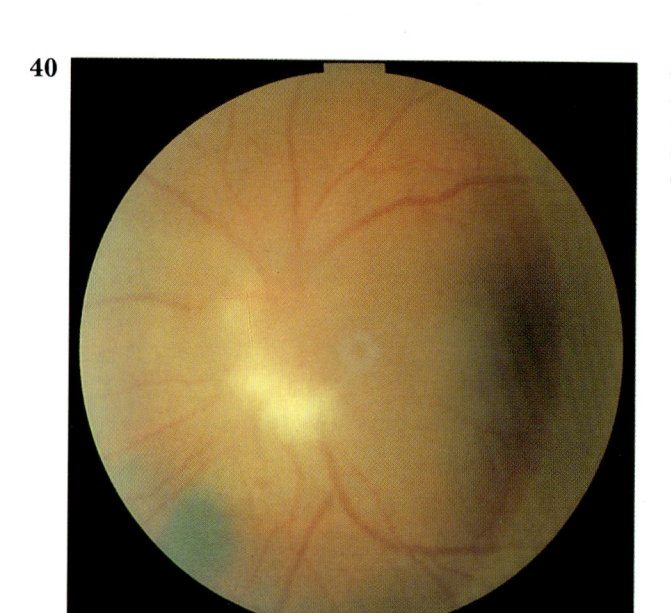

40 Toxoplasmic papillitis. A 42-year-old patient with a dense vitreitis overlying active toxoplasmosis inflammation of the optic nerve head. This obligate intracellular organism has a predilection for neural tissue, especially the optic papilla.

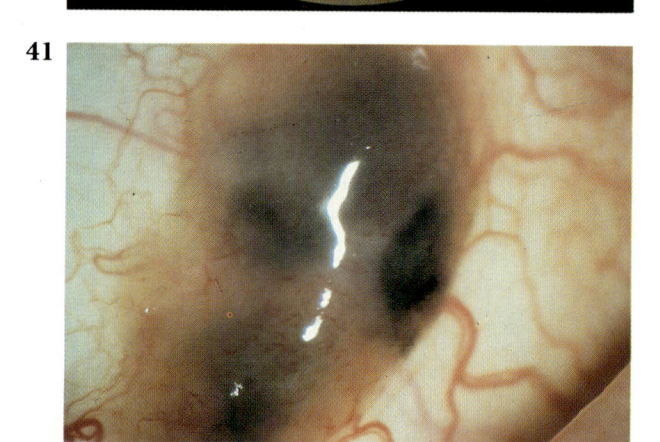

41 Malignant melanoma. Gross enlargement of conjunctiva with surrounding episcleritis in a patient who has mechanical blood vessel inflammation due to an infiltrating conjunctival malignant melanoma.

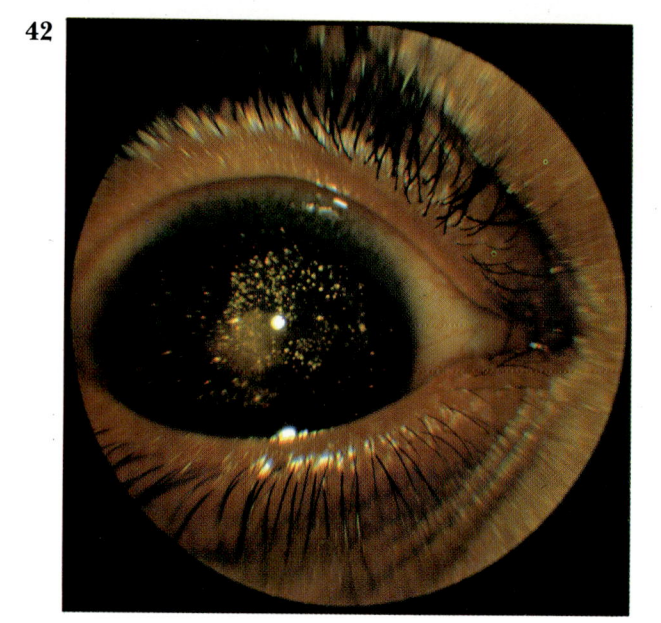

42 Hemophthalmitis. Seeming anterior segment inflammation with very lucent particles in the anterior chamber actually representing hemophthalmitis caused by trauma and not an inflammation. Note the dense white cataract as a consequence of the trauma in this 13-year-old black girl who was hit in the eye with a baseball bat.

43 Posterior subcapsular cataract. Typical posterior subcapsular cataract that developed as an iatrogenic side effect of steroid treatment for chronic iridocyclitis in a patient with ankylosing spondylitis.

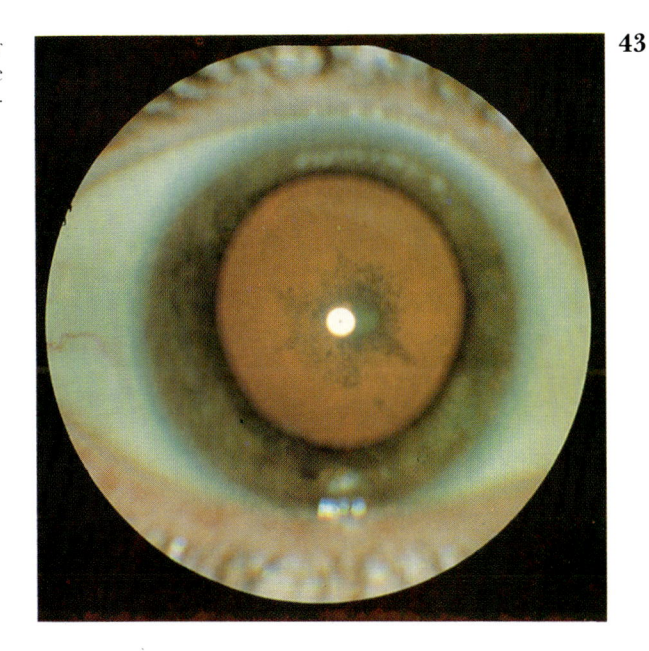

44 Filamentary keratitis. A 32-year-old black woman suffering from systemic sarcoidosis and secondary dry eye syndrome demonstrates filamentary keratitis of the cornea. The cornea is stained prominently with fluorescein.

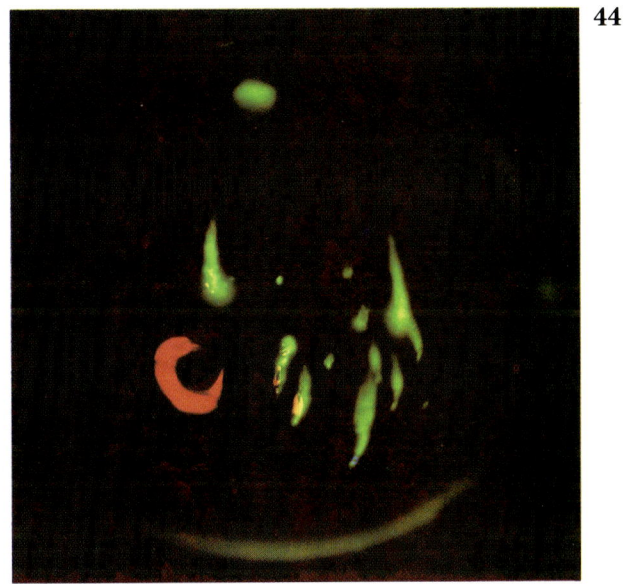

45 Interstitial keratitis. Same patient as Figure 44 with sarcoidosis demonstrating interstitial keratitis noted deep to the slit beam in the cornea. The differential diagnosis for intestinal keratitis that often accompanies uveitis includes the systemic syndrome of syphilis, leprosy, tuberculosis, mumps, herpes simplex and zoster.

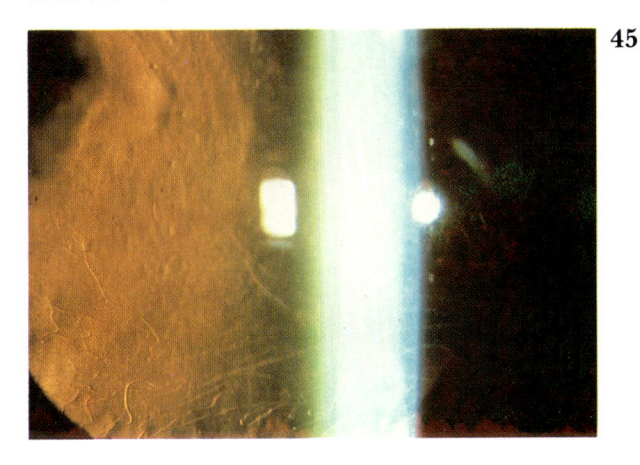

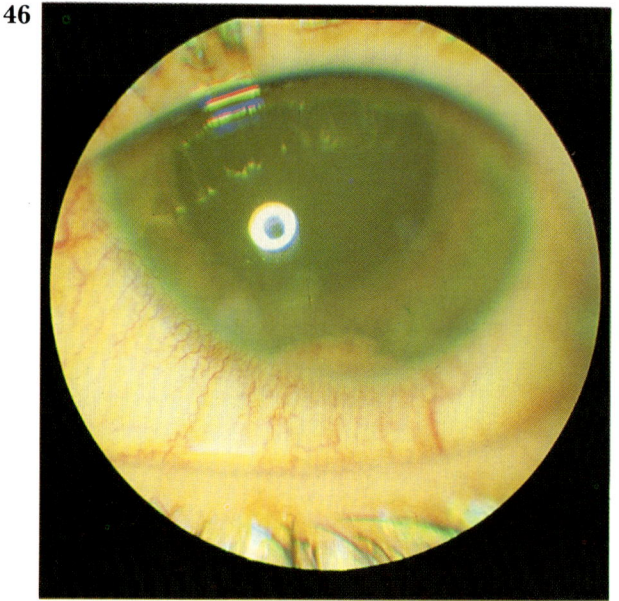

46 Berlin's nodule. Inflammatory nodule in the inferior angle and iris speckled with petechiae and fringed by limbal flush. It is called a Berlin's nodule in the classical literature describing this finding in systemic sarcoidosis. It is an iris nodule not unlike a Busacca nodule but located in the chamber angle.

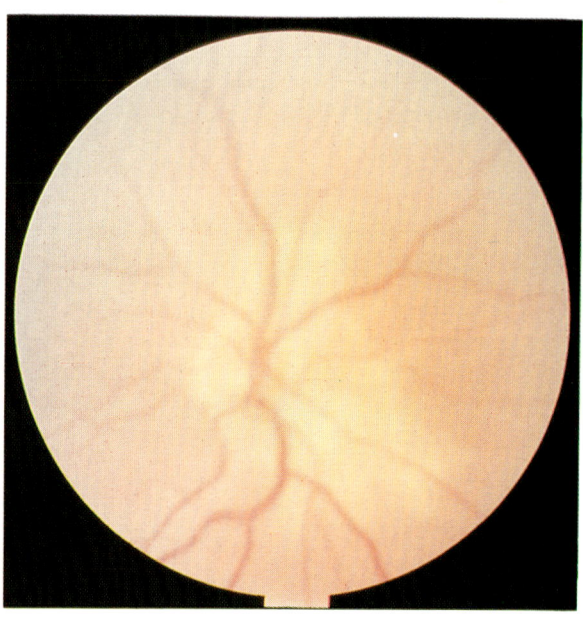

47 Sarcoid nodule. Sarcoid nodule on the optic papilla in a 32-year-old white woman with established pulmonary sarcoidosis.

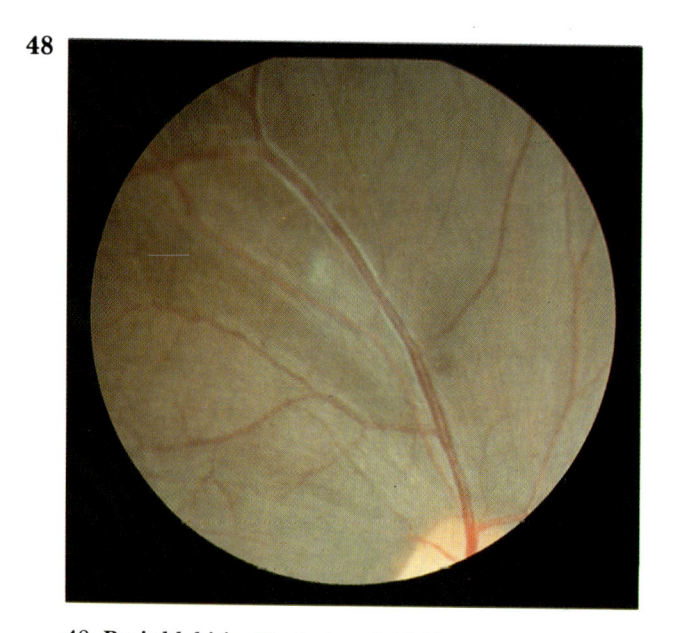

48 Periphlebitis. Typical periphlebitis in the fundus of this 23-year-old black woman with systemic sarcoidosis. Notice the beaded appearance of the retinal veins as highlighted by the perivascular cuffing.

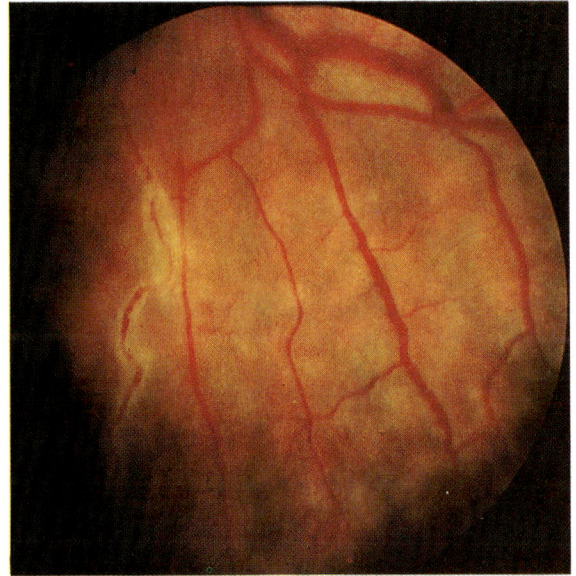

49 Necrotizing vasculitis. Focal necrotizing vasculitis in a patient with Behçet's syndrome; however, the differential diagnosis for such a vasculitis would include all the panuveitides such as sympathetic ophthalmia, Vogt–Koyanagi–Harada disease, syphilis, tuberculosis, all of the collagen-vasculoses, sarcoidosis, and if there were a retinal inflammation adjacent to it, toxoplasmosis.

50 Profound retinal infarction secondary to vasculitis in a patient with Behçet's disease. This infarction might be seen as the natural progression of events from the focal vasculitis in Figure 49.

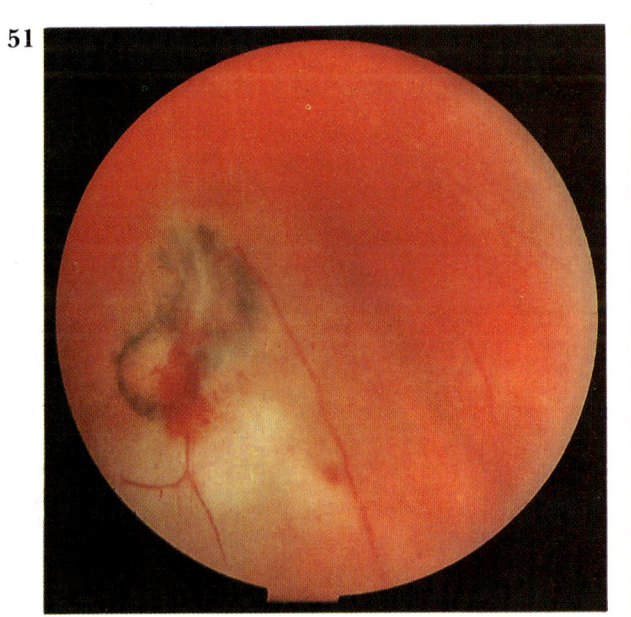

51 Focal hemorrhage in the retina and into the overlying vitreous caused by the necrotizing vasculitis associated with reactivating toxoplasmosis. This patient has an initial pigmented but inactive toxoplasmosis scar with a satellite activating with white intraretinal and epiretinal inflammation adjacent to it.

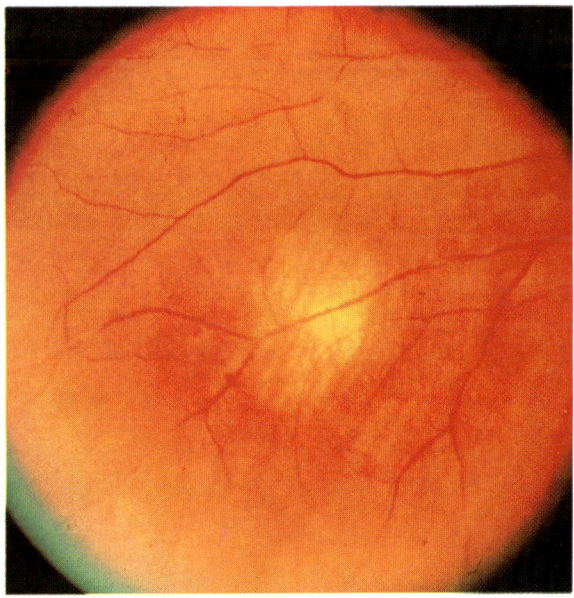

52 Inactive vasculitis in a 42-year-old patient with Behçet's disease. Retinal pigment epithelial dropout in the area of a previous vasculitis is the consequence of her relapsing inflammatory systemic condition.

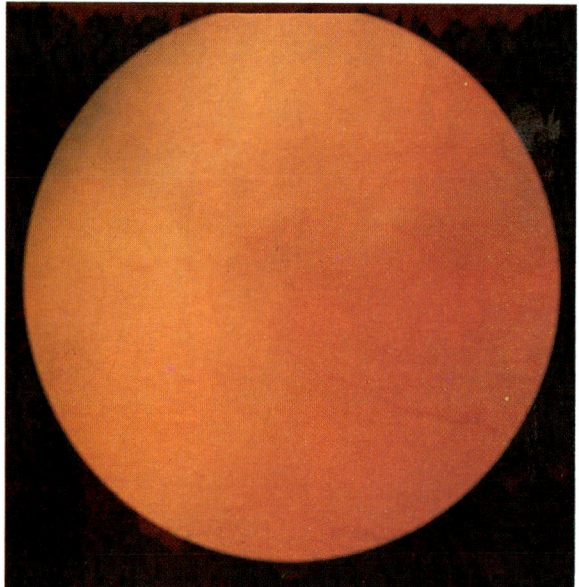

53 Obscured retinal detachment. Patient with vitreitis and underlying white retina that may be mistaken for inflammation in the retina. Actually, retinal detachment is present and obscured by the vitreous haze from the hemorrhage encapsulated in it. There is a horseshoe tear at the 11 o'clock position in the billowed-up retina that discloses the diagnosis for the cellular concentration in the vitreous.

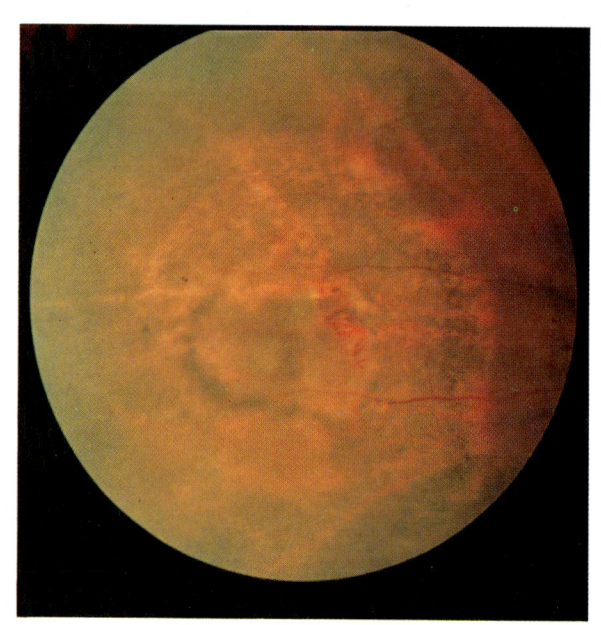

54 Vitreous hemorrhage. Cellular infiltration of the vitreous thought to be due to intraocular inflammation but was actually caused by retinal tear. The tear has its own pigmented demarcation line posterior to it.

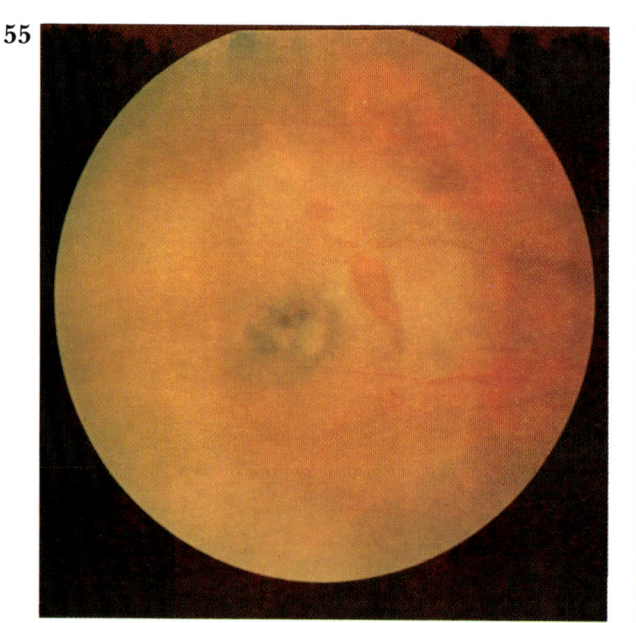

55 Retinal tear with its adjacent retinal pigment epithelial hyperplasia and demarcation line after cryopexy, now outlining the elongated morphology of this retinal rip.

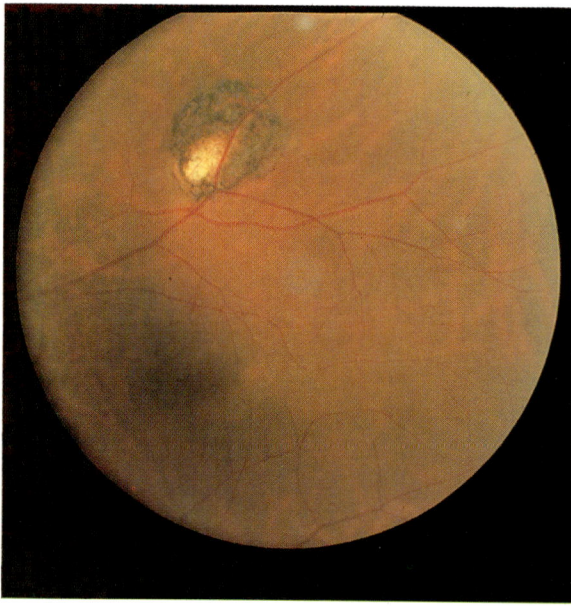

56 Inactive toxoplasmosis scar. Hypopigmented central core of a hyperpigmented lesion deep to a retinal vessel that represents an inactive toxoplasmosis scar.

57 Recurrent toxoplasmosis. Sequential hypopigmented and hyperpigmented scar marching from the superior aspect of the retina inferiorly down toward the macula and ending in a now inactive scar, kissing into foveolar fixation, caused by recurrent toxoplasmosis.

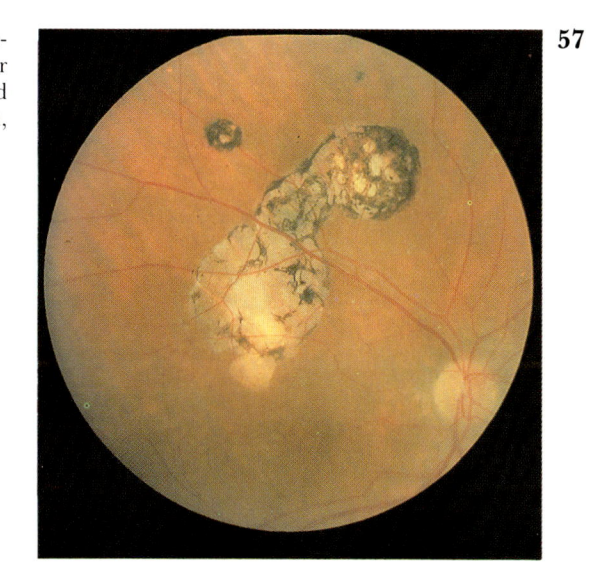

58 Large, white excrescence of inflammation in and under the retina in this nine-year-old boy representing Coats' disease which is a pseudo-inflammation and the white inflammatory material represents lipid and cholesterol, some in crystal form. The differential diagnosis for such a lesion would include *Toxocara canis* and retinoblastoma.

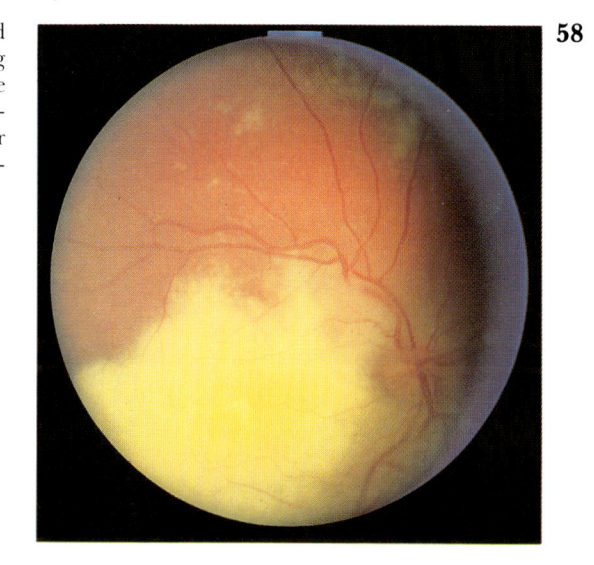

59 Disorganized retinal architecture with central abscess highlighted by a fibrous band leading to the optic papilla in a youngster with *Toxocara canis* infestation. Such a constellation of signs should not be confused with toxoplasmosis, an isolated retinitis that does not cause such an overwhelming disorganization of intraocular morphology. The fibrous band leading from the peripheral abscess to the optic papilla is a characteristic clinical sign ascribed to toxocariasis.

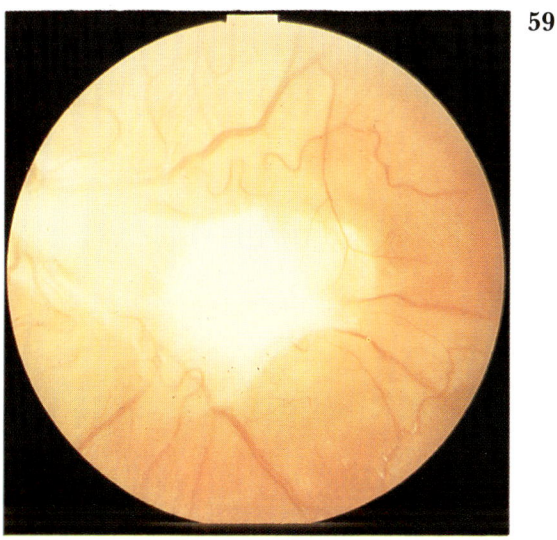

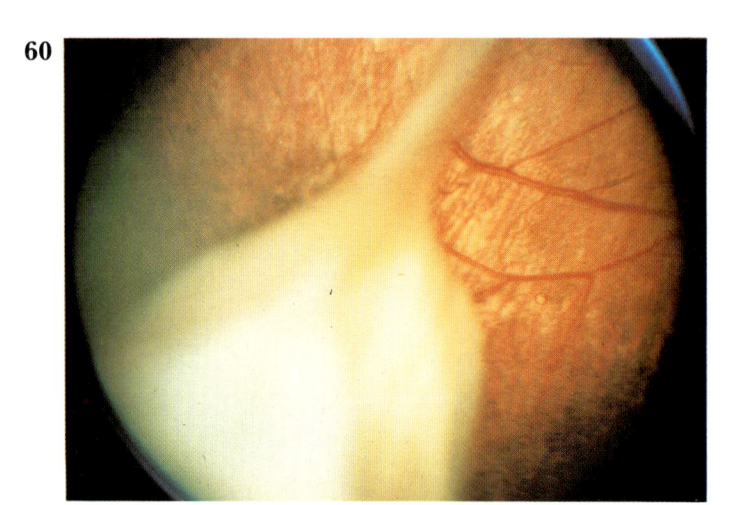

60 Toxocara canis. Very peripheral white abscess in a patient with *Toxocara canis* infestation with relatively clear vitreous demonstrating the late and inactive phase of this disease. Note the prominent band extending from the fibrous abscess and ultimately connecting to the optic papilla.

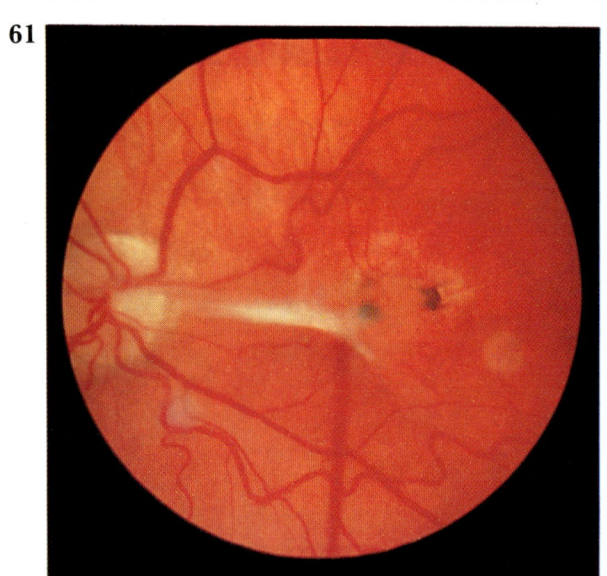

61 Toxocara canis. Nine-year-old child with minimal resultant inflammation from *Toxocara canis* infestation in the macula. Note the prominent fibrous band leading to the optic papilla and the disturbance of the arcade morphology. The vessels leading from the optic disc and radiating out to the temporal periphery are very tortuous in character.

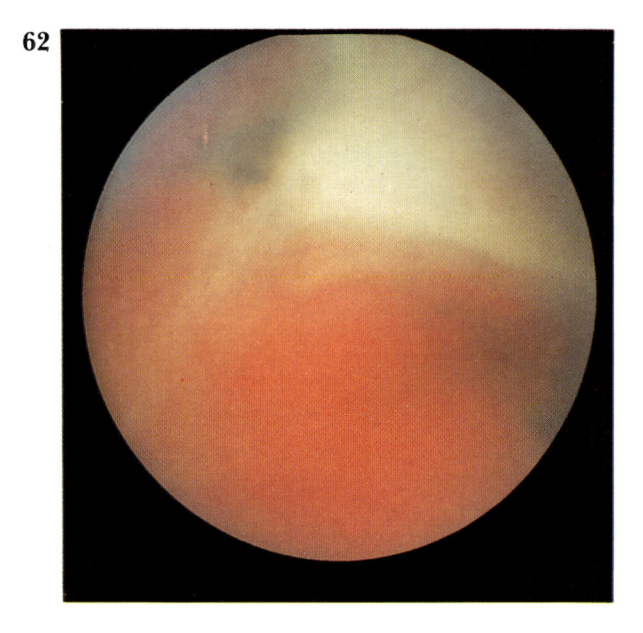

62 Acute toxocariasis infestation with endophthalmitis and vitreous haze overlying the abscess forming below it. The band extends from the most prominent highlighted white area of the abscess to the optic nerve head.

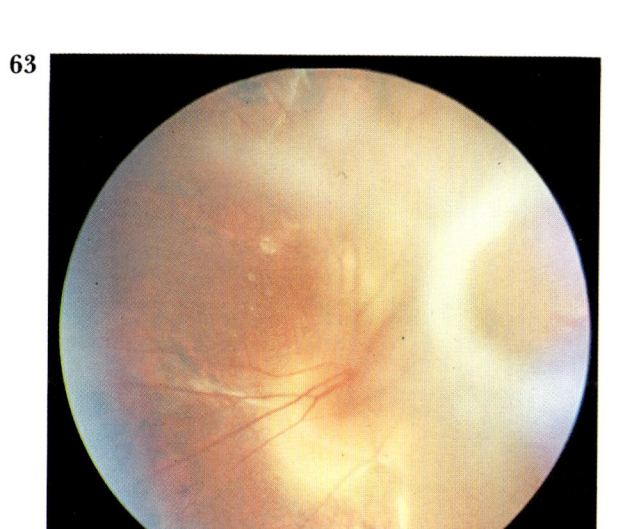

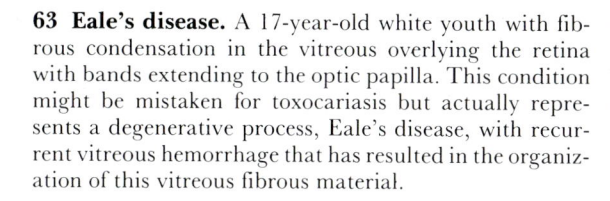

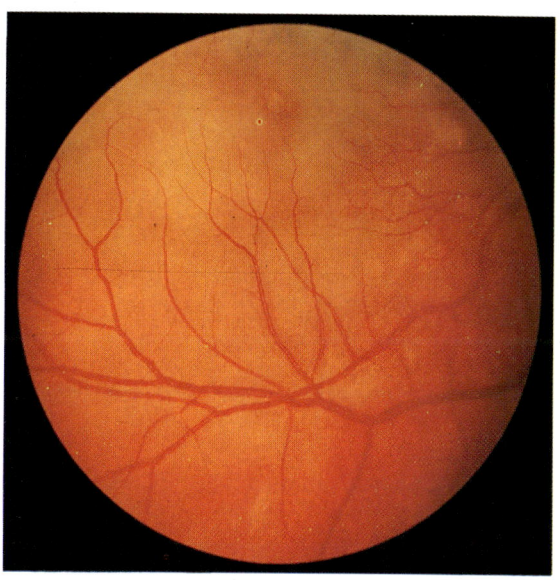

63 Eale's disease. A 17-year-old white youth with fibrous condensation in the vitreous overlying the retina with bands extending to the optic papilla. This condition might be mistaken for toxocariasis but actually represents a degenerative process, Eale's disease, with recurrent vitreous hemorrhage that has resulted in the organization of this vitreous fibrous material.

64 Acute multifocal posterior plaquoid epitheliopathy. A 24-year-old white woman with white retinal and subretinal lesions representing acute multifocal posterior plaquoid epitheliopathy. Note that this is a deep retinal inflammation and that the vessels coursing over the area of white inflammation are relatively undisturbed in their morphology. This is an epithelitis of the retinal pigment epithelium. There may be few or no cells in the overlying vitreous.

65 Coccidioidomycosis choroiditis. Another patient with deep retinal inflammation which might be confused with acute multifocal posterior plaquoid epitheliopathy, but actually represents a coccidioidomycosis choroiditis. This patient also suffers from meningitis caused by the fungus infection. This fungus infection is endemic to the Southwest and is usually spread through pulmonary infection.

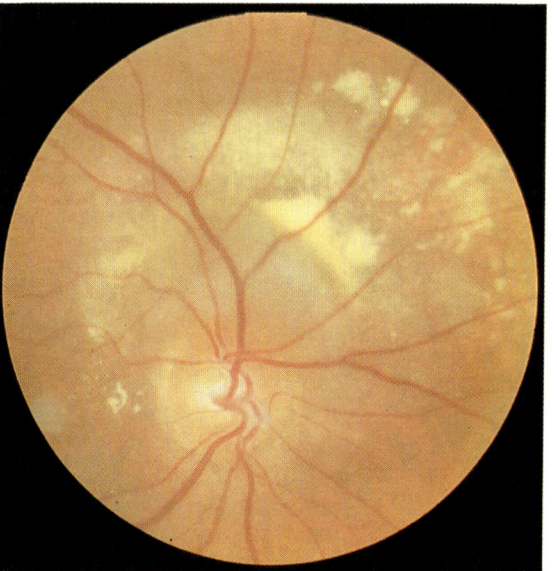

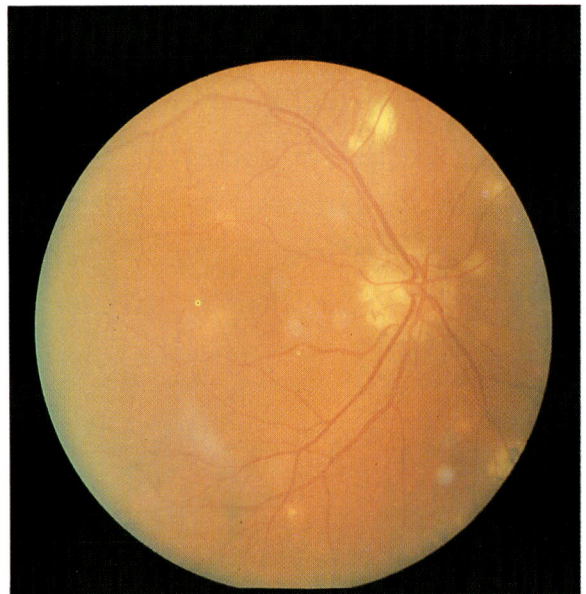

66 Diffuse focal choroidal infiltrates with some vitreous cellularity in patient with acute ocular histoplasmosis syndrome. In this specific instance, there is no subretinal neovascular membrane.

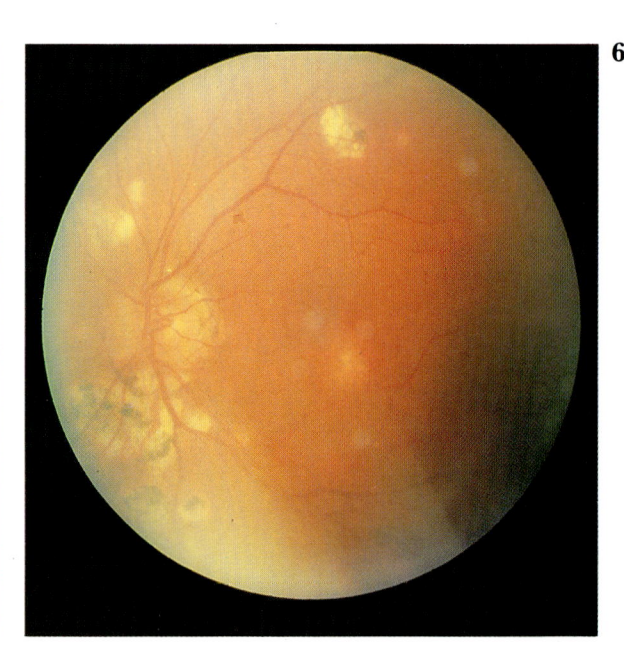

67 Ocular histoplasmosis. Fellow eye of patient with ocular histoplasmosis syndrome with subretinal neovascular membrane inferior to the fovea in this left eye. Note the myriad retinal pigment epithelial scars, some of which are hypopigmented and some of which are hyperpigmented. Not all peripheral 'punched-out' lesions of ocular histoplasmosis are hypopigmented.

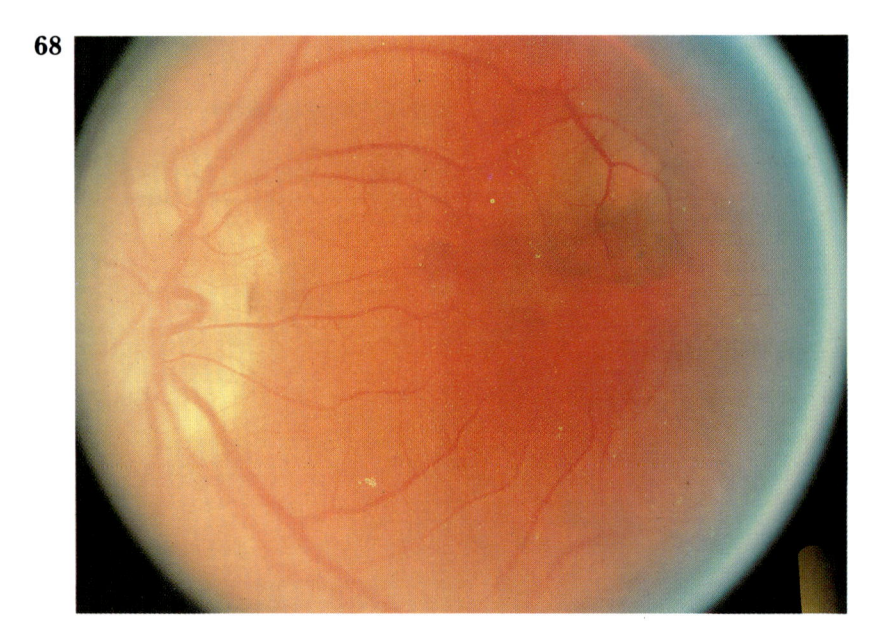

68 Subretinal neovascular membrane. More typical subretinal neovascular membrane in patient with ocular histoplasmosis syndrome. Note the gray-green coloration of the net under the retinal pigment epithelium with the hemorrhage formation nasal to it. Also note the peripapillary depigmentation in this patient as part of the histoplasmosis triad.

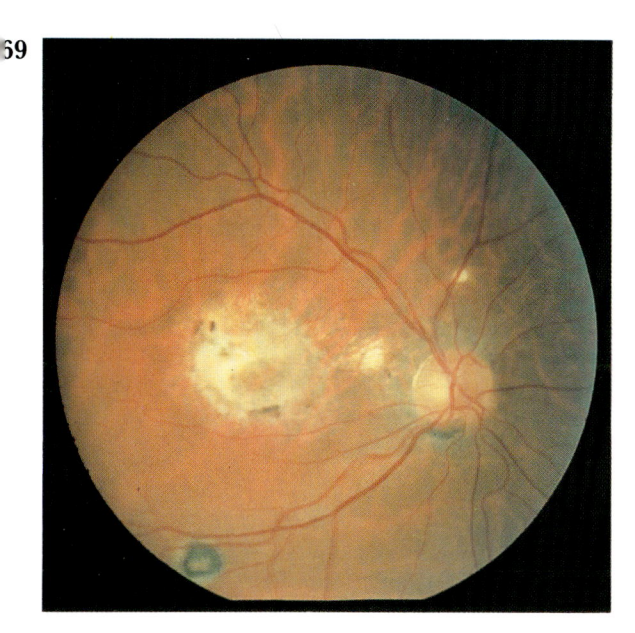

69 Old scarred-up macular disciform lesion from subretinal neovascular membrane in this 24-year-old patient with ocular histoplasmosis syndrome. The entirety of the triad can be seen in this wide-angle photograph including the macular scar, the peripapillary pigmentary changes, and peripheral 'punched-out' lesions, two of which are hypopigmented and one of which is hyperpigmented with retinal pigment epithelial hypertrophy.

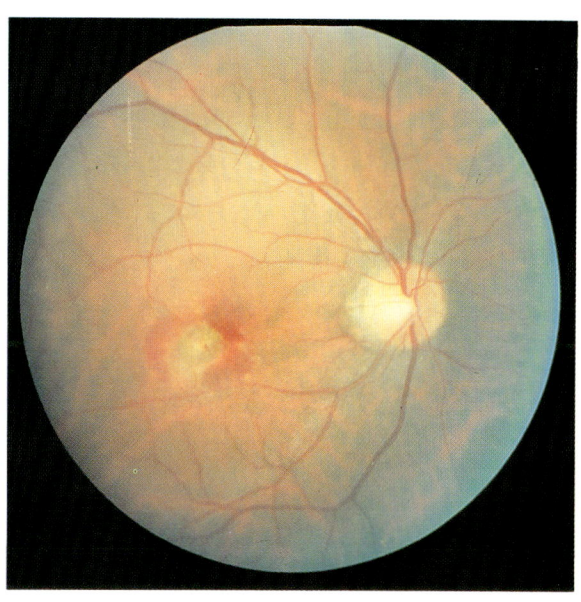

70 Acute hemorrhaging subretinal neovascular membrane in a 23-year-old Chinese man that is highly suspect for ocular histoplasmosis syndrome, but in this eye there are no peripheral 'punched-out' lesions or any peripapillary pigmentary disturbances.

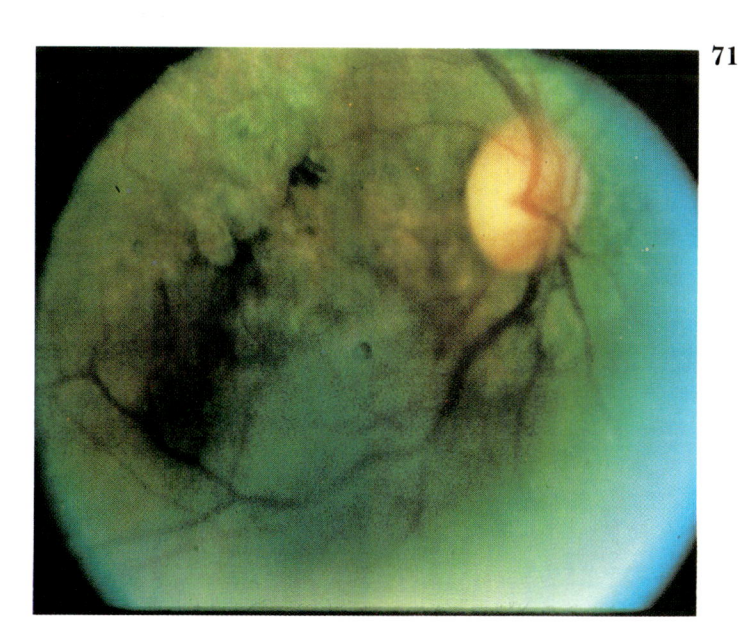

71 Harada syndrome. Profound retinal pigment epithelial disturbance throughout the whole posterior pole in this patient with alternating areas of hypopigmentation and hyperpigmentation, all of which is caused by pigment migration in the Vogt–Koyanagi–Harada syndrome. It is a consequence of repeated serous detachment of the retina with its irritative component to the retinal pigment epithelium.

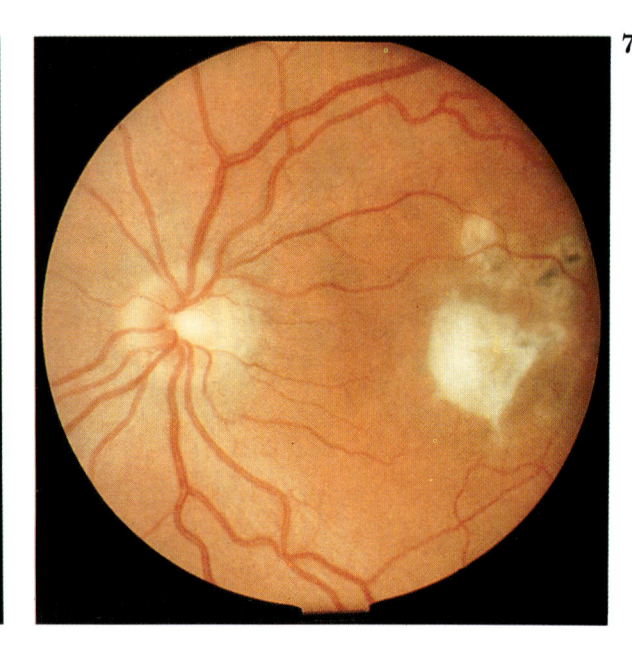

72 Harada syndrome. A 40-year-old Mexican man with Vogt–Koyanagi–Harada disease who demonstrated multiple areas of retinal pigment epithelial disturbance but, more importantly, a chronic subretinal fibrosis and permanent scarring from recurrent serous detachment of the retina.

73 Behçet's disease. A 23-year-old white woman with scarred subretinal neovascular membrane as a consequence of ciliary circulation vasculitis due to Behçet's disease. Subretinal neovascular membranes can occur in many of the inflammatory conditions where it is assumed that a break in Bruch's membrane is occurring due to inflammation in the deep retinal layers, as in several types of choroiditis and retinal-choroiditis (i.e., toxoplasmosis, histoplasmosis, coccidioidomycosis).

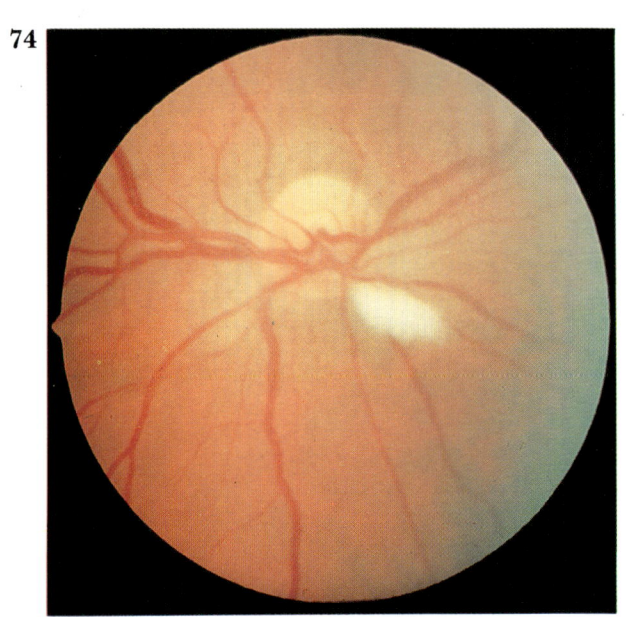

74 Myelinated nerve fibers. A 32-year-old white woman sent in for a focus of retinitis adjacent to optic papilla, thought to be toxoplasmosis but representing myelinated nerve fibers evident upon contact lens examination. There are no cells in the vitreous overlying this lesion.

75 Retinoblastoma. A 19-year-old white man who was refused entrance into the Coast Guard because he was noted to have 'inflammation in and in front of the retina.' This lesion, which looks like crumpled cottage cheese curds, represents a regressed retinoblastoma. The cellular material in the vitreous overlying it is the typical seeding of retinoblastoma as seen in younger children with active tumors. This inactive tumor represents one of the two forms of regressed retinoblastoma. The other is referred to as 'fish flesh'.

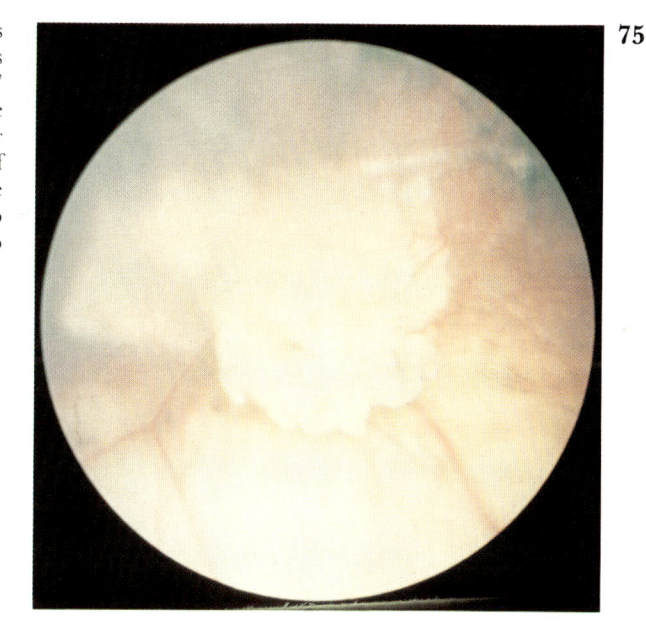

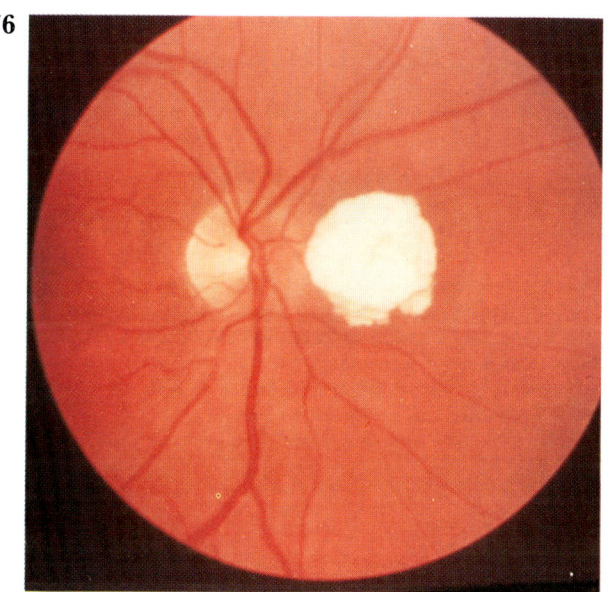

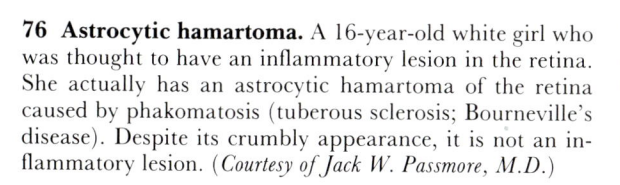

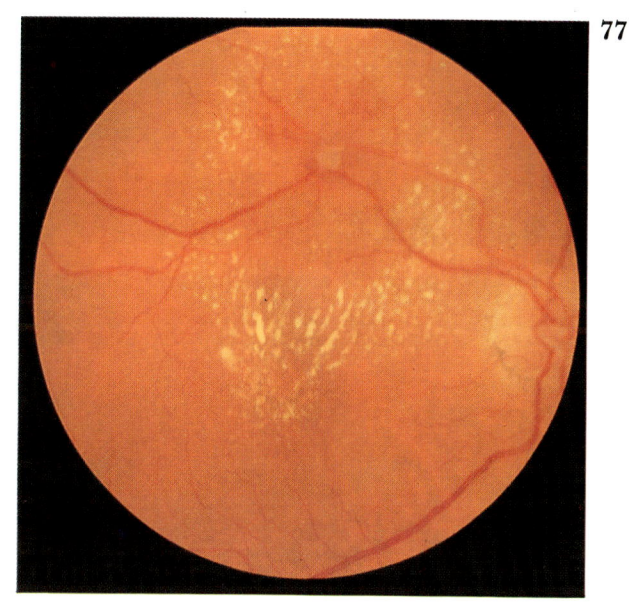

76 Astrocytic hamartoma. A 16-year-old white girl who was thought to have an inflammatory lesion in the retina. She actually has an astrocytic hamartoma of the retina caused by phakomatosis (tuberous sclerosis; Bourneville's disease). Despite its crumbly appearance, it is not an inflammatory lesion. (*Courtesy of Jack W. Passmore, M.D.*)

77 Macroaneurysm. A 45-year-old white man with systemic hypertension was thought to have a focus of inflammation in the retina and choroid with surrounding exudate. In fact, this lesion is a macroaneurysm with surrounding exudative material in the retina.

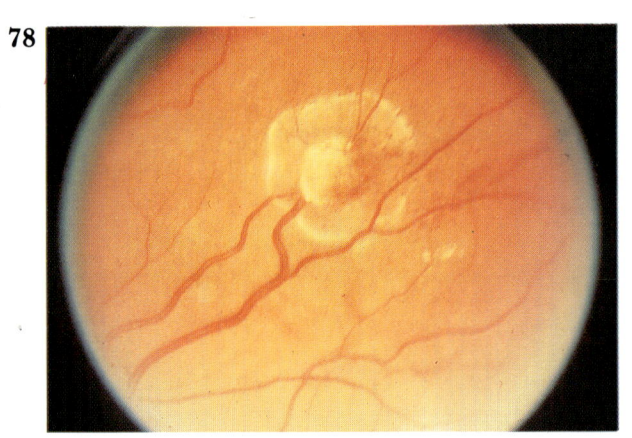

78 Retinal angioma. A 30-year-old white man with angioma of the retina thought to be a focus of inflammation. On fluorescein angiography it lights up in the early arterial phase as a diffuse lightbulb excrescence of the retina. Such an angioma in the periphery is but a form-fruste of the Von Hippel–Lindau syndrome. Note the large feeder vessels coursing into the retinal angioma.

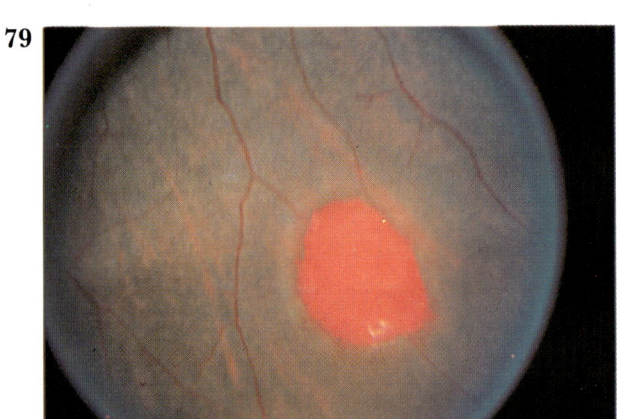

79 Sickle 'salmon patch'. The red-looking inflammatory lesion in the peripheral retina of this 11-year-old black girl is actually a salmon patch of neovascularization from sickle-cell disease. This neovascularization lights up intensely on fluorescence angiography but was initially thought by her referring ophthalmologist to be an inflammatory lesion. The underlying hematologic disorder was only discovered after referral because of the fundus picture. It is important to remember that black patients with sickle disease may have only sickle trait and yet have the full-blown retinopathy seen in a patient with S-S or S-C disease.

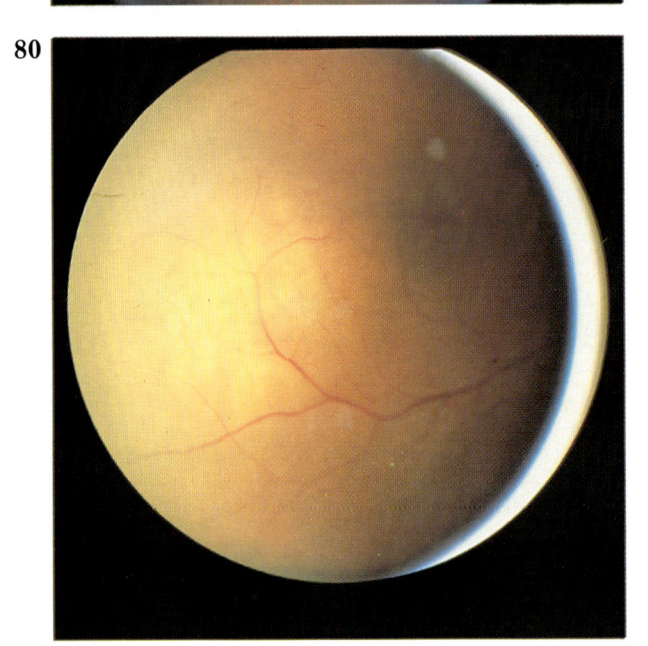

80 Metastatic bronchogenic carcinoma. This 54-year-old white man was thought to have a choroiditis because there are cells overlying this lesion in the vitreous. However, this lesion represents a metastatic bronchogenic carcinoma of the lung that had some vitreous cells overlying it. It shrunk away after radiation therapy.

81 Serous detachment. This 45-year-old white woman has a large shifting retinal detachment temporal to the macula in this right eye. This condition was thought to be inflammatory because there were overlying cells in the vitreous, and there was copious shifting fluid suggestive of a serous detachment of a Vogt–Koyanagi–Harada syndrome.

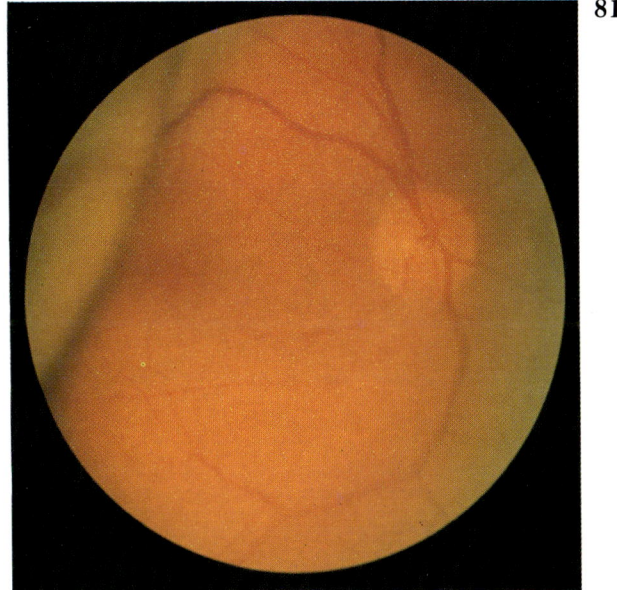

82 Malignant melanoma. More careful observation of the shifting fluid in this serous detachment of this 45-year-old white woman will demonstrate in this enlargement photo the focus of malignant melanoma of the choroid underlying the detachment in the superior aspect of this photograph.

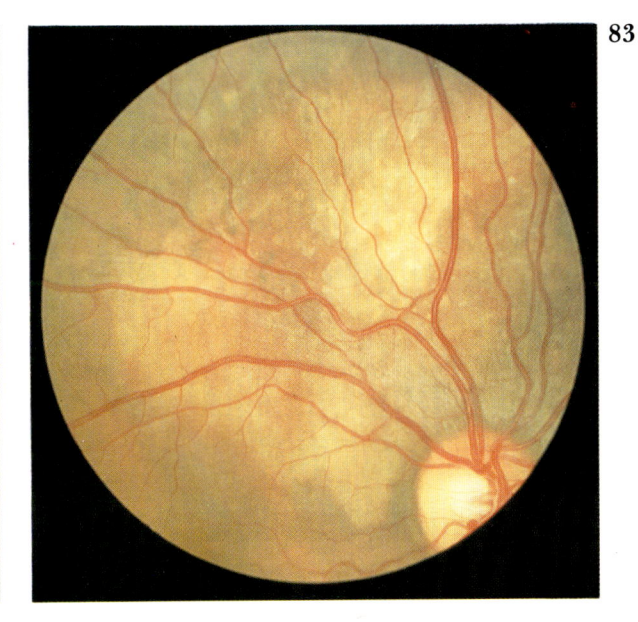

83 Osseous choristoma. This 22-year-old white woman who on first observation might be thought to have retinal pigment epithelial changes either from prior serous detachment of the retina as seen in Vogt–Koyanagi–Harada disease or foci or choroiditis seen in tuberculosis, coccidioidomycosis or a frank choroidal infiltration from malignancy, actually has osseous formation under the retina by both ultrasonography and CAT scan. This is a case of osseous choristoma in a young woman as has been reported by Gass *et al*. Such osseous formation under the retina is probably not inflammatory in nature but may be due either to degenerating choroidal hemangioma that may be subclinical or due to some irritative or metamorphosing phenomenon in the retinal pigment epithelium. (*Courtesy of Howard Schatz, M.D.*)

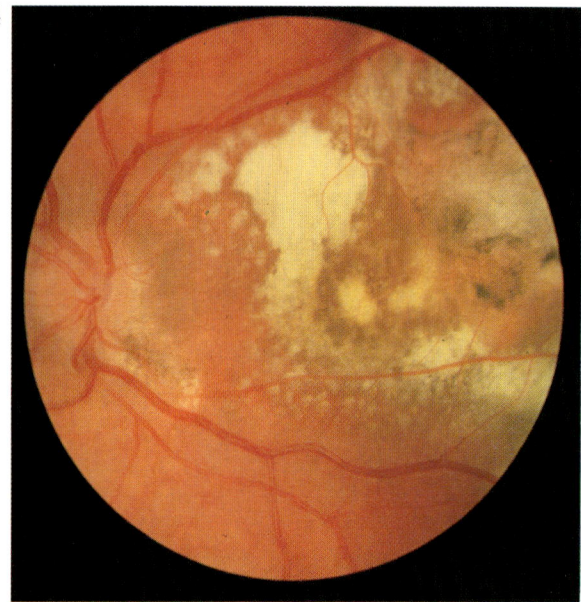

84 Coats' Disease. A 10-year-old white boy with hypopigmentary and hyperpigmentary changes under the retina in the macula region. Shifting fluid suggests Coats' disease in this youngster with lipid and cholesterol crystals and deposits floating under the retina.

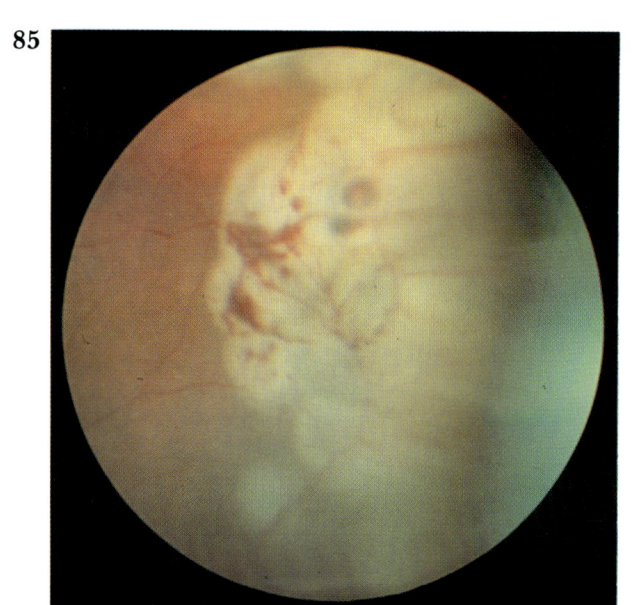

85 Coats' disease. As in Figure 84 where Coats' disease caused serous detachment in the retina in a 10-year-old boy, this 13-year-old boy who had serous detachment of the retina delimited by laser treatment nevertheless demonstrates the typical lightbulb telangiectases on the surfaces of an abnormal retina where the Coats' disease processes were already beginning to hemorrhage.

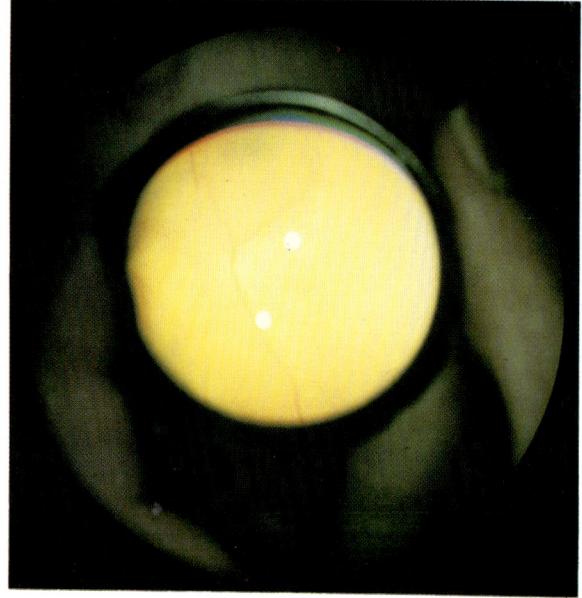

86 Coats' disease. A nine-year-old white boy with total serous detachment of the retina and cells in the vitreous overlying it from Coats' disease. Such a presentation might simulate the active endophthalmitis form of *Toxocara canis* and needs to be differentiated from it. In such a case, it is most helpful to find lightbulb telangiectases (as in Figure 85) in the peripheral retina to corroborate the suggestion of Coats' disease.

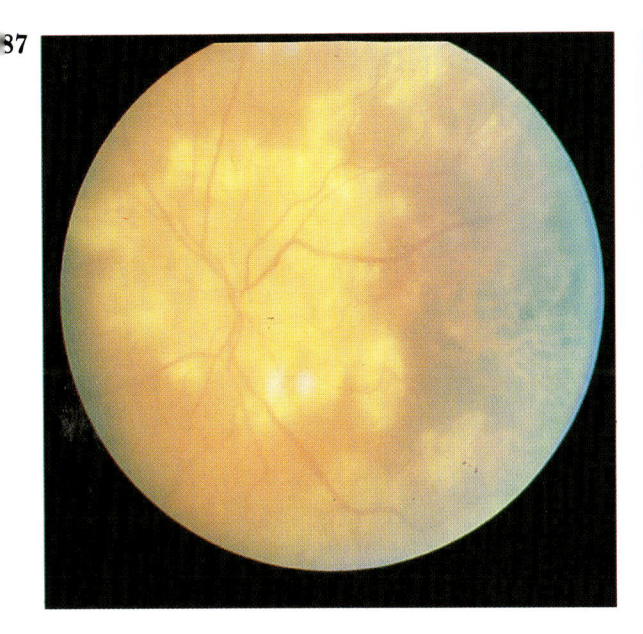

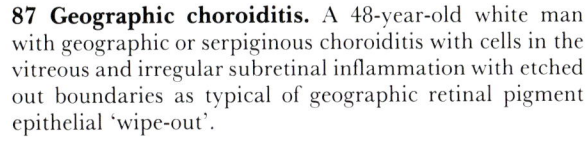

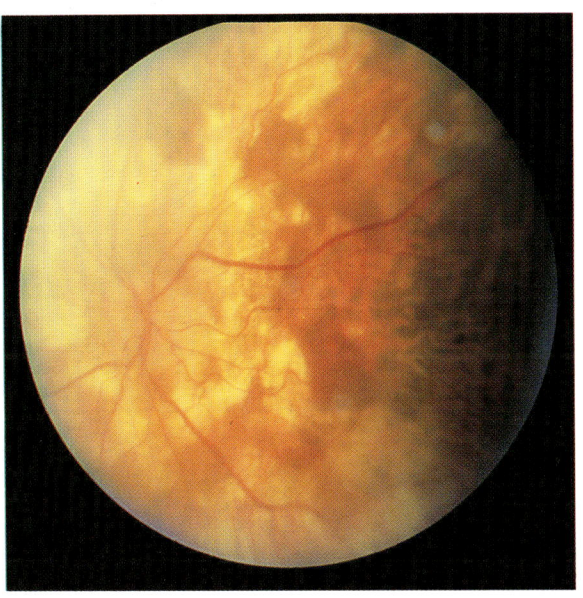

87 Geographic choroiditis. A 48-year-old white man with geographic or serpiginous choroiditis with cells in the vitreous and irregular subretinal inflammation with etched out boundaries as typical of geographic retinal pigment epithelial 'wipe-out'.

88 Geographic choroiditis. Later photograph of same patient as in Figure 87 where the geographic changes have extended further out from the disk superiorly and inferiorly to demonstrate even more retinal pigment epithelial 'wipe-out'.

89 Angioid streaks. A 23-year-old white woman with similar retinal pigment epithelial changes, scalloped and irregular edges underneath the retina demonstrating 'wipe-out' of the retinal pigment epithelium but closer observation will reveal that these changes represent angioid streaks circumferential around the disk and invading the macula with scarring from subretinal neovascular formation. This degenerative phenomenon due to breaks in Bruch's membrane is part of a pseudoxanthoma elasticum syndrome, quite different from the inflammatory nature of geographic choroiditis as noted in the previous photographs.

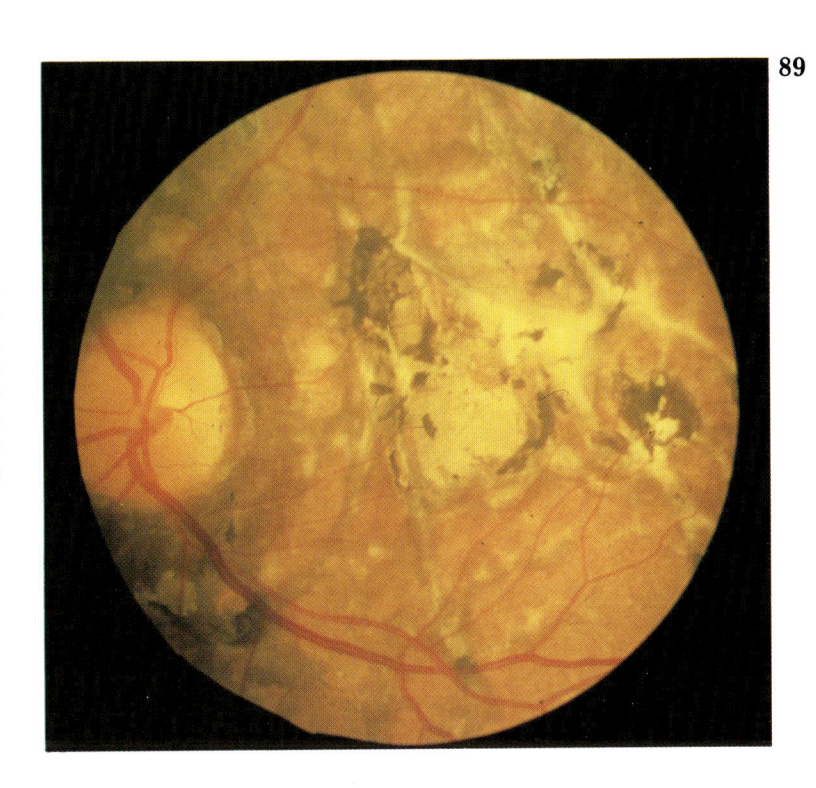

35

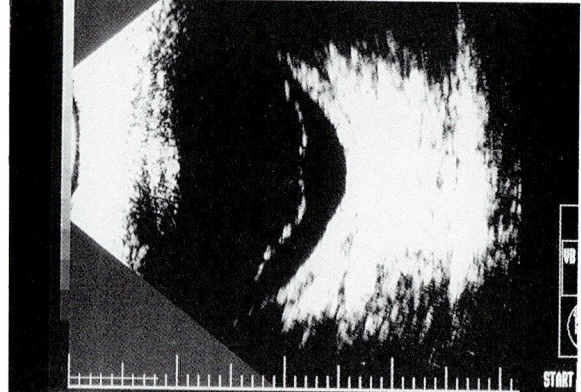

90 Panophthalmitis cataract. A 56-year-old male with panophthalmitis cataract whose B-scan ultrasound demonstrates retinal detachment.

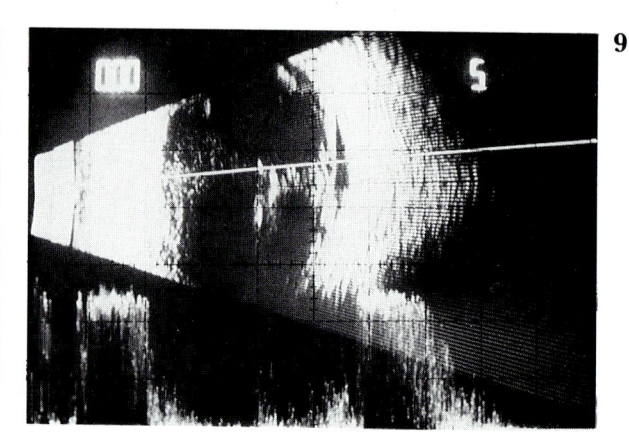

91 Traction retinal detachment. A 17-year-old white male with uveitis whose dense cataract is demonstrated in the anterior portion of this B-scan ultrasound, demonstrating a traction retinal detachment as noted by the large echographic stalk in the center of the vitreous attached to the retinal echoes peeling from the back surface of the eye.

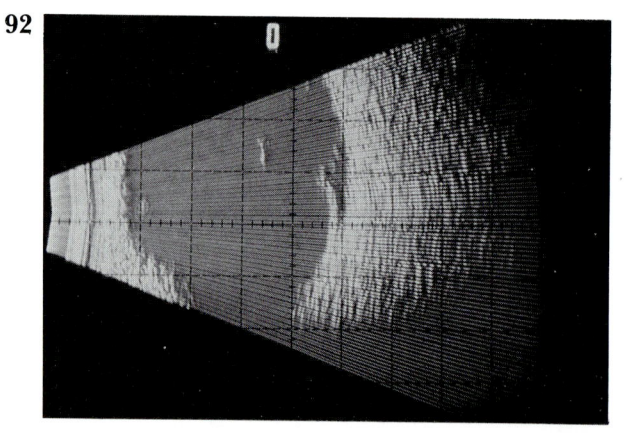

92 Behçet's disease. A 34-year-old Indian male with Behçet's disease whose cataract precluded a view of this traction retinal detachment as noted on B-scan ultrasonography.

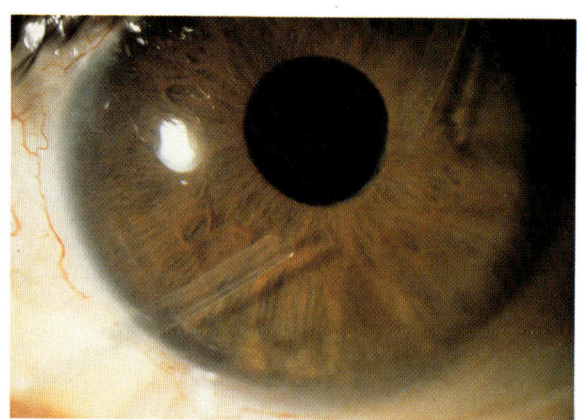

93 Molteno implantation. A 42-year-old Pakistani male who underwent Molteno Seton implantation to control the uveitic glaucoma of Behçet's disease.

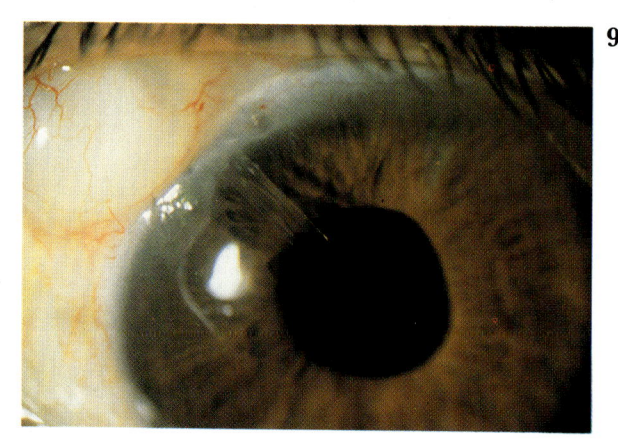

94 Molteno implanatation. Note bleb from Molteno implantation in a 27-year-old patient with Vogt–Koyanagi–Harada syndrome uveitic glaucoma.

Rheumatoid Arthritis

While rheumatoid arthritis is not usually an arthritis-associated uveitis syndrome (like ankylosing spondylitis, Reiter's syndrome, and juvenile rheumatoid arthritis), it can be a contiguous cause of iridocyclitis when it occurs in association with a scleritis or episcleritis. Some of the very severe melting syndromes such as keratomalacia may occur near the limbus and can secondarily stimulate a secondary iridocyclitis (**98, 100**). Dry eye syndrome or keratitis sicca is most commonly associated with rheumatoid arthritis (**95, 96**).

Rheumatoid arthritis is a chronic progressive polyarthritis which occurs three times more commonly in women than in men. The average age of onset is 30 to 40 years. There is a familial tendency and joint deformities are the rule. Keratitis sicca, scleritis, and sclero-keratitis are the main ophthalmic manifestations, but a troublesome, nongranulomatous iritis may occur with these conditions in rare cases.

There are many extra-articular manifestations of rheumatoid arthritis which include pericarditis, pleuritis, nodular pulmonary disease, interstitial fibrosis of the lungs, muscle atrophy, lymphadenopathy, splenomegaly, and rheumatoid nodules. Interestingly, the vasculitis which is seen with peripheral neuropathy is not a feature found in the retina. The cutaneous manifestations of this disease include purpura splinter hemorrhages, skin infection due to vascular necrosis (**143**), ulceration, and digital gangrene (**142**).

RHEUMATOID ARTHRITIS

Definition:
- Secondary iridocyclitis (usually episcleritis)
- Primary corneal melt (ischemia)

Presentation:
- Iridocyclitis
- Nongranulomatous

Investigation:
- Positive RA latex
- ESR
- Joint Xray

Therapy:
- Local intensive steroids
- Periocular
- Short course high-dose systemic steroids
- Antimetabolites
- Cyclosporine

Prognosis:
- Sometimes good
- Sometimes poor

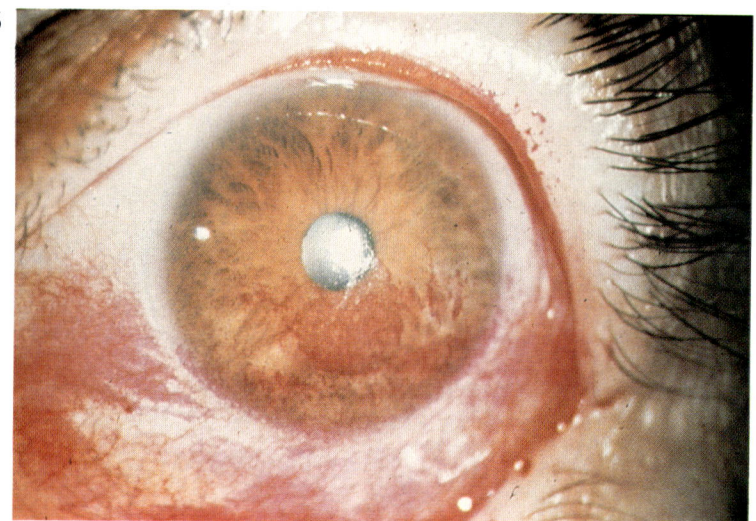

95 Typical dry eye syndrome demonstrated by rose Bengal staining of the cornified epithelium of the conjunctiva in the corneal limbus.

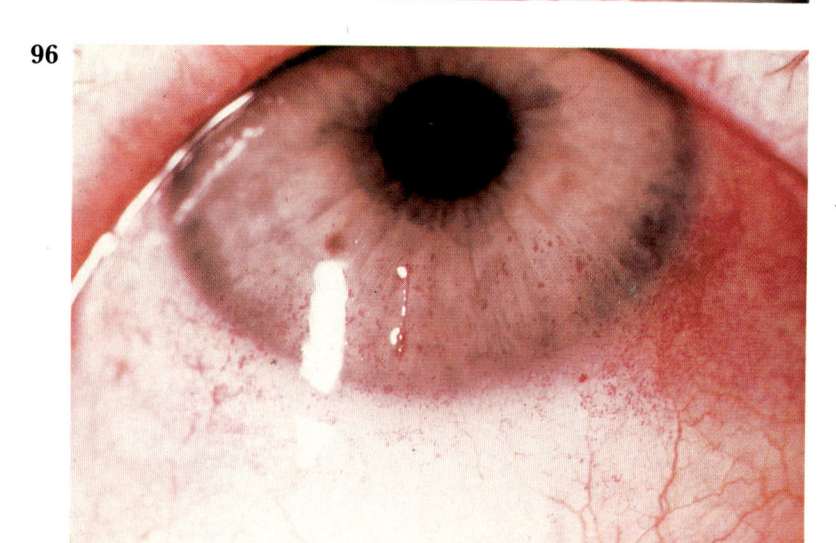

96 Filamentary keratitis may be a prominent manifestation secondary to keratitis sicca as seen here with a filament of the inferior cornea, highlighted by rose Bengal staining in the conjunctiva in and around the limbus.

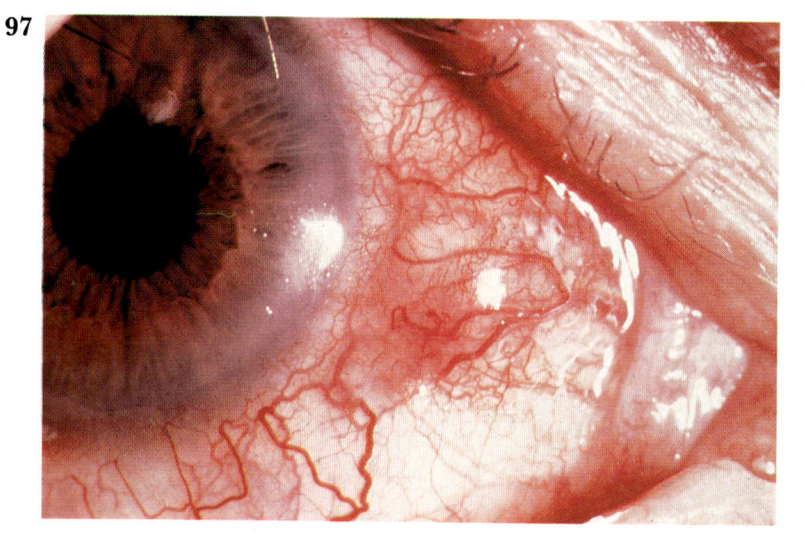

97 Nodular scleritis occurring near the limbus is a cause of secondary iritis.

98 A corneal melt with secondary iridocyclitis is a common manifestation in rheumatoid arthritis as noted by the limbal ulcer seen here.

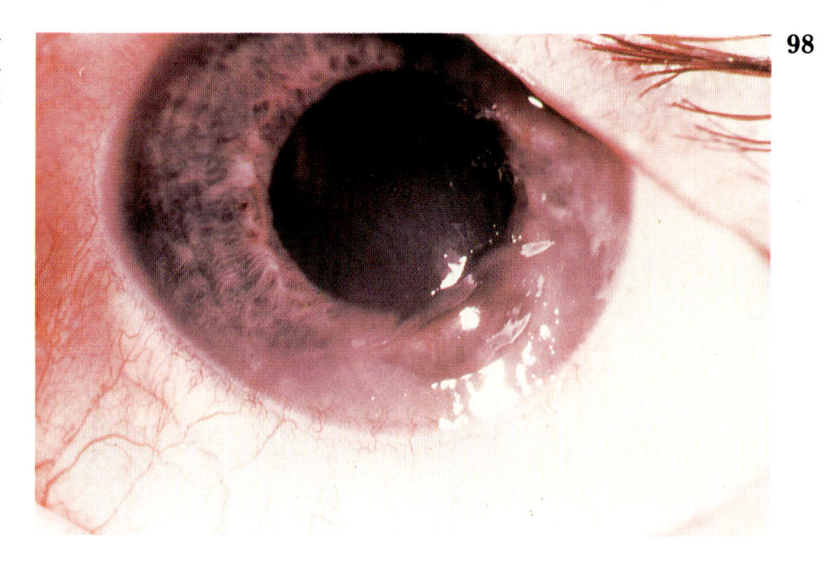

99 Episcleritis and scleritis. An intensely injected conjunctiva, episclera, and sclera is the rule with a diffuse rheumatoid scleral uveitis.

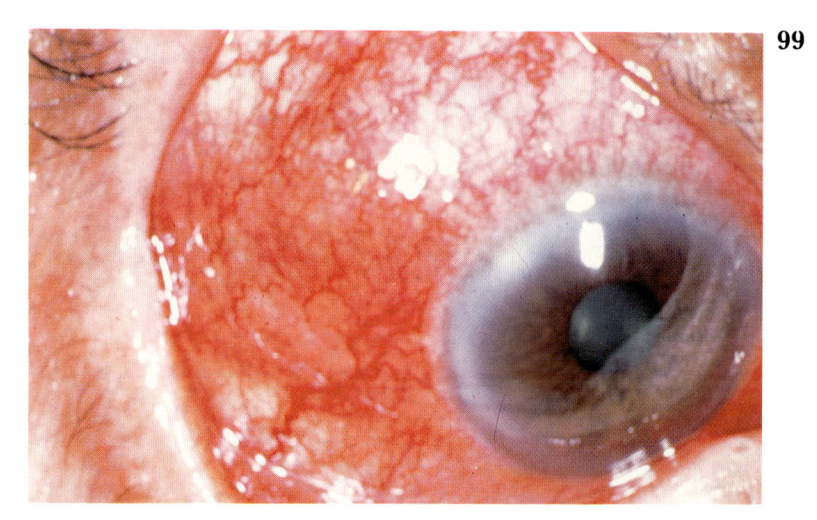

100 Profound keratomalacia perforans is demonstrated with almost no residual sclera remaining and compounded by a profound uveitis with a cloudy cornea. This scleral-corneal melting is not amenable to surgical repair because there is no anterior tissue into which a possible scleral graft can be sewn. (*Courtesy of Wills Eye Hospital, Residents' Teaching Collection.*)

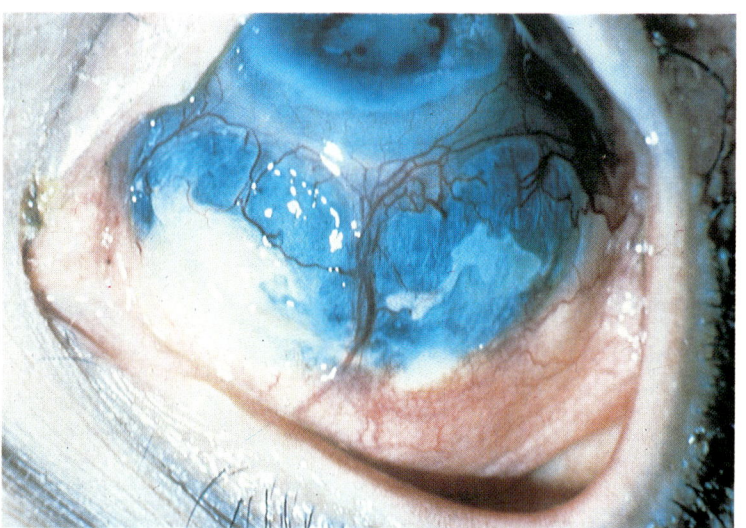

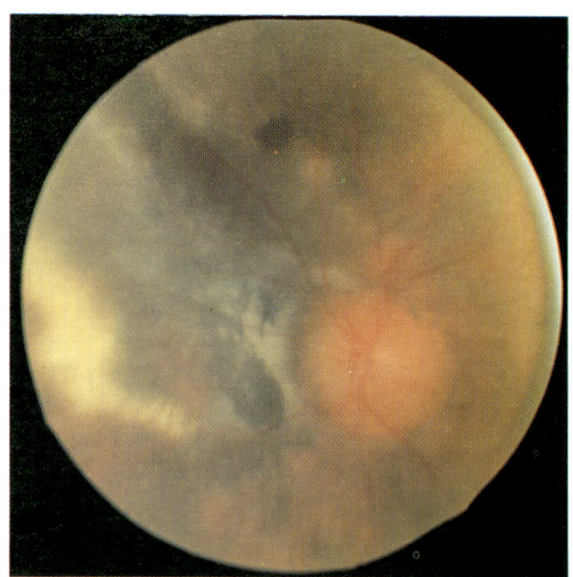

101 Uveal effusion. Fundus of patient with uveal effusion due to posterior nodular scleritis caused by rheumatoid disease. These cases may frequently be confused with malignant melanoma of the choroid when associated with serous retinal detachment.

Juvenile Rheumatoid Arthritis

Juvenile rheumatoid arthritis is not a children's variety of adult rheumatoid arthritis. It is a different disease which may be a chronic and progressive crippler of children. Onset is usually from 2 to 4 years of age; the disease rarely manifests itself before the age of 6 months. It is more common in young girls than boys. Iridocyclitis and associated ocular complications of cataract and glaucoma are frequently significant causes of blindness in these children and may overshadow the acute initial episode of arthritis over a long period. Because cataract or cyclitis can occur in a white quiet eye much as with pars planitis, accurate classification of this syndrome is essential.

There are three distinct types of juvenile rheumatoid arthritis: Still's disease, polyarticular juvenile rheumatoid arthritis, and monoarticular or pauci-articular rheumatoid arthritis. Paradoxically, ocular inflammation is rare when the systemic disease is most severe, and it is the monoarticular or pauci-articular variety of juvenile rheumatoid arthritis that has the most severe forms of ocular complications. Frequently the systemic illness may be so mild as to escape detection, but ocular complications may occur in up to 25% of the patients with the monoarticular or pauci-articular variety of juvenile rheumatoid arthritis.

Still's disease is the classic febrile severe illness with large joint involvement, lymphadenopathy, splenomegaly, and is a systemic illness which may be confused with mononucleosis. It may only have occasional iridocyclitis with apparent ocular manifestations. The polyarticular type of juvenile rheumatoid arthritis accounts for 50% of the children with this disease. Still's disease is usually seen in young children but few have ocular involvement.

The patients who may have mild or no history of monoarticular or pauci-articular arthritis but who do have the signs of iridocyclitis (**103**) with synechiaed pupils, secondary glaucoma, cataracts, and more importantly, band keratopathy (**104**) as a presenting sign, usually have juvenile rheumatoid arthritis until proven otherwise. The iridocyclitis is essentially nongranulomatous, although small and fine keratic precipitates are usually present. It is typically indolent and the eye is usually neither injected nor painful. For these reasons iridocyclitis may go unnoticed by family physicians and parents until the vision is so reduced that it may even be discovered by a routine eye examination. Posterior segment inflammation is very unusual, but choroiditis has been noted and vitreous floaters may be common. When a child presents with such a quiet white eye with band keratopathy, synechiae, and vitreous cells, *Toxocara canis* must be ruled out. Pars planitis usually presents in older children and frequently does not have synechiae or band keratopathy. Children with juvenile rheumatoid arthritis are usually seronegative for rheumatoid factor and positive for antinuclear antibody.

JUVENILE RHEUMATOID ARTHRITIS

Definition:
- Chronic iridocyclitis

Presentation:
- Iridocyclitis
- Nongranulomatous

Investigation:
- ANA
- ESR
- Pediatric rheumatologic consultation

Therapy:
- Medium strength mydriatic/cycloplegic agent, at least night time, even in remission
- More frequent mydriatic/cycloplegics during exacerbations
- Periocular steroids
- Systemic steroids during exacerbations
- Some patients do well on low-dose chronic systemic steroids
- Cyclosporine contraindicated
- Antimetabolites usually are contraindicated

Complications:
- Cataracts
- Band keratopathy
- Phthisis bulbi

Prognosis:
- Variable

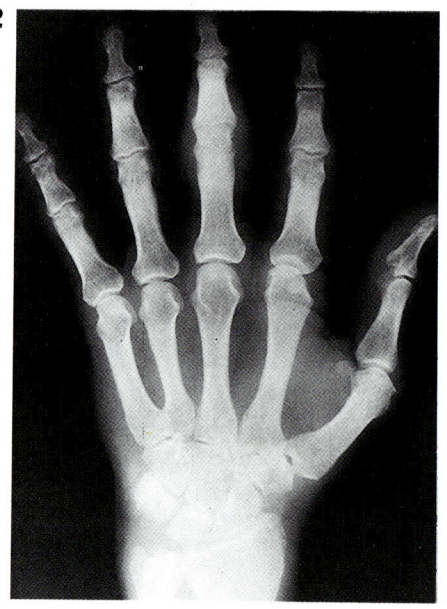

102 Monoarticular arthritis in the hand of a small child with juvenile rheumatoid arthritis and concomitant iridocyclitis, cataract, and synechiae.

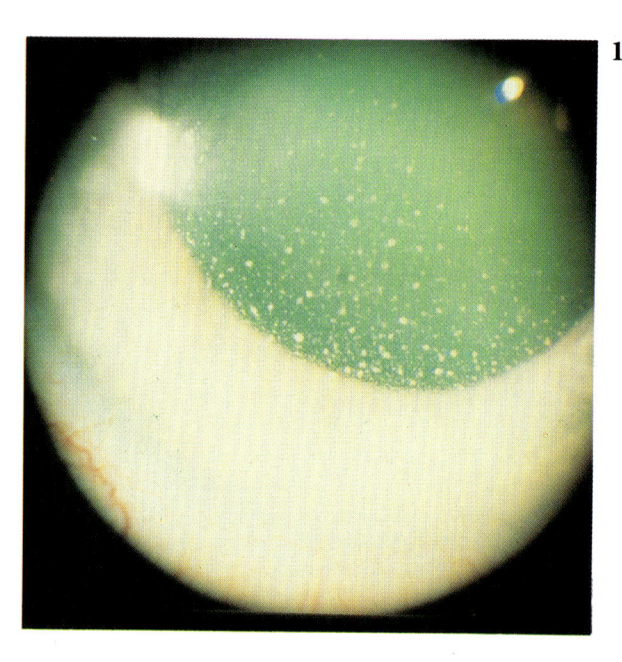

103 Small, fine, white KP in a child with early cataract formation and iridocyclitis with a juvenile rheumatoid arthritis picture.

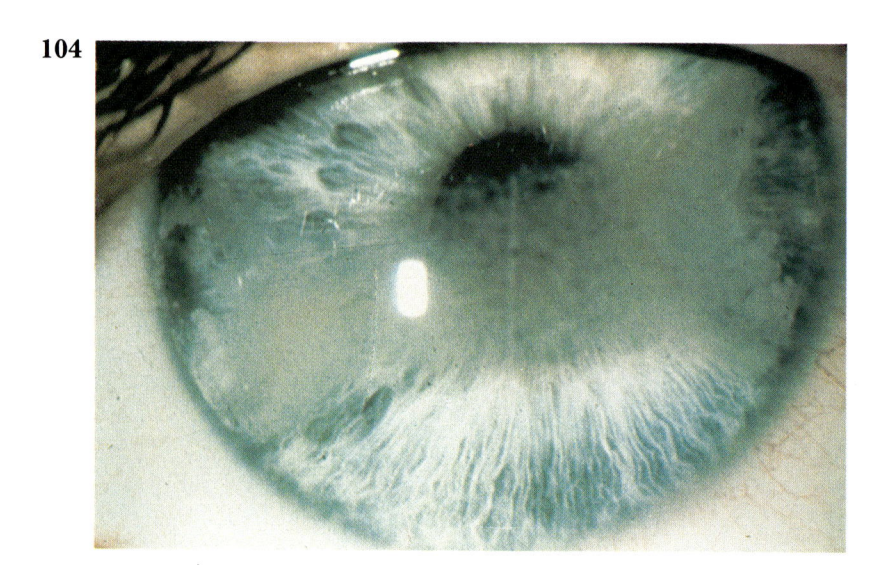

104 Band keratopathy in an otherwise white, singularly quiet eye in a child with juvenile rheumatoid arthritis who has ongoing quiet iridocyclitis.

105 Dense white cataract and synechiae in patient with monoarticular juvenile rheumatoid arthritis.

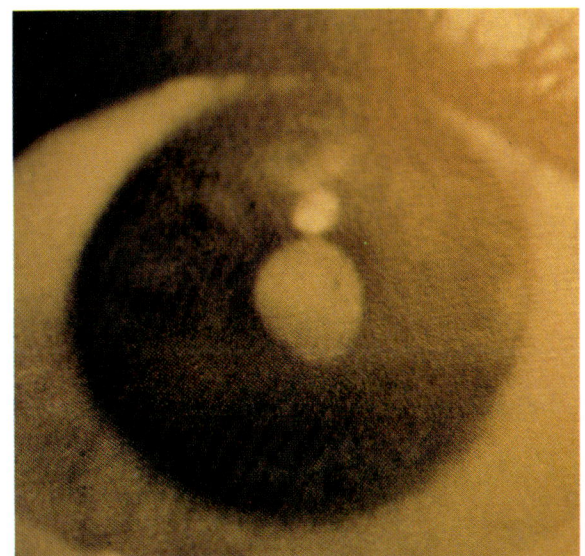

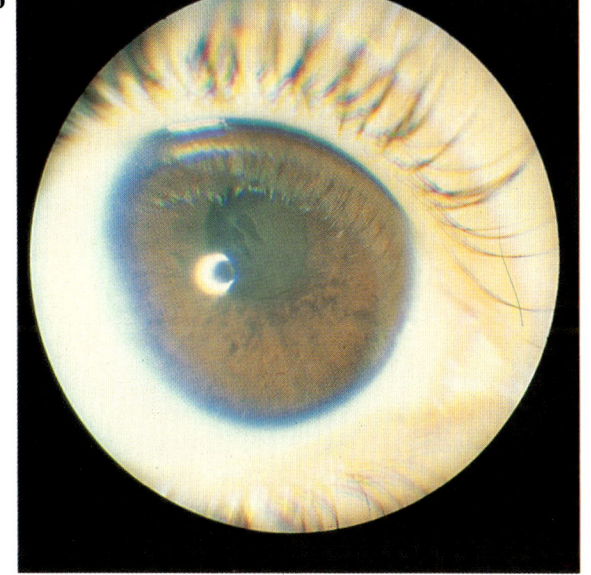

106 Cyclitic membrane formed after cataract surgery in child with juvenile rheumatoid arthritis. In former times these eyes were considered poor candidates for cataract surgery; however, with the advent of pars plana vitrectomy techniques, these eyes may be successfully operated on for cataract and cyclitic membrane. Many avoid the development of phthisis bulbi.

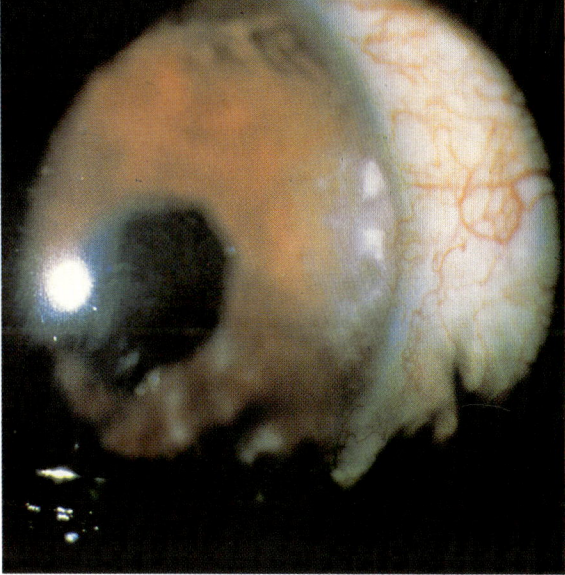

107 Recurrent flare-up of intense iridocyclitis with large white KP in a 24-year-old woman who suffers from constant, typical low-grade iritis secondary to juvenile rheumatoid arthritis. Note the 'early' band keratopathy changes temporally.

Ankylosing Spondylitis

Ankylosing spondylitis occurs most frequently in young men in their 20s and 30s. The eye disease may be unilateral but often occurs in both eyes, although almost never concurrently. Iridocyclitis may precede clinical joint disease in these patients.

In most patients recurrent iridocyclitis of the acute, intermittent variety is the rule. About half of all patients whose Xrays show evidence of ankylosing spondylitis are asymptomatic. Therefore, sacroiliac Xrays of all men with recurrent iridocyclitis, regardless of systemic complaints, is a worthy undertaking.

The HLA b27 antigen is positive in over 90% of patients, while the sedimentation rate is often elevated during an acute attack of spondylitis and tests for rheumatoid factor are negative.

ANKYLOSING SPONDYLITIS

Definition:
- Acute intermittent iridocyclitis

Presentation:
- Iridocyclitis
- Nongranulomatous

Investigation:
- HLA b27
- ESR
- Sacroiliac joint Xrays

Therapy:
- Intensive local steroids
- Pupillary dilatation
- Periocular steroids, if severe
- No R_x between attacks

Complications:
- Cataracts
- Posterior synchiae
- Glaucoma
- Rarely: phthisis bulbi

Prognosis:
- Good
- Poor, if chronic

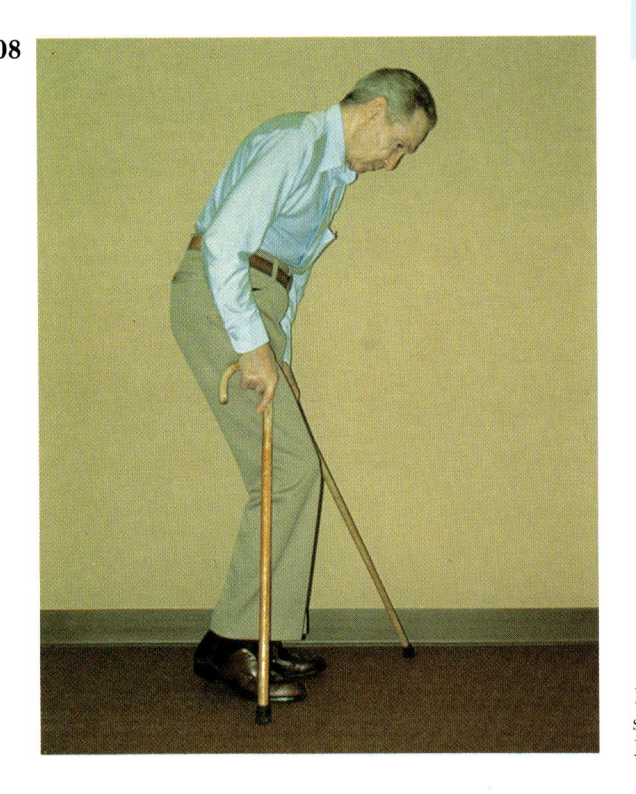

108 Marie–Strümpell spine. Man with ankylosing spondylitis demonstrating a typical stooped posture of the Marie–Strümpell spine.

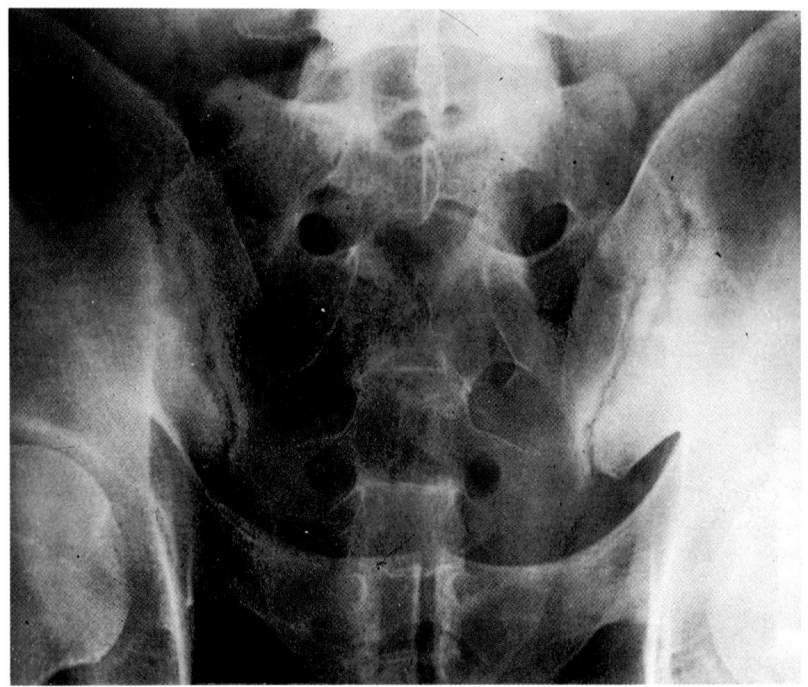

109 Sacroiliac sclerosis. Sacroiliac Xrays show sclerosis and blurring of the margins of the sacroiliac joints in patient with ankylosing spondylitis. (It is worthy to note that in early spondylitis a technetium scan may be more sensitive than Xray and may be positive in the absence of typical Xray changes.)

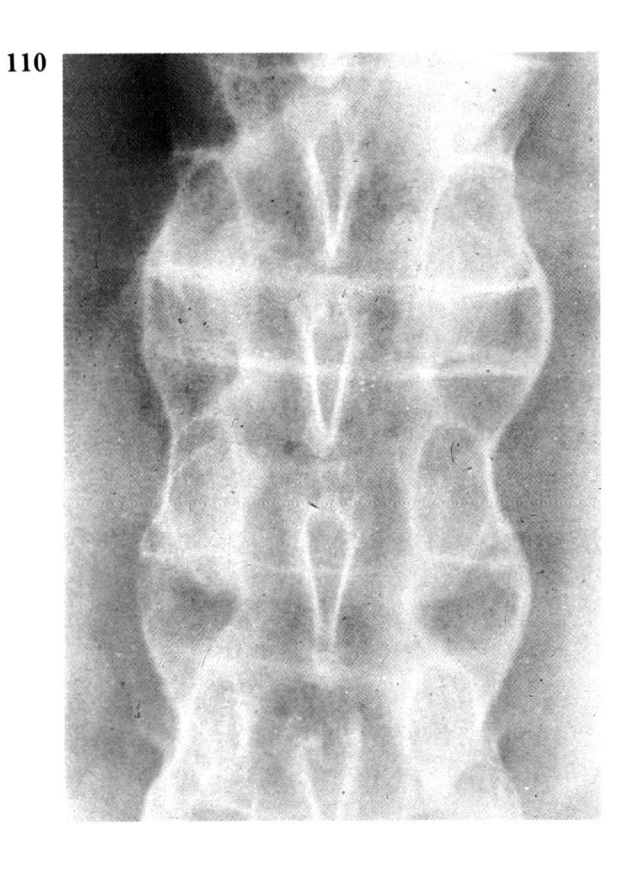

110 Typical bamboo spine in patient with advanced ankylosing spondylitis.

Reiter's Disease

This syndrome occurs most often in men and consists of a nonspecific urethritis with polyarthritis and conjunctivitis followed by recurrent iridocyclitis. There may be cutaneous mucosal lesions which may confuse the syndrome with Behçet's disease. Most patients are between 20 and 40 years of age.

The first ocular sign may be conjunctivitis which occurs in up to a third of the cases (**111**). The ocular signs that follow most often are iritis and recurrent iridocyclitis. There may be severe pain, photophobia, diminished vision, synechiae, KP, and large numbers of cells in the anterior chamber and the anterior vitreous. Keratitis and episcleritis may also occur.

The systemic signs of Reiter's syndrome are nonspecific urethritis and cystitis which can lead to chronic prostatitis and recurrent urinary tract inflammations. The arthropathic manifestations of Reiter's disease are usually inflammation of the large weight-bearing joints, particularly ankles and knees, and there seems to be some late overlap with ankylosing spondylitis. A cutaneous inflammation of keratoderma blenorrhagica may occur in less than 10% of cases. The mucosal lesions affecting the mouth and genitalia occur in 25% of patients.

REITER'S DISEASE

Definition:
- Acute intermittent iridocyclitis

Presentation:
- Iridocyclitis
- Nongranulomatous

Investigation:
- HLA b27 (positive 80%)
- ESR
- Xrays
- Rheumatologic consultation

Therapy:
- Intensive local steroids
- Pupillary dilatation

Complications:
- Cataracts
- Posterior synechiae
- Glaucoma
- Rarely: phthisis, if chronic

Prognosis:
- Excellent (often begins with papillary conjunctivitis)

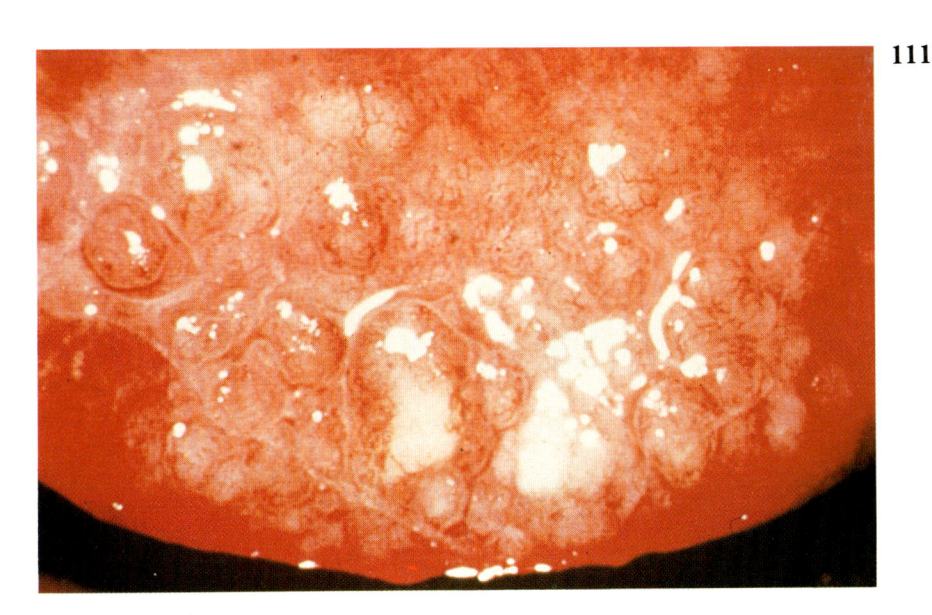

111 Large papillary conjunctivitis in a 12-year-old patient with Reiter's disease.

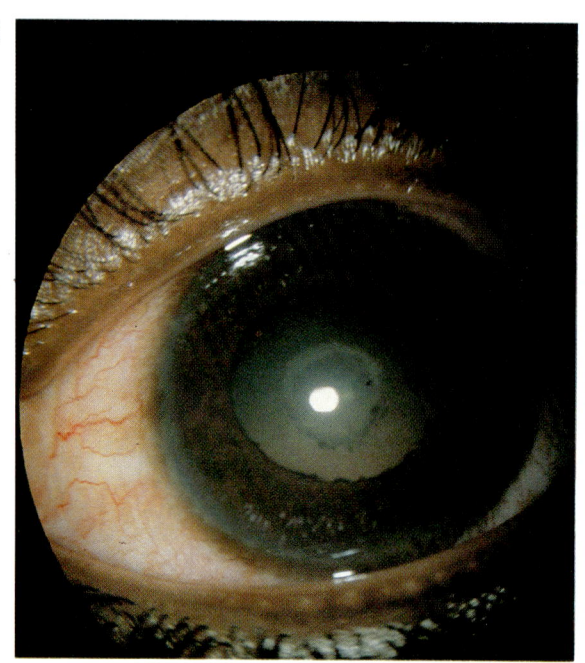

112 Synechiaed pupil. A 19-year-old black patient with Reiter's disease demonstrating a dilated pupil with Voissus' ring from which he had synechiae for 360° on the anterior lens capsule.

Sarcoidosis

Sarcoidosis is a multisystemic disease whose histologic hallmark is a noncaseating granuloma. Vasculitis and, more specifically, phlebitis (**123**) are common accompaniments to the histologic features of this disorder. Sarcoidosis accounts for between 3 to 10% of all cases of uveitis. Between 25 and 50% of patients with systemic sarcoidosis develop uveal inflammation. The most common manifestation is iridocyclitis, but many different intraocular and extraocular structures may be involved.

Sarcoidosis is seen most commonly in Scandanavia and along the Atlantic Gulf coasts of the USA. In the USA this type of inflammation occurs in black patients 10 times more frequently than in whites, women outnumbering men 2 to 1. HLA b8 has been reported to occur more often in sarcoid patients than in the general population. Although sarcoidosis has been reported in children and the elderly, it is most likely to occur in young and middle-aged patients. For the majority of patients, ocular disease remains active for only several years while less than 10% develop a chronic form of the disease for longer than this.

Systemic sarcoidosis involves the parenchyma of the lungs in 80% of patients. Hilar adenopathy (**113**), involving the large lymph nodes draining the lungs, may be seen in over 75% of patients, many of whom will be asymptomatic. Gallium scan of the head (**114, 115**) and thorax will often demonstrate enlarged glandular tissue in the lacrimal area, as well as the salivary glands, and the adenopathy of the hilar region. Angiotensin converting enzyme (ACE) should also be obtained, but may be positive in the presence of other granulomatous diseases. Skin manifestations of sarcoidosis are seen in approximately a third of patients (**116, 117**), while hepatomegaly will occur in only 15% of patients. One should carefully scan the eyelids and the conjunctiva (**118**) with double eversion of the lids for sarcoid nodules, which may be of great benefit in yielding the histologic hallmark of noncaseating granuloma. However, blind biopsy of the conjunctiva is considered fruitless.

A severe recurrent iridocyclitis occurs most frequently. Choroiditis and retinal vasculitis are often present and almost exclusively manifest as periphlebitis. The iridocyclitis is often characterized by large mutton-fat granulomatous KP (**119, 120**), dense posterior synechiae, peripheral anterior synechiae, and marked cell and flare in the anterior chamber. The complications of this may be an acute or chronic secondary glaucoma or band keratopathy, cataract, and granulomatous nodules on the iris surface, at the pupillary margin, in the stroma (**121**), and in the angle (Busacca, Koeppe, Berlin's nodules). Characteristically, many of these iris nodules become vascularized.

Sarcoidosis may manifest itself in the posterior segment of the eye but not unless it is accompanied by anterior segment inflammation. Round, yellow-gray lesions found in the choroid resolve, usually leaving a choroidal scar. When the retina itself is involved, there are usually exudates around the retinal vessels, predominantly on the venular side, described as 'candle wax drippings'. Snowball opacities in the vitreous cavity are usual and may be confused with those found in pars planitis. The optic nerve may be involved with a granuloma (**122**), causing resultant visual field defects in the central vision. Cystoid macular edema may be a complication of the inflammation due to chronic phlebitis of the posterior segment of the eye.

SARCOIDOSIS

Definition:
- Granulomatous inflammation

Presentation:
- Anything (great mimicker): iritis, vasculitis, granulomata
- Granulomatous

Investigation:
- Chest Xray
- Skin test (anergy to TBC, mumps, etc.)
- Conjunctival biopsy
- ESR
- Consultation
- ACE (serum angiotensin converting enzyme)
- Serum lysozyme
- Gallium scan
- Serum proteins
- Serum and urinary calcium, phosphorus, PO4
- Xray (hands, feet)
- Kveim test

Therapy:
- Local steroids
- Periocular steroids
- Treat recurrent iridocyclitis
- Treat chronic iridocyclitis
- Treat active choroiditis lesions with systemic steroids covered by antituberculous therapy (for instance INH)

Prognosis:
- Variable

Noncaseating epithelioid cell tubercle is the characteristic histologic hallmark of sarcoidosis. The epithelioid cells probably derive from macrophages and often contain intermingled lymphocytes and multinucleated giant cells: Langerhan's cells. Schaumann bodies are characteristic inclusions found in the cytoplasm of the giant cells that are accompaniments of other acidophilic bodies. The necrosis that is usually associated with tuberculosis is not found in sarcoidosis.

Infiltration of the glandular tissue of the lacrimal gland may produce a nonpainful firm swelling in the supratemporal quadrant of the orbit and may be a common finding in patients with generalized systemic sarcoidosis. Other types of extraocular involvement include keratitis sicca and nodular infiltrations in both the bulbar and palpebral conjunctiva, which when recognized may offer a high yield for diagnostic biopsy. Corneal involvement in sarcoidosis is usually secondary to attendant hypercalcemia, and band keratopathy may sometimes be seen, as an end-stage uveitis, *T. canis*, and end-stage glaucoma.

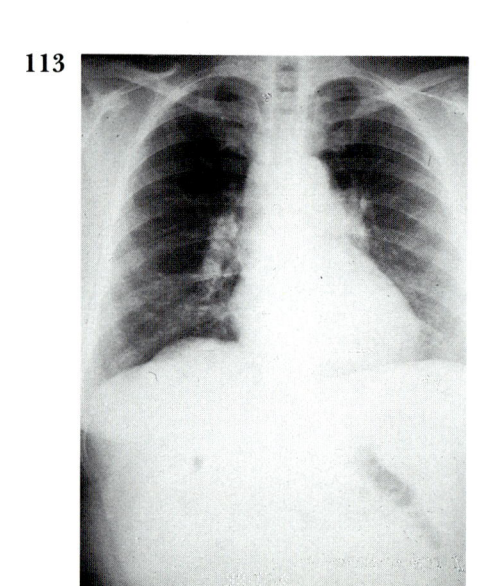

113 Chest Xray of a patient with sarcoidosis demonstrating prominent hilar adenopathy.

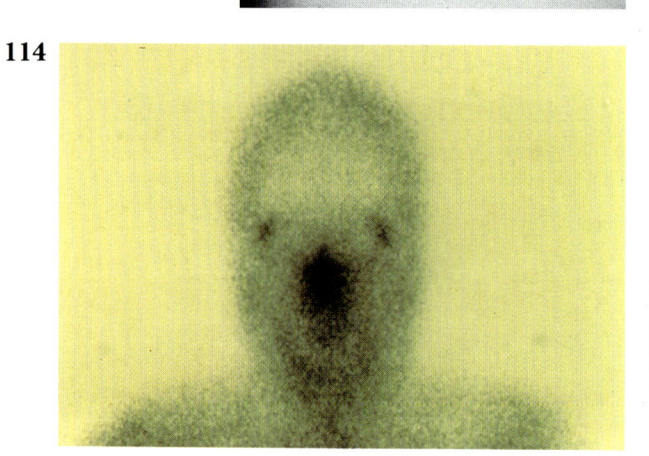

114 Gallium scan of the head in a patient with sarcoidosis demonstrates uptake in the area of lacrimal and salivary glands.

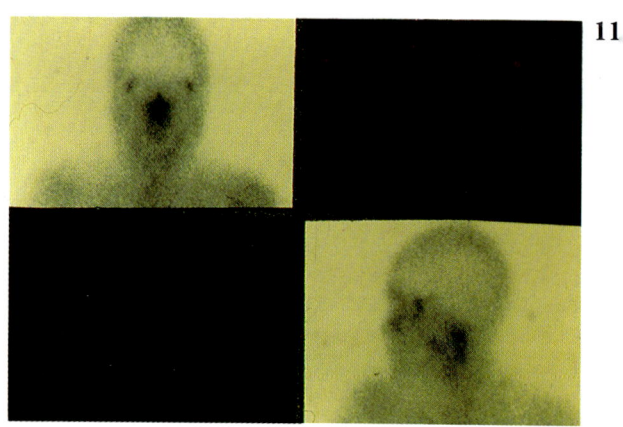

115 Gallium scan of a patient with sarcoidosis who demonstrates prominent uptake of lacrimal glands, salivary glands and lining of the nasal and pharyngeal mucosa.

116 Distinct sarcoid nodules are noted in the lower lid and the maxillary skin of this patient.

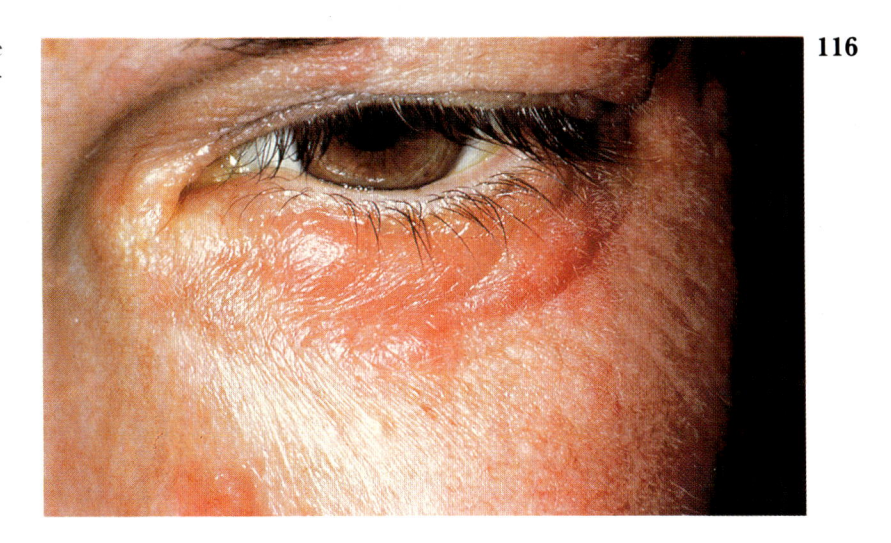

116

117 Large sarcoid granuloma at the upper canthus in this this 32-year-old black man. The raised, rubbery, and reddish lesion of 'lupus pernio' is the specific cutaneous lesion noted in sarcoidosis.

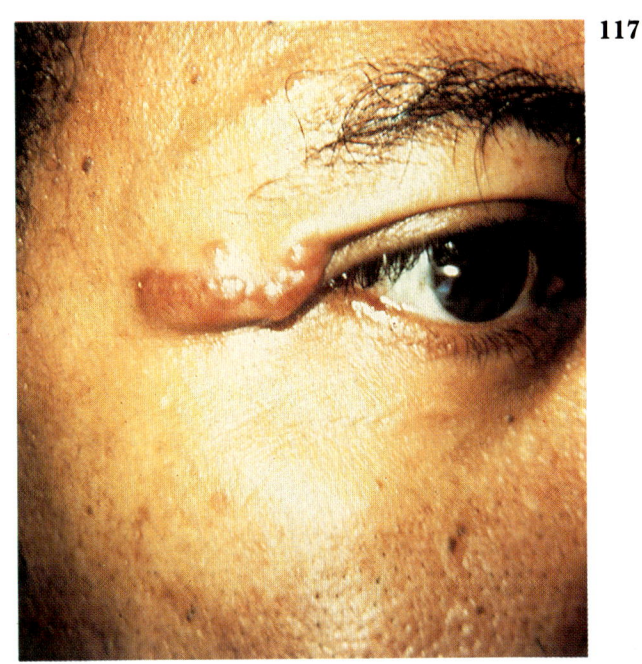

117

118 Grayish-white sarcoid granuloma hugs the palpebral and bulbar conjunctiva of the lower lid which will yield a diagnostic noncaseating granuloma. (*Courtesy of G. Richard O'Connor, M.D.*)

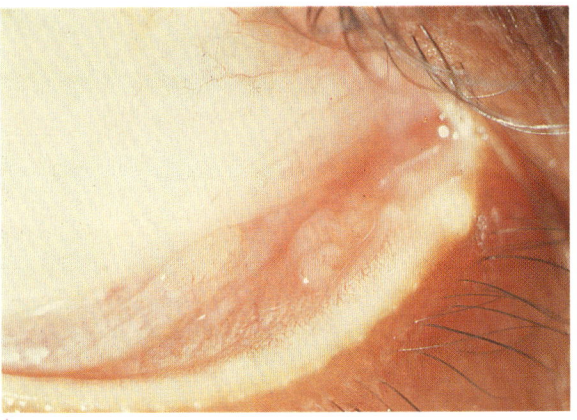

118

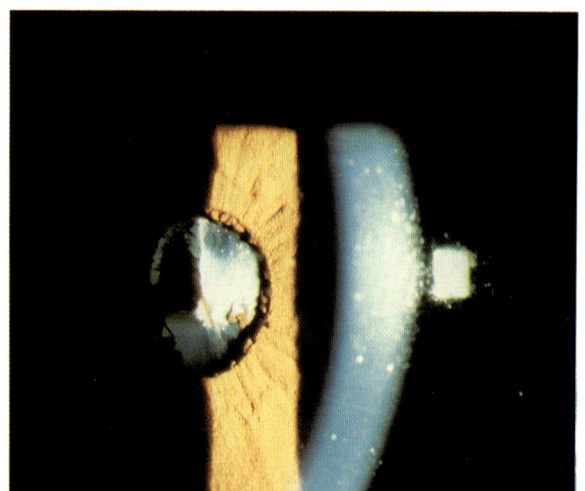

119 Peripheral anterior synechiae and cataract development in patient with round mutton-fat KP.

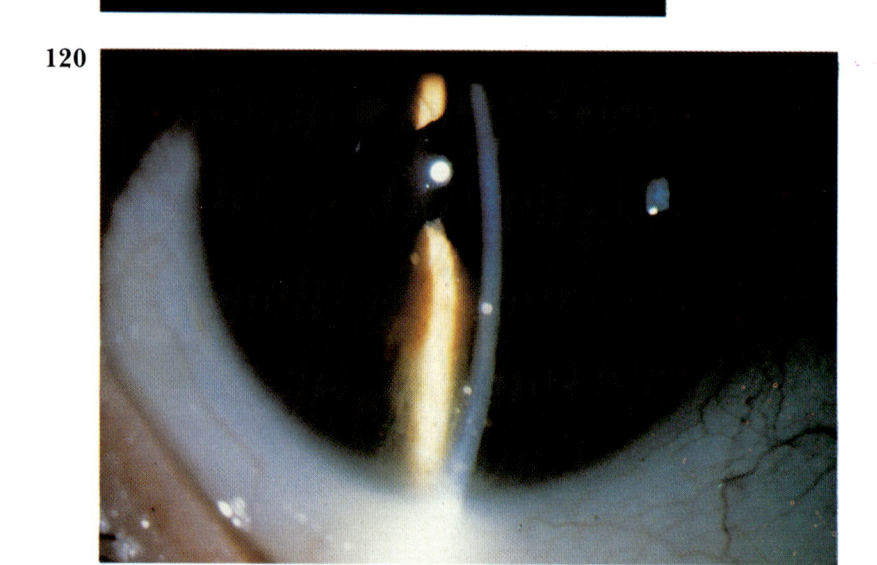

120 Mutton-fat KP in patient with almost inactive iridocyclitis from sarcoidosis.

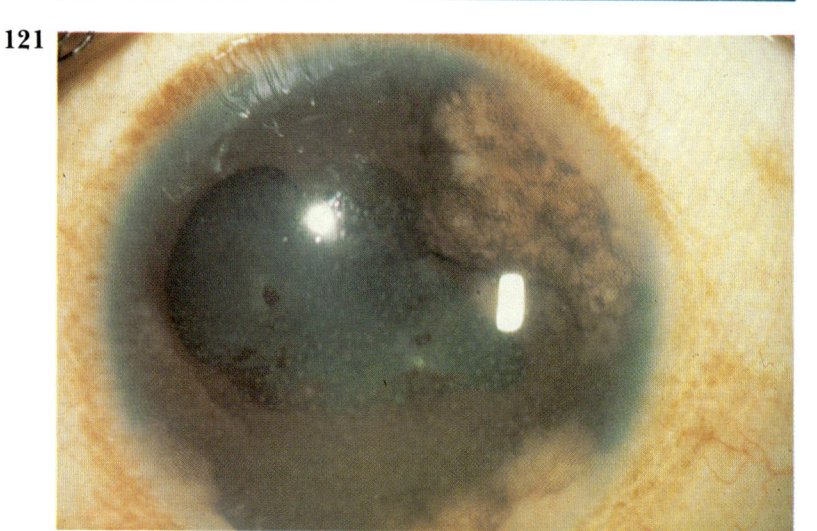

121 Giant iris stromal nodule in patient with a profound sarcoid iridocyclitis with extensive synechiae formation. (*Courtesy of Jonathan Belmont, M.D.*)

122 Fluffy white enlargement of the optic nerve due to papillitis secondary to sarcoidosis in a young black man. (*Courtesy of Jonathan Belmont, M.D.*)

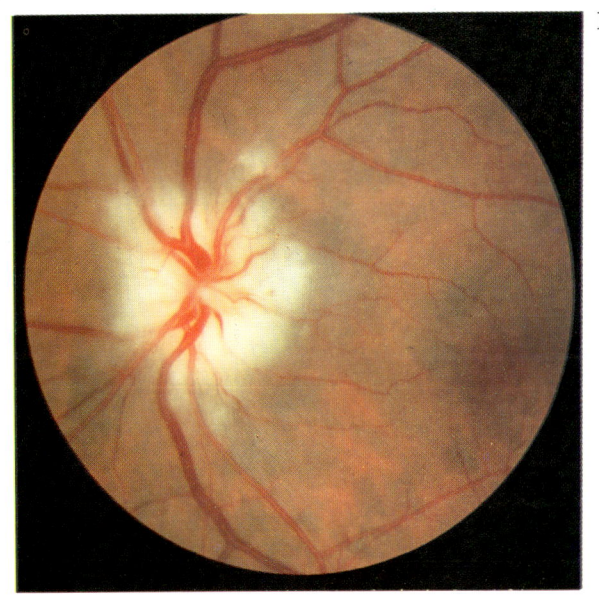

123 Typical 'candle wax drippings' in patient with a phlebitis that is characteristic of sarcoid involvement of the posterior pole.

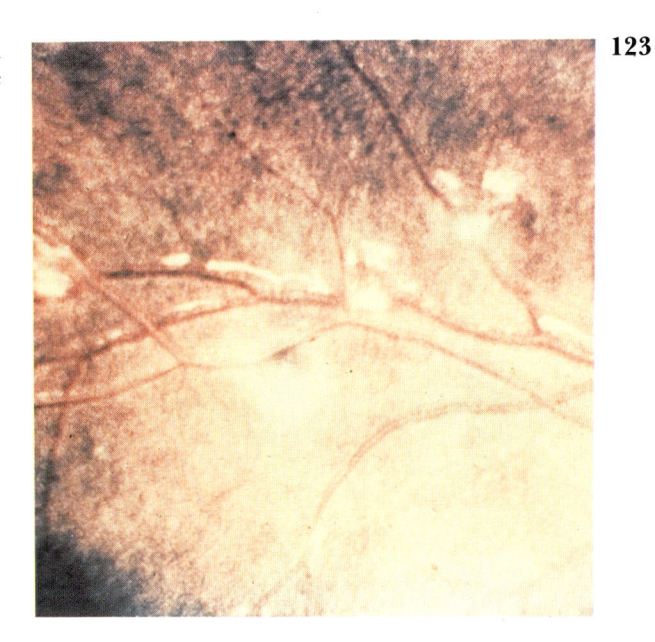

Acquired Immune Deficiency Syndrome (AIDS)

Human Immunodeficiency Virus (HIV) is a retrovirus and has RNA as its genome. It can affect all types of human cells but much of its pathology is secondary to infection of the T-cell helper inducer cells. Since the T-cell is crucial for the cell-immediated immune response, infection and immobilization of this cell causes a severe immunosuppression in the host. This results in opportunistic infection which may be seen in the eye. AIDS is the most severe manifestation of HIV infection and occurs at a point when the immune system is rendered incompetent by the HIV infection and opportunistic organisms such as *Pneumocystis carinii*, *Cryptococcus neoformans*, cytomegalovirus, *Toxoplasma gondii*, candidiasis, or unusual malignancies such as Kaposi's sarcoma (**127**), may be seen.

The noninfectious retinopathy of AIDS may be caused by interaction between viral antigens and antibodies that circulate in the blood, but this has not been shown. The retinopathy presents as cotton wool spots (**128**) without active infection and these are due to infarction of the nerve fiber layer of the retina. Focal microvascular dilatation may occur in the tissues adjacent to these infarctions. Usually these infarctions in the nerve fiber layer are in the order of one-quarter to one-half of a disc diameter in size and they may be distinguished from infectious retinitis by the fact that they do not enlarge and do not have cells in the vitreous overlying them (**129**). The morphology distribution of these lesions tends to change and they may even disappear over a period of time. This form of retinopathy occurs in 25% to 90% of AIDS patients and much less frequently in patients with Aids-Related Complex (ARC) or asymptomatic HIV infection.

The presence of a P24 antigen, a surface HIV antigen in the blood, may also increase as the disease advances and this may be related in time to the advancement from the cotton wool spot type retinopathy to actual infection in the retina with an opportunistic organism. The reoccurrence in the general population of syphilis (**131, 132**) occurring in conjunction with AIDS cannot be over emphasized, and one should be careful to also screen patients for tuberculosis as well as the candida and cryptococcus. Both acute necrotizing herpes zoster retinitis (**126**) and herpes simplex retinitis have also been reported in patients with AIDS. These viral infections presenting as a necrotizing vasculitic-type retinopathy may be difficult to differentiate clinically from cytomegalovirus retinitis (**130**). However, autopsy studies have demonstrated that greater than 95% of viral retinitis in AIDS is a result of CMV infection.

In times past patients with CMV retinitis had been immunosuppressed by cancer treatment, organ transplantation with exogenous immunosuppression from the steroids, cyclosporine or the immune incompetence of the newborn. CMV infection was first recognized in 1947 as a congenital infection in immunosuppressed infants. With the advent of organ transplantation and chemotherapy, CMV retinitis became more common in adults. It is projected that there will be 50,000 cases of cytomegalovirus retinitis in 1992 as a result of AIDS alone.

AIDS (ACQUIRED IMMUNE DEFICIENCY SYNDROME)

Definition:
- Acquired immune deficiency syndrome caused by retrovirus infection (RNA only)
- Associated opportunistic infections:
  CMV
  Toxoplasmosis, syphilis, cryptococcus, tuberculosis, pneumocystis
  Other herpetic infections

Presentation:
- Iridocyclitis
- Retinal cotton-wool infarction early
- Retinitis late, vasculitis, necrosis

Investigation:
- HIV testing
- P24 surface antigen (advanced disease)

Therapy:
- Gancyclovir (CMV)
- Foscarnet (CMV)
- Peripheral retinal photocoagulation (to prevent retinal detachment)
- Acyclovir (herpetic infection)

Complications:
- Retinal detachment frequent with CMV
- Retinal necrosis frequent with CMV

Prognosis:
- Poor

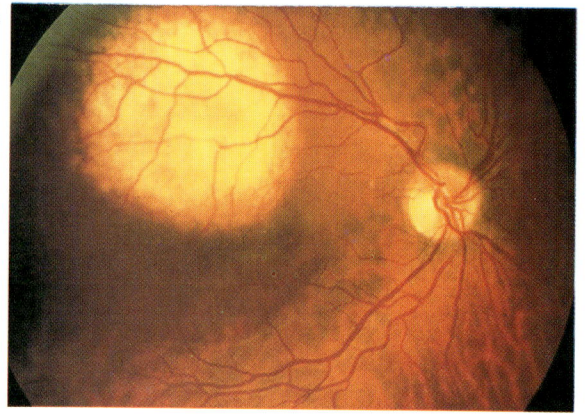

124 Fundus demonstrating *Pneumocystis carinii* **choroiditis** which developed concurrent with pneumonitis in a patient with AIDS. (*Courtesy of C.Y. Lowder, M.D., and D.M. Meisler, M.D., Cleveland Clinic Foundation, Cleveland, Ohio.*)

Therapy for cytomegalovirus retinitis in the past was limited to reducing the exogenous immunosuppression of patients. With the advent of gancyclovir (DHPG) and foscarnet patients may now be treated. Gancyclovir is viral static, both *in vitro* and *in vivo*. Therapy with 5 mg/kg intravenously twice daily will result in upwards of 80% of patients having a clinical response in 10 to 14 days. Acyclovir is not sufficiently active against CMV infection. Recurrences are common in AIDS patients because of the underlying persistent immunosuppression. In others, recurrences may not occur. Maintenance regimens are being tested for AIDS patients, keeping them on 5 mg/kg intravenously once daily for 5 to 7 days per week which may prolong the mean time until relapse. Maintenance doses lower than 25 mg/kg/wk have been associated with a higher relapse rate. Foscarnet has been shown to prolong the patient's life on average 4 months longer than those treated with ganciclovir. Induction with 60 mg/kg/8 hours for 14 days is followed by maintenance doses between 90 mg/kg/day to 120 mg/kg/day. Serum creatinine, calcium, magnesium, and hemoglobin must be followed closely for toxic effects. While the visual loss which occurred due to active infection may not improve after treatment (because of retinal necrosis), macular edema often resolves. The main complication of gancyclovir toxicity is white cell suppression in the marrow, and white cell counts need to be checked on a weekly basis.

125 *Pneumocystis carinii* **choroiditis** and concurrent pneumonitis in another patient. (*Courtesy of C.Y. Lowder, M.D., and D.M. Meisler, M.D., Cleveland Clinic Foundation, Cleveland, Ohio.*)

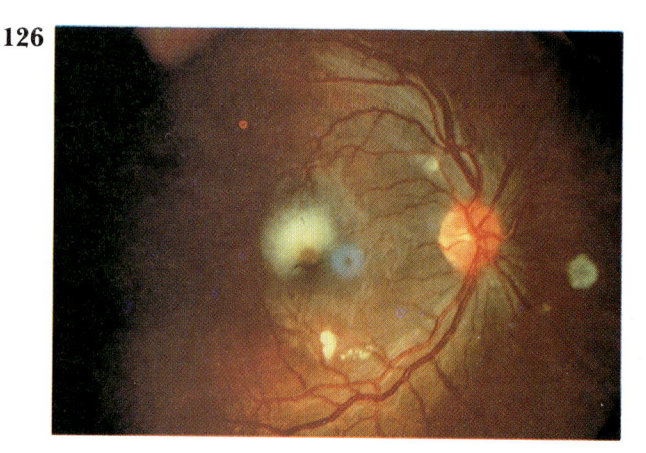

126 Varicella-zoster chorioretinitis. A 21-year-old black male presenting with metamorphopsia demonstrates opportunistic varicella-zoster chorioretinitis, bilaterally, and in the framework of AIDS. Herpes zoster virus cultured from vitreous biopsy. (*Courtesy of S.S. Weismann, M.D., Manhattan Eye, Ear and Throat Hospital, New York.*)

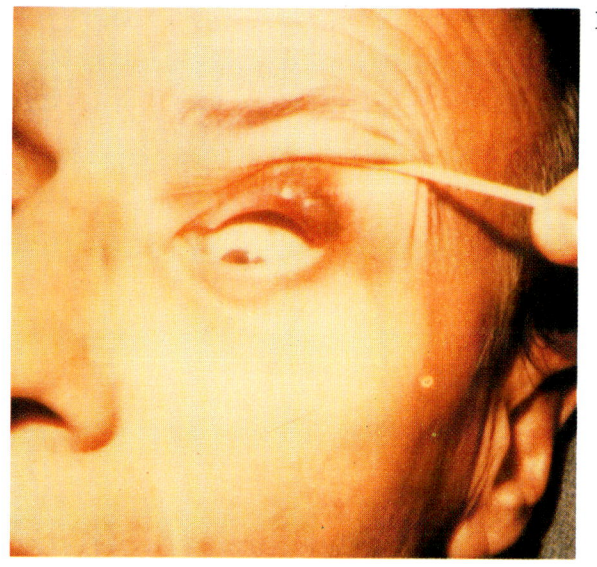

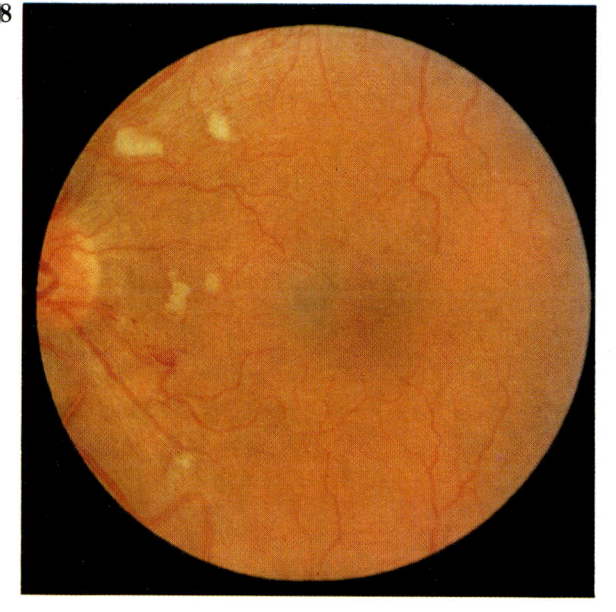

127 Kaposi's sarcoma. A 32-year-old white male demonstrates Kaposi's sarcoma as seen in AIDS syndrome in left upper eyelid.

128 Cotton wool exudation. A 22-year-old white male demonstrating a cotton wool exudation in the nerve fiber layer of the retina as earliest manifestation of AIDS.

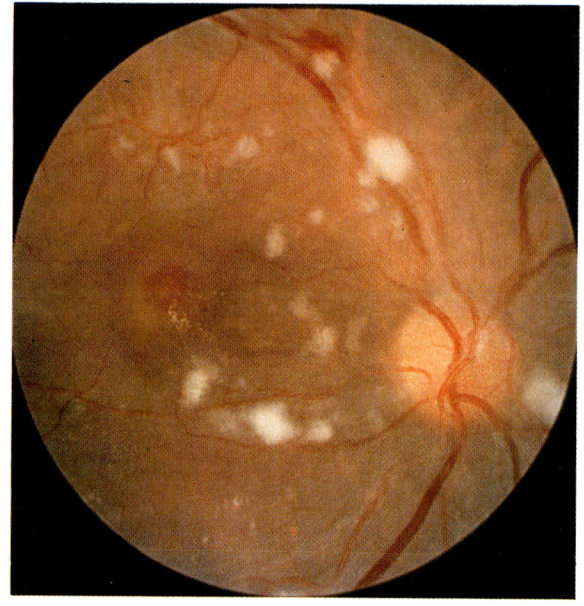

129 More advanced cotton wool exudation in the nerve fiber layer with few internal limiting membrane dot hemorrhages indicative of AIDS.

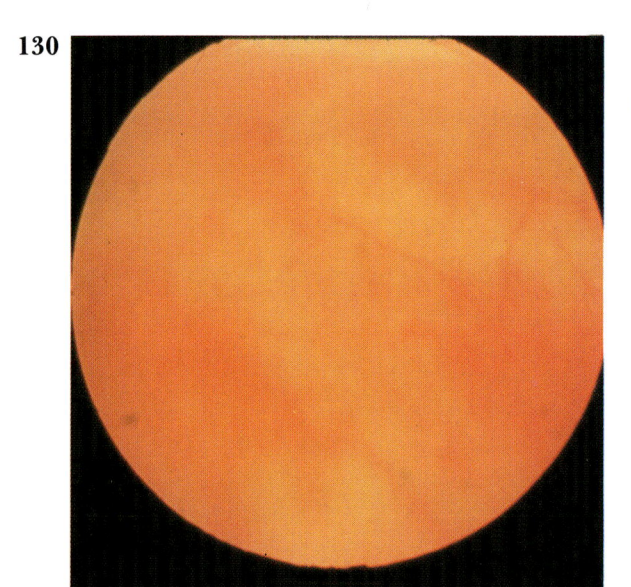

130 Cytomegalic inclusion disease infection. Cheesy exudation admixed with hemorrhage in the retina of a patient with AIDS indicative of the retinopathy of cytomegalic inclusion disease infection (CMV).

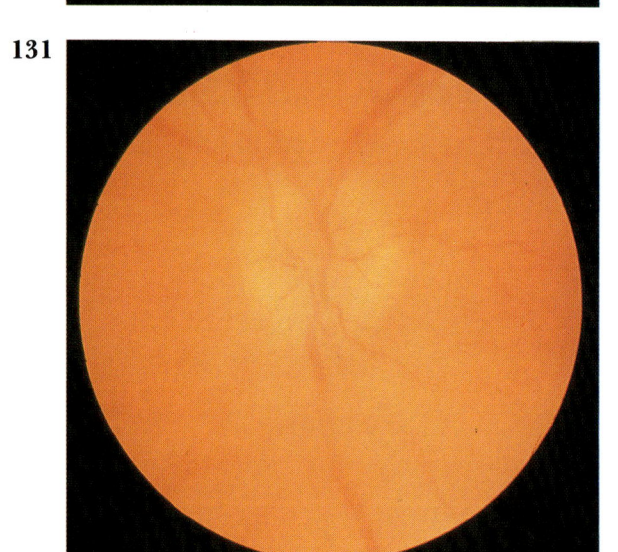

131 Acute syphilitic infection. A 27-year-old professional white male who demonstrates papillitis as a consequence of acute syphilitic infection seen in the framework of AIDS discovered during workup.

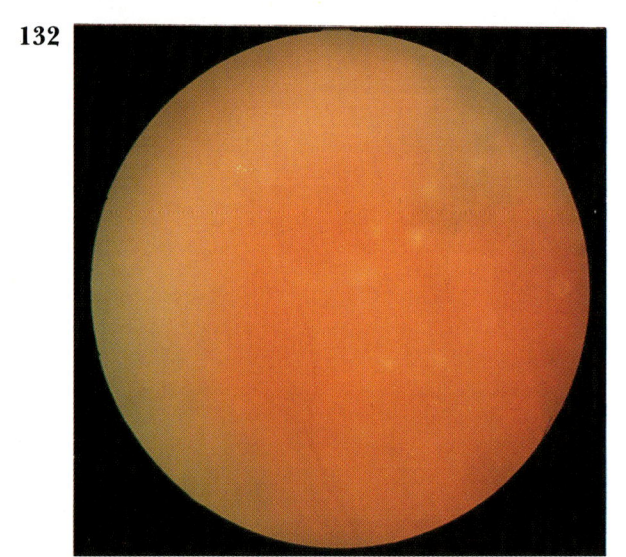

132 Acute syphilitic infection. Peripheral retina of same patient (Figure 131) who demonstrates small, white focal choroidal infiltrates due to acute syphilitic infection all of which resolved on systemic intravenous penicillin.

Lyme Disease

Lyme disease is a tick-borne (**137**) spirochetal disease caused by an organism similar to the treponema causing syphilis. It produces early and late manifestations in many organ systems. Infection with the *Borrelia burgdorferi*, first identified in 1982, produces prominent symptoms and signs in the skin, heart, joints, nervous system, as well as neuro-ophthalmologic (**135**) and ocular abnormalities. Ophthalmologic manifestations of Lyme disease include conjunctivitis, periocular edema, iridocyclitis, panophthalmitis, choroiditis, optic disk swelling (**134**), macular edema, pseudotumor cerebri, optic neuritis, as well as optic neuropathy. Episcleritis and conjunctivitis have been associated with each report of ocular inflammation. While conjunctivitis has been observed in approximately 11% of cases, very severe manifestations have been reported which include choroiditis with exudative retinal detachment, iritis, which progressed on antibiotic treatment to vitritis, and panophthalmitis requiring pars plana vitrectomy, the consequence being phthisis and monocular blindness. In the latter case, although *Borrelia burgdorferi* was not cultured from the initial surgical vitrectomy specimen, it was identified microscopically among the vitreous debris after enucleation of the globe. Stromal-keratitis has been identified in eight patients with positive Lyme titers. One of them also had a positive FTA-ABS, suggesting either a diagnosis of syphilis or concurrent infection. It is to be noted in the literature that a positive Lyme titer, the consequence of Lyme disease, can very rarely produce a positive VDRL but is never responsible for a positive FTA-ABS. It is important to note that papilledema is observed in association with the meningoencephalitis of Lyme disease, occasionally presenting as well with elevated intracranial pressure and transient visual obscurations. Facial palsies, diplopia and cranial nerve deficit have repeatedly been reported with Lyme disease in the literature.

Lyme disease usually begins in the Summer, less often during Spring or Fall, but only rarely in Winter. This is due to the timing of the tick-borne infection and the tick's need for blood meals. While it has been reported worldwide with especially extensive neurological manifestations of the disease in Europe, Lyme disease has been reported in 43 American states. Most cases have clustered in a few endemic areas, mainly the Northeast, Minnesota, Wisconsin, and the West Coast. The pathognomonic criteria for diagnosis of Lyme disease includes a circular rash (**136**) which develops into erythema migrans following the tick bite. It enlarges, and as the center clears, it forms an erythematous annular lesion that is painful and itchy. The untreated lesion usually lasts several weeks but can recur for up to a year. Unfortunately, the rash may not be seen on half of the patients who present with confusing manifestations of ocular or neurological disease which have been ascribed to Lyme disease.

The serologic evidence for Lyme disease may include the enzyme-linked immunoadsorbent assay (ELISA) and the indirect immunofluorescent antibody (IFA). Both of these tests measure the IgM and IgG in patients' serum reacting with *Borrelia burgdorferi*. A serum dilution greater than 1:256 is considered positive. Many patients who present with confusing ophthalmologic and neurologic signs may be considered to be suffering from Lyme disease. They may not be aware of a pre-existing bite of a tiny tick or having had a history of erythema migrans, The Cen-

---

LYME DISEASE

Definition:
- Acute or chronic infection

Presentation:
- Conjunctivitis
- Iridocyclitis
- Choroiditis
- Phthisis bulbi
- Optic nerve inflammation

Investigation:
- IFA
- ELISA (check both IgG and IgM)
- May be negative in early disease and in cases treated early
- Medical consultation

Therapy:
- Doxycycline (vibramycin and others), 100 mg b.i.d.
- Amoxicillin (250 to 500 mg b.i.d.)
- Penicillin G (IV), 224 million units per day (IV)
- Ceftriaxone (IV), 2 g/day (IV)

Complications:
- Papilledema
- Optic perineuritis
- Disc edema
- Keratitis
- Neuritis (3rd and 4th nerves)

Prognosis:
- Good, if treated early
- Poor, if treated late

ter for Disease Control in Atlanta lists the current definition of Lyme disease to include any of the following:

- A patient who lives in an endemic area with erythema migrans within 30 days of exposure to tick bite.
- A patient exposed in an endemic area without erythema migrans and has involvement of one organ system in a positive laboratory test.
- A patient without a history of exposure to a tick bite, but has erythema migrans as well as involvement of two organs.
- A patient without exposure in an endemic area but with erythema migrans and positive serology.

The disease progresses through three stages. Stage I (infection) includes the dermatologic manifestation of erythema migrans, lymphadenopathy, fever- and influenza-like symptoms which may include headache, stiff neck, nausea and includes the initial ophthalmologic presentation of conjunctivitis, photophobia and episcleritis. Stage II (dissemination) includes erythema chronicum migrans, lymphocytoma, cardiac abnormalities which include palpitations, arrythmia, heart block and even mild choroiditis, as well as arthritis and arthralgias. Disease in this stage may progress in a neurologic manner to include meningitis with papilledema, craniofacial neuritis and neuroinflammation, painful radiculopathy and encephalitis. It is during Stage II of the disease that most of these significant ophthalmologic features of Lyme disease occur, such as iritis or iridocyclitis, uveitis (**133**), retinitis, pars planitis, choroiditis, endophthalmitis and the neurologic manifestations of optic disk swelling, optic disk pallor, optic disk inflammation, Horner's syndrome and even Argyll Robinson pupil. Stage III, or the late immunological disease, includes chronic acrodermatitis atrophicans, as well as a chronic rheumatologic manifestation, along with fatigue and encephalomyelitis, a demyelination syndrome suggesting multiple sclerosis, as well as late stromal-keratitis in the eye, episcleritis and orbital myositis have been reported. The treatment of Lyme disease is oral tetracycline, 250 mg four times a day, or doxycycline, 100 mg twice a day for 10 to 30 days. For children in whom tetracycline is contraindicated, amoxicillin or penicillin B is recommended, and in cases of penicillin allergy, erythromycin proves effective. Stage II Lyme disease may call for intravenous ceftriaxone, 2 g per day for two weeks or longer. Oral doxycycline may be substituted. The use of corticosteroids in Lyme disease is still controversial. They have been helpful in treating choroiditis and arthritis and certain neurologic sequelae, but a high incidence of failure to antibiotic treatment has been reported in patients previously treated with steroids.

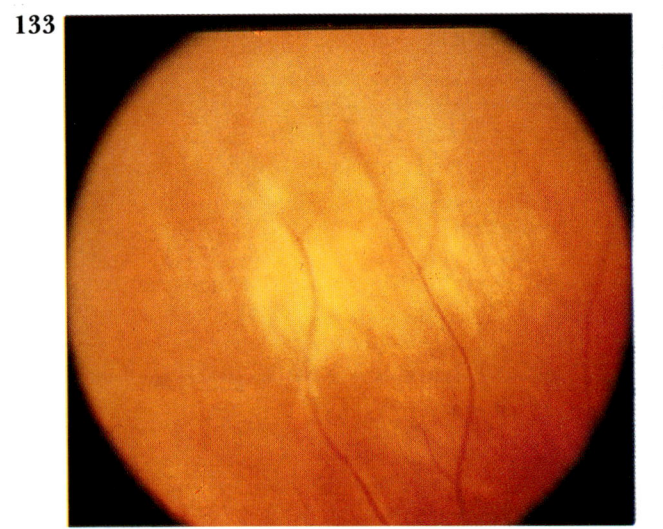

133 Retinal vascular sheathing with vasculitis and a positive Lyme titer at 1-64 in a 26-year-old white female. The patient was treated with 300 mg doxycycline daily for 2 months with clearing of her uveitis.

134 Hemorrhagic papillitis in a 28-year-old white female with Lyme disease.

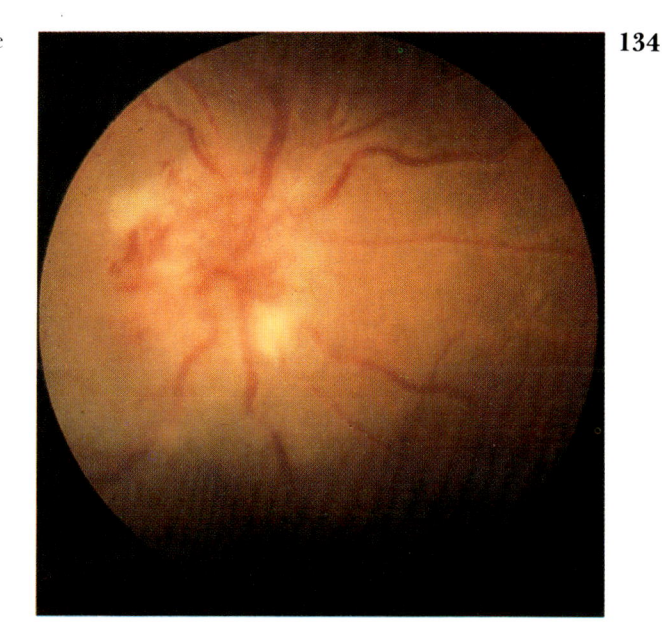

135 Multiple small foci. IRI scan of brain demonstrating multiple small foci of increased intensity in the cerebral white matter consistent with multiple sclerosis or acute infection with Lyme disease. The patient also developed a right partial third-nerve palsy.

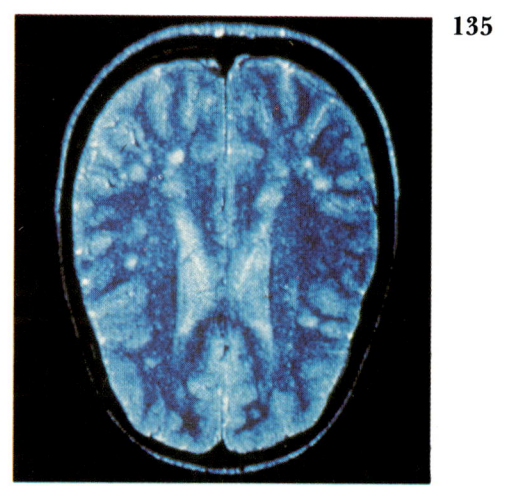

136 Typical concentric erythema migrans dermal lesion ('bull's eye') of Lyme disease. (*Courtesy of the Center for Disease Control, Atlanta, Georgia.*)

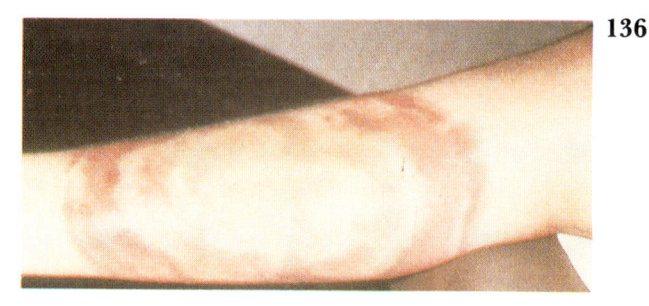

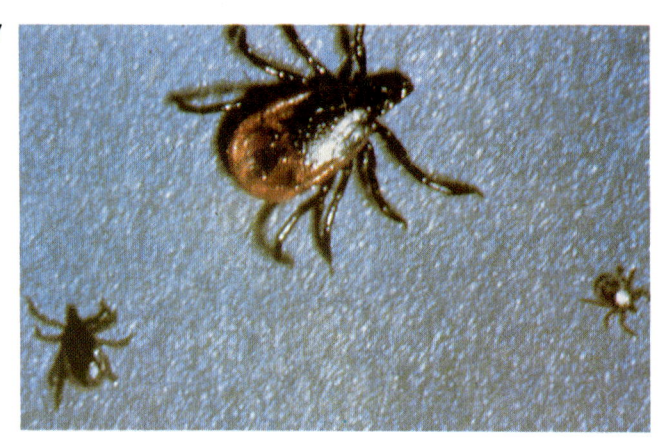

137 *Ixodes dammini* tick, the common deer tick known to carry the Lyme disease spirochete. The largest tick shown is the adult, the nymph is the intermediate size which is roughly the size of a sesame seed, and the larva is about the size of a sand grain. (*Courtesy of the Center for Disease Control, Atlanta, Georgia.*)

Syphilis

Syphilis, at one time overdiagnosed if not misdiagnosed as a common cause of uveitis, became rare when brought under antimicrobial control. Recently, due to the worldwide resurgence of venereal disease, there is a fully documented increase in syphilitic ocular disease. For this reason syphilis must still be considered in the differential diagnosis of uveitis, and the FTA-ABS is the most sensitive indicator for syphilis infection. Occasionally, when syphilis has only been partially treated or in cases of central nervous system syphilis, the FTA-ABS is positive and the VDRL is negative.

Congenital syphilis is usually manifested by the 'salt and pepper fundus' inflammation of the retinal pigment epithelium, with its concomitant typical corneal lesions and pale optic nerve. Acquired syphilis causes various types of ocular inflammation including iris nodules, iridocyclitis that may be severe and unresponsive to corticosteroid therapy, and in some cases, large keratic precipitates. An indolent, progressive type of iridocyclitis should alert the clinician to the possibility of this newly resurgent disease. Papillitis may be the manifestation of systemic syphilis infection (**131**). Diffuse chorioretinitis, choroiditis (**132**), and particularly vasculitis (**138**) are additional complications that may occur later in the disease or may be clinical signs indicating steroid-unresponsive uveitis. Any or all of these ocular inflammatory signs may be associated with the skin lesions of secondary syphilis including maculopapular rash, usually found on the palms and the soles.

These ocular forms of syphilis gradually worsen and progress from initial iridocyclitis to the whole spectrum of syphilitic eye disease and are often accompanied by vasculitis of the posterior pole.

Current treatment suggests systemic therapy of 24 million units of intravenous penicillin; the ocular inflammation is treated with steroids. Penicillamine, to enhance penicillin absorption, is advocated by some authorities.

SYPHILIS

Definition:
- Acute or chronic infection

Presentation:
- Presents as anything (mimicker as with sarcoidosis)
- Granulomatous

Investigation:
- VDRL
- FTA-ABS
- MHTPP
- LP
- HIV test necessary in conjunction
- Medical consultation

Therapy:
- Systemic penicillin; current regimen 24 million units intravenous, treat ocular inflammation with steroids

Complications:
- Cataracts
- Glaucoma
- Macular scarring
- Optic nerve dysfunction and scarring
- Phthisis

Prognosis:
- Variable
- Sometimes refractory to full treatment

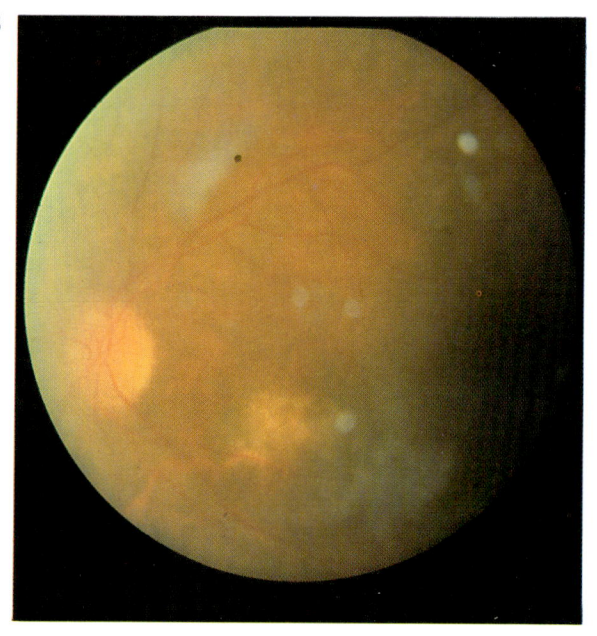

138 Leutic choroiditis and vasculitis. Fundus of patient with lesion of exudative choroiditis and areas of vasculitis seen along the major vessels. Central nervous system syphilis is documented on serology from spinal fluid examination. (*Also see* ***131, 132, AIDS*** *chapter, page 58.*)

Collagen Vascular diseases *(Connective Tissue Inflammation)*

The collagen vasculoses, which include lupus erythematosus, polyarteritis nodosum, Wegener's disease, and chronic relapsing polychondritis, represent systemic inflammatory disorders that may produce a vasculitis in the posterior pole of the eye (**144, 145, 147, 148**). This retinal and/or choroidal vasculitis may simulate Behçet's disease, Vogt–Koyanagi–Harada disease, syphilis, tuberculosis, etc.

The ocular findings include butterfly eruptions and purpuras on the lids and maxilla as well as telangiectasis and true vasculitis. Keratitis sicca may be present in about a third of the patients. Corneal punctuate epithelial keratitis as well as deep disciform keratitis may be presenting signs caused by photophobia, lacrimation, and ocular discomfort. Nodular necrotizing scleritis may be a prominent part of this disease as it is especially in rheumatoid arthritis. Cotton wool spots called cytoid bodies may appear in the retina in up to 20% of patients (**139**). These are the consequences of occlusive vasculitis of the nerve fiber cell layer in the retina (**140, 141**). The term 'cytoid bodies' should be reserved for the histological finding of this phenomenon rather than the clinical presentation of cotton wool exudates, which occur as infarction of the nerve fiber layer in the retina where Wallerian degeneration of the neurons develops. Papilledema may also be a prominent finding in these systemic inflammations.

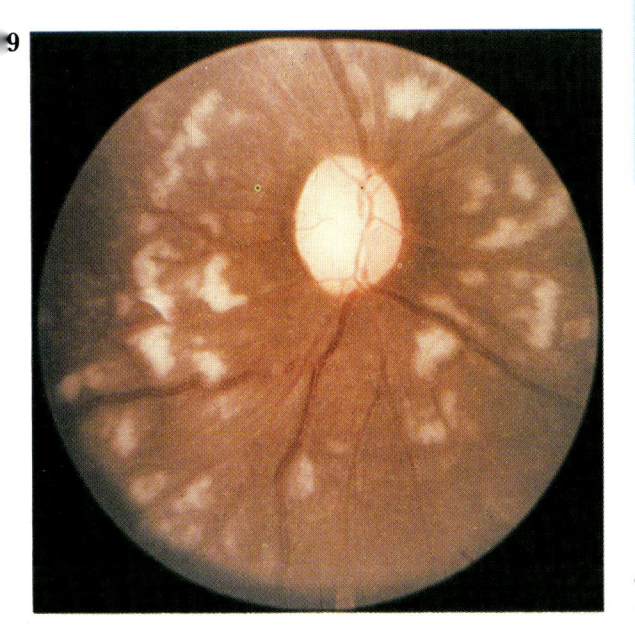

CONNECTIVE TISSUE DISEASE

Definition:
- Systemic vasculitis with tissue disorders including arthralgias and arthritis

Presentation:
- Iridocyclitis
- Scleritis
- Vitritis
- Retinitis
- Vasculitis
- Nongranulomatous

Investigation:
- FA
- ANA
- ESR
- Lupus anticoagulation
- PTT
- Serum immune complexes (Raji)

Therapy:
- Periocular steroids
- Systemic steroids
- Immunosuppressant agents (chlorambucil, cytoxan)
- Cyclosporine

Complications:
- Retinal ischemia
- Chronic retinitis and vasculitis
- Nerve ischemia
- Infarction of retina

Prognosis:
- Fair

139 Diffuse cotton wool infarcts in the nerve fiber layer of the retina with optic pallor in a young patient with lupus erythematosus.

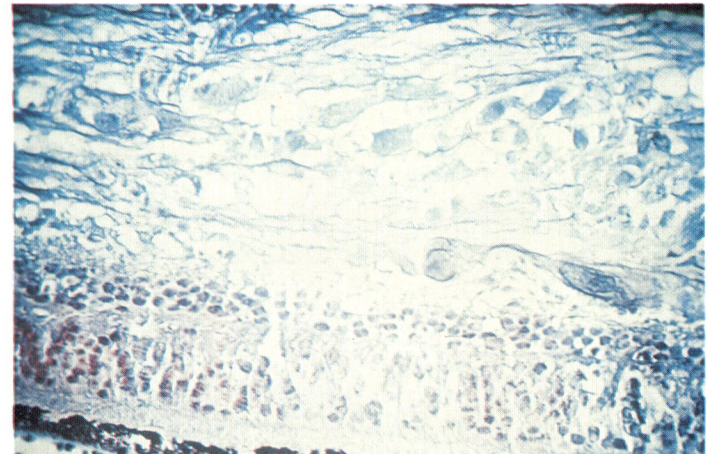

140 Cytoid bodies are noted as the rounded up basophilic staining areas in the nerve fiber layer of the retina.

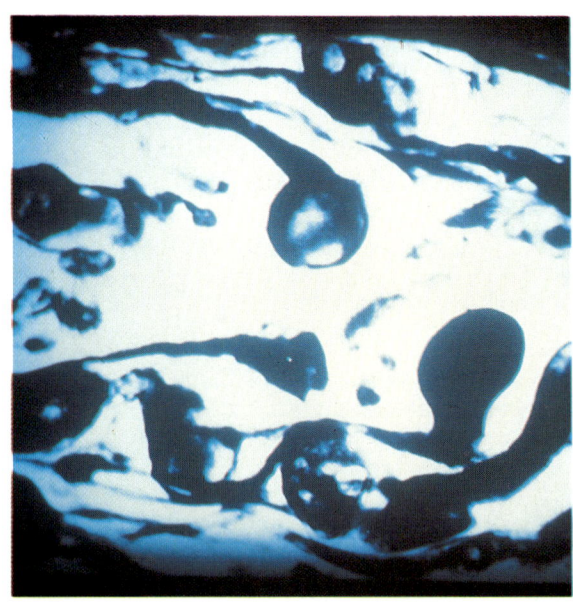

141 Cytoid bodies. Enlargement of these lollipop-shaped Wallerian degenerations of the axons in the nerve fiber layer of the retina or so-called cytoid bodies.

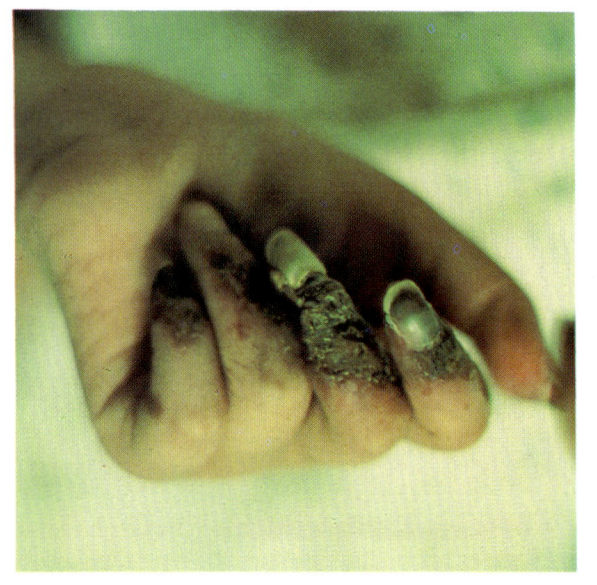

142 Occlusive vasculitis. Extreme presentation of gangrene due to an occlusive necrotizing vasculitis in the fingers (Raynaud's phenomenon) of a patient with lupus erythematosus.

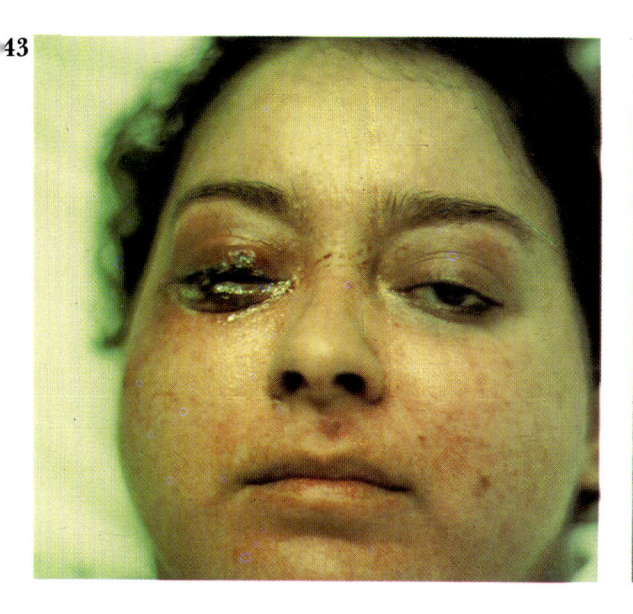

143 Necrotic vasculitis. Same patient as Figure 142 showing necrotic occlusive vasculitis on upper and lower lid of the right eye.

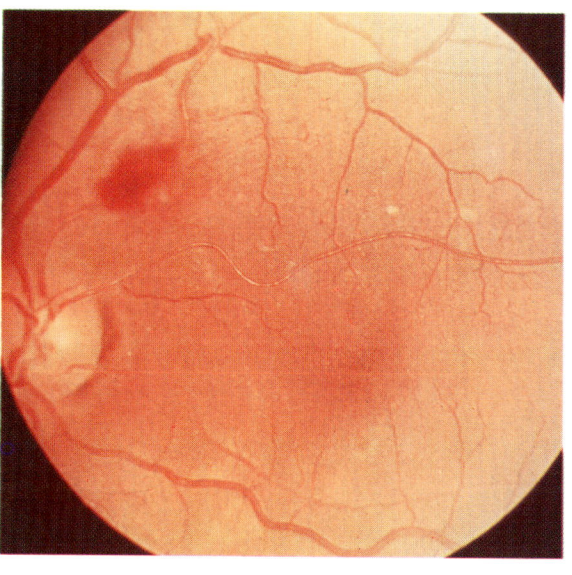

144 Mixed picture of hemorrhagic hypertensive retinopathy with vasculitis in patient with polyarteritis nodosum with systemic hypertension.

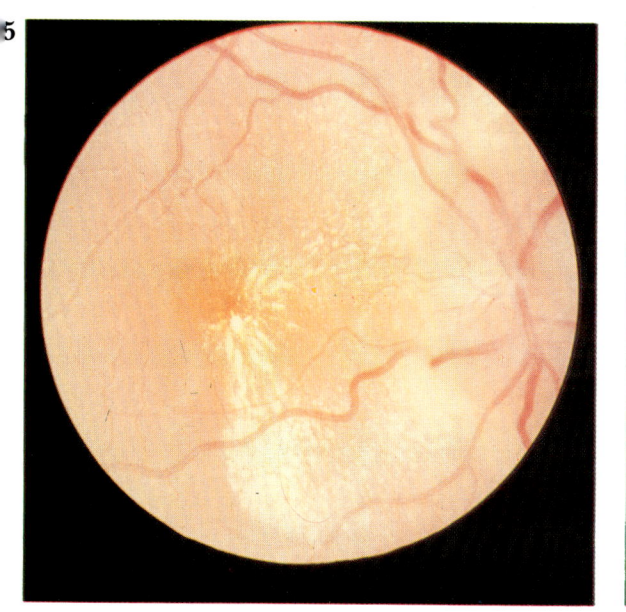

145 Diffuse vasculitis. A 12-year-old white girl with lupus erythematosus showing diffuse vasculitis along with hypertensive retinopathy and macular star. Note swelling of the optic nerve head.

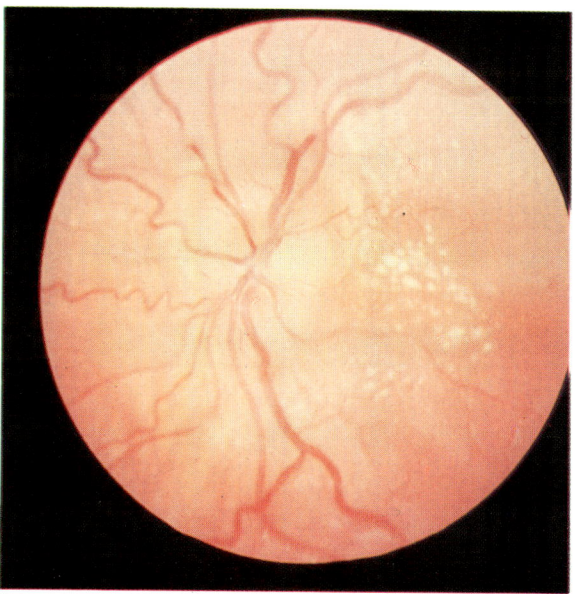

146 Exudative retinopathy. The fellow eye of patient with mixed picture of hypertensive and exudative vasculitic retinopathy secondary to inflammatory vessel changes as well as hypertension from chronic renal disease.

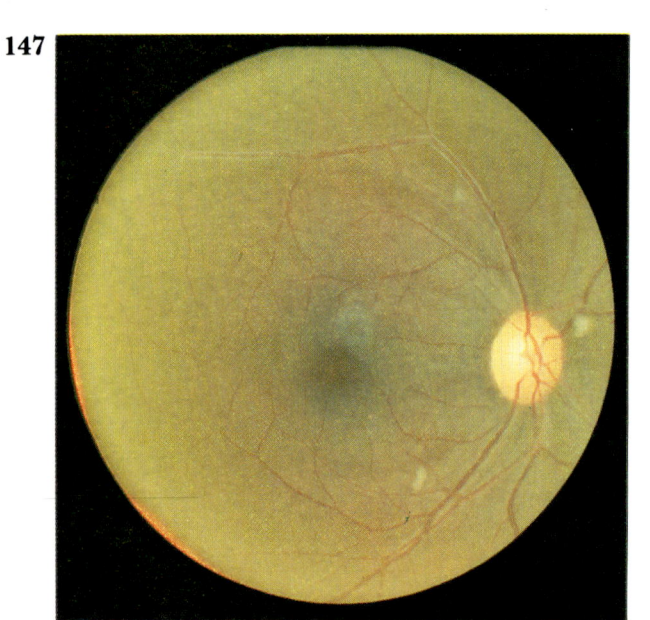

147 Focal, discrete cotton wool infarcts in the nerve fiber layer of retina of a 24-year-old black woman with systemic lupus erythematosus who also demonstrates a profound vasculitis.

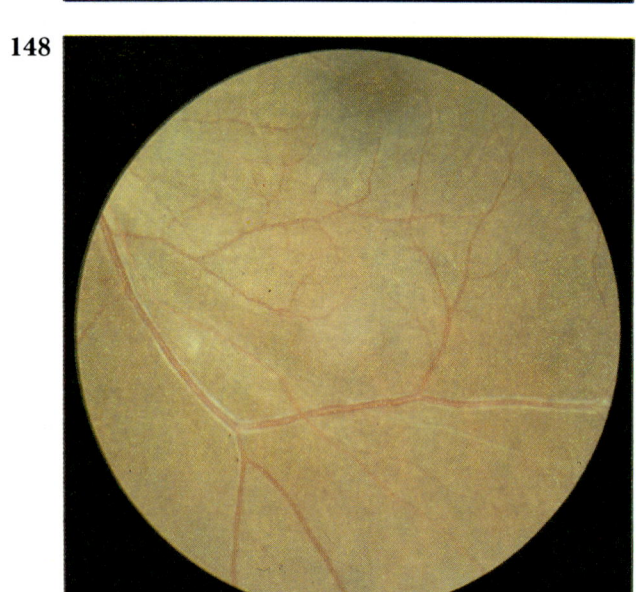

148 Perivascular sheathing. Same patient as Figure 147, with a higher magnification of the perivascular sheathing as a prominent manifestation of vasculitis.

Vogt–Koyanagi–Harada Syndrome

Vogt–Koyanagi–Harada syndrome is the true clinical brother of sympathetic ophthalmia because this type of panuveitis affects the iris, ciliary body, and choroid and may manifest all of the same clinical signs. It appears to be an autoimmune reaction to melanin or uveal pigment since the ocular as well as the central nervous system (uveo-encephalitis) signs all occur where melanosomes are present as in the chorda tympani (middle ear inflammation), choroidal plexus (meningitis), and the base of the hair shaft (poliosis may be a very common sign). The dysacusis may be manifest by tingling or deafness. Alopecia areata with poliosis (**151**) and vitiligo (**149, 151, 153, 154**), often the hallmarks of this disease, are common depigmented findings. Late findings of central nervous system vasculitis may include coma, paresis, disorientation, psychosis, and other underlying signs that may be diagnosed by abnormal electroencephalograms. Aside from the anterior segment ocular disease appearing as a typical granulomatous iridocyclitis and vitritis, diffuse choroiditis with serous detachments of the retina are a common form of the disease and may occur in the absence of the anterior segment inflammation (Harada's syndrome). The foci of choroiditis tend to include vasculitis in a focal fashion as well as the overall serous detachment of the retina as a late consequence of that blood vessel inflammation. The very typical ocular signs of Vogt–Koyanagi–Harada diseases such as iridocyclitis, pigment mottling of the retinal pigment epithelium where previous serous detachment has occurred (**159**), poliosis, and vitiligo around the eyes may occur in the absence of any systemic complaints whatsoever.

The disease appears to have a predilection for the more pigmented races, especially Orientals. In Japan, Vogt–Koyanagi–Harada disease and Behçet's disease account for 25% of all cases of uveitis seen. The Harada's variety of Vogt–Koyanagi–Harada, in which only serous detachment of the retina occurs as an inflammatory manifestation in the absence of anterior inflammation, appears to be more common in Spanish-speaking peoples.

Fluorescein angiography of Vogt–Koyanagi–Harada disease is highly characteristic and may be very helpful to establish the diagnosis (**156**). Choroiditis appears to block the vessels early, affect late leakage as in any typical vasculitis, and there is usually a marked accumulation of fluid in the subretinal space when serous detachments of the retina are occurring. The mottling of the retinal pigment epithelium so typical after serous detachments appears as a blocked hypofluorscence on fluorescein angiography.

VOGT–KOYANAGI–HARADA

Definition:
- A systemic inflammation with vasculitis in the retina, exudative detachment of the retina with choroiditis, etc.

Presentation:
- Iridocyclitis
- Choroiditis
- Exudative retinal detachment
- Retinal vasculitis
- Granulomatous
- Poliosis, ? Vitiligo

Investigation:
- Lumbar puncture during attacks
- Fluorescein angiogram
- Medical consultation
- Skin and hair follicles biopsy for absence of melanocyte
- HLA BW22J
- HLA LDWa (Japan)
- HLA GR4
- HLA DQw3 (Western)

Therapy:
- Intensive local systemic steroids
- Periocular steroids
- Low-dose local or systemic steroids in chronic cases
- Immunosuppressive agents (chlorambucil)
- Cyclosporine

Complications:
- Cataract
- Glaucoma
- Optic nerve dysfunction
- Retinal vasculitis
- Retinal necrosis
- Phthisis

Prognosis:
- Mixed, depending on character of case
- Especially its chronicity is related to inflammatory activity
- Cataract surgery well tolerated
- All surgery poorly tolerated in cases chronically active

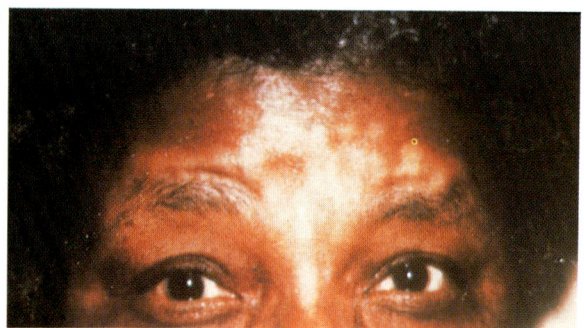

149 Facial vitiligo in a 56-year-old black female as part of her syndrome of Vogt–Koyanagi–Harada disease.

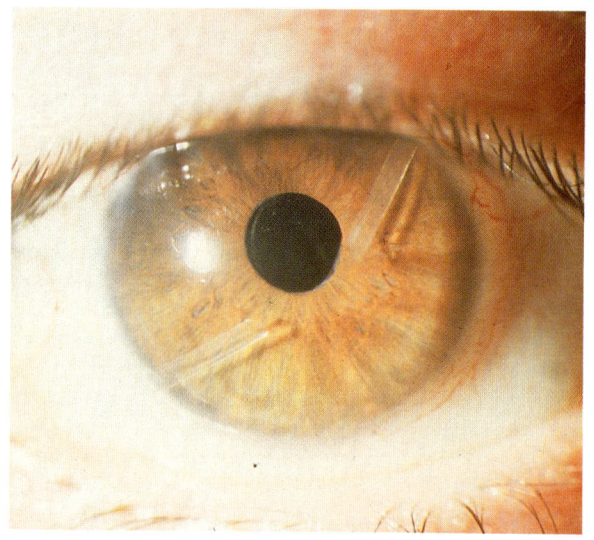

150 Vogt–Koyanagi–Harada disease uveitis in patient who underwent two Molteno Seton implants to control uveitic glaucoma.

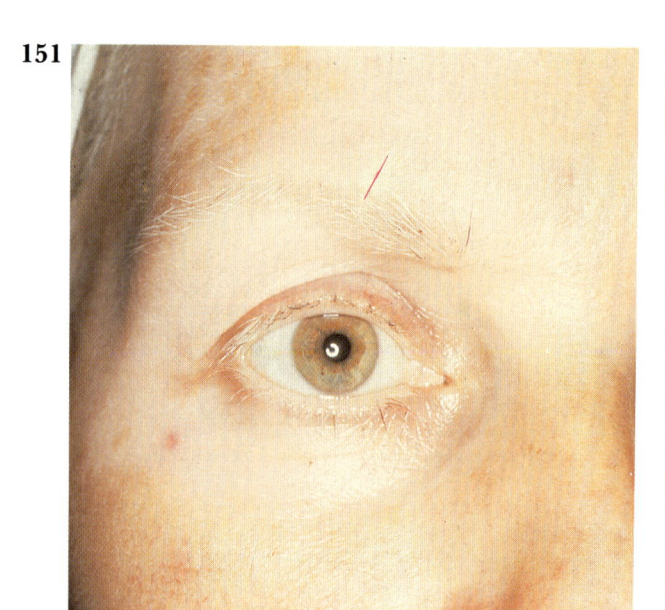

151 Facial vitiligo and poliosis (whitening or depigmentation of lashes) in patient with Vogt–Koyanagi–Harada disease.

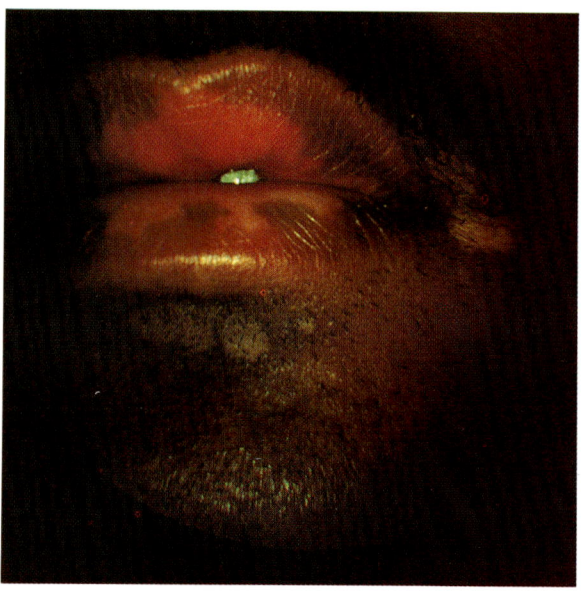

152 Vitiliginous changes on the lips and perioral skin of a black patient with Vogt–Koyanagi–Harada disease.

153 Vitiliginous changes on the thumb and hands of patient with Vogt–Koyanagi–Harada disease.

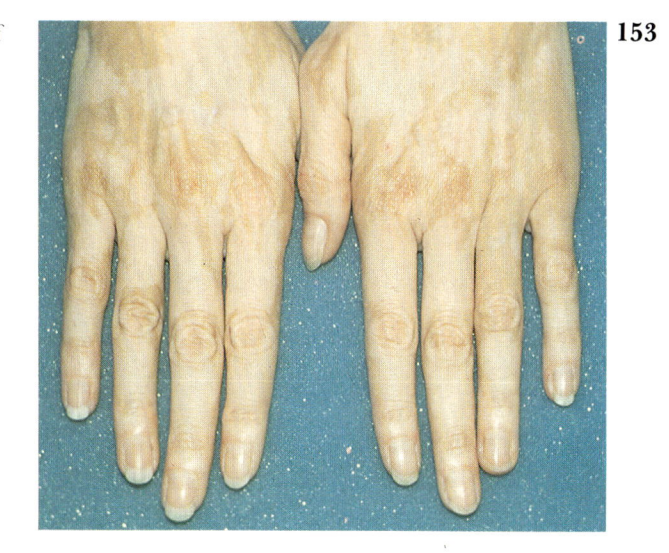

154 Vitiliginous changes on foot of patient with Vogt–Koyanagi–Harada disease.

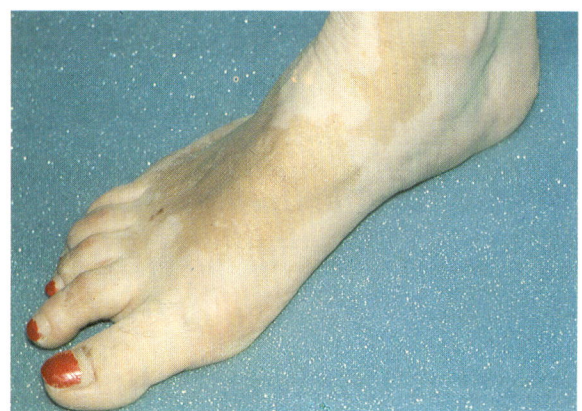

155 Prominent patchy multifocal choroidal leakage in patient with Harada syndrome which is a pattern very characteristic of this disease.

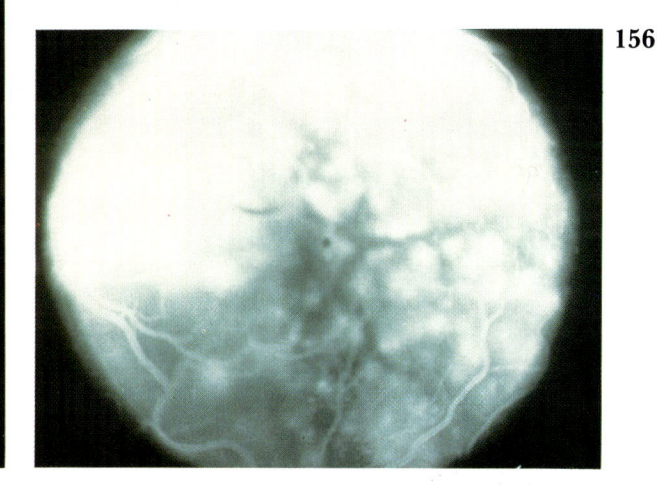

156 Fluorescein angiogram of Vogt–Koyanagi–Harada disease demonstrates multiple pinpoint leakage sites at the level of the retinal pigment epithelium, which coalesce.

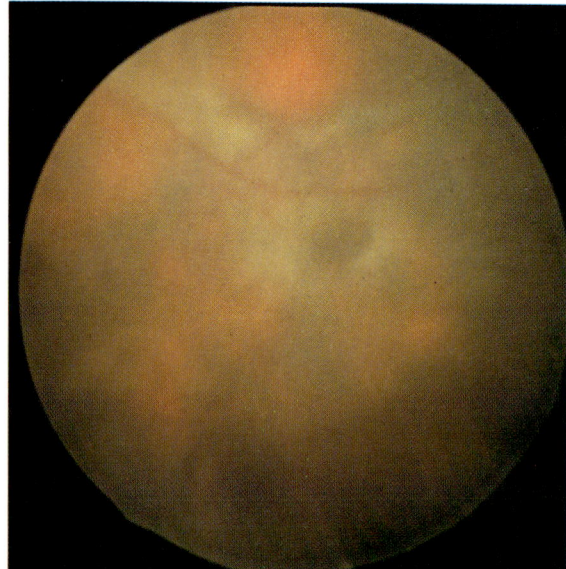

157 Serous detachment of the retina in patient with Vogt–Koyanagi–Harada disease with underlying choroidal scarring.

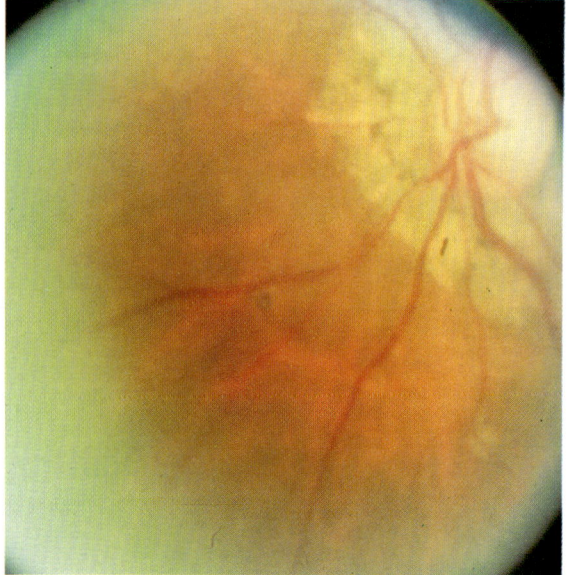

158 Inactive inflammation in patient with Vogt–Koyanagi–Harada disease showing areas of scarred retinal pigment epithelium in and around the optic nerve head and focal areas of similar retinal pigment epithelium disturbance peripherally.

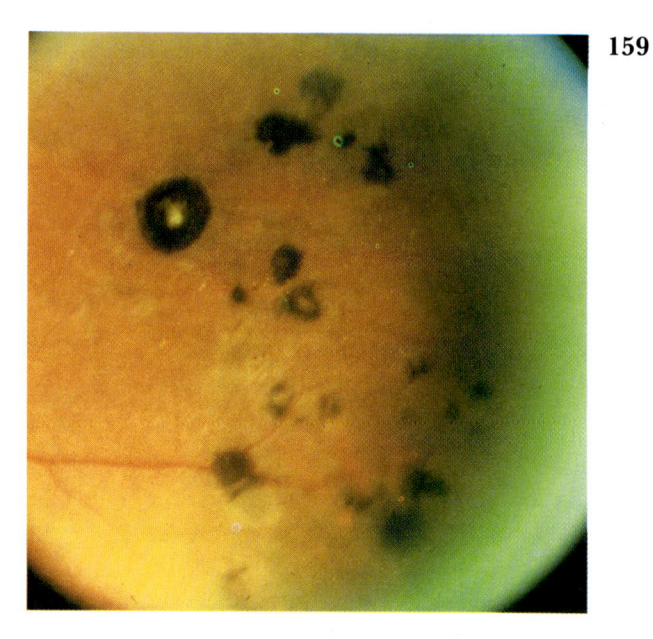

159 Areas of clumped and discrete hyperpigmentation of the retinal pigment epithelium surrounded by areas of retinal pigment epithelial atrophy from patient with recurrent serous detachment of the retina with Vogt–Koyanagi–Harada disease

160 Dense vitritis. Patient with acute inflammation from Vogt–Koyanagi–Harada disease in both the anterior and posterior segment of the eye. The vitiritis is so dense that it gives the appearance of a cataract.

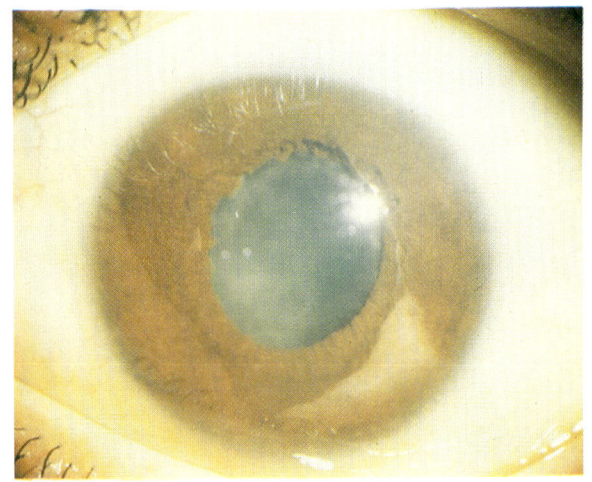

All of the clinical signs of Vogt–Koyanagi–Harada disease are similar to sympathetic ophthalmia, including the vitiligo, poliosis, alopecia, and dysacusis. Sympathetic ophthalmia is also a granulomatous panuveitis that may occur as early as two to four weeks after a penetrating or very profound blunt injury to an eye in which uveal pigment is presumably disturbed. It may occur up to 20 years after such an injury. There is a profound iridocyclitis and vitritis, and disseminated yellow-white nodules may be seen in the fundus (Dalen–Fuchs). These nodules are inflammations in the retinal pigment epithelium itself where the pigment is phagocytosed by epithelioid cells. In the presteroidal era useful vision was only achieved in 50% of eyes with sympathetic ophthalmia, but now better than 90% can be saved with combinations of steroidal and nonsteroidal anti-inflammatory agents.

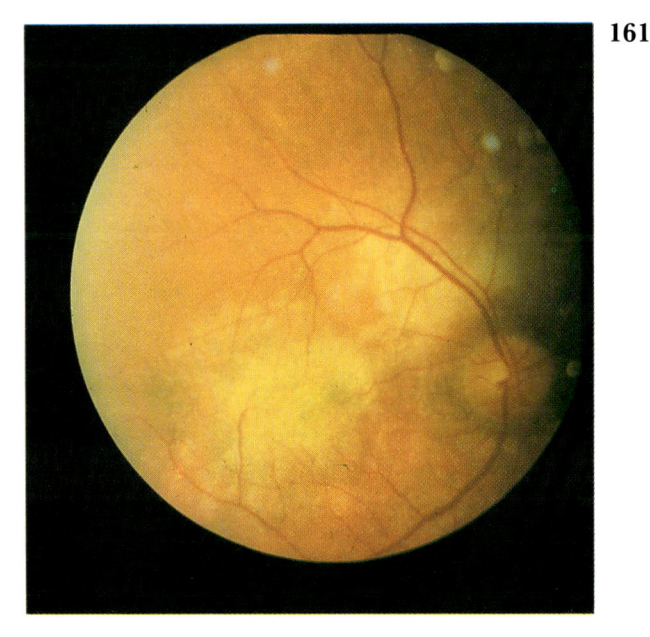

161 Resolved serous detachment of the retina in patient with only minimal vasculitic changes from Vogt–Koyanagi–Harada disease resulting in scarring of the retinal pigment epithelium under the retina but with preservation of 20/30 vision.

Uveal Effusion

The uveal effusion syndrome has been described by Schepens and Brockhurst as an insidious, progressive, non-reghmatogenous detachment of the retina, choroid and ciliary body with dependent fluid. It may be found in association with post-operative hypotony, scleral buckling procedures, scleritis and other inflammatory states. The disease has been described in middle-aged men whose eyes show little or no external inflammation and very little intraocular inflammation. A few of the patients have mild cellular infiltration in the vitreous gel. The syndrome may be accompanied by headache and neck stiffness. Cerebrospinal fluid examinations have shown elevations of the fluid protein with a mild pleocytosis. Otherwise, the patients are healthy with no abnormalities of pigmentary changes in the skin, hair, dysacusis, etc. Treatment of the uveal effusion with corticosteroids has been ineffective, and attempts at drainage of the subretinal fluid have been followed by rapid reformation of fluid in the same location. Pathogenesis of this disease is unknown.

Fluorescein angiographic study demonstrates a stasis in the choroidal vasculature and it is suspected that the fluid leaks from the choroid into the subretinal space. On resolution of the detachment, retinal pigment epithelial window defects are noted with pigment mottling (**164**).

UVEAL EFFUSION

Definition:
- Acute exudative detachment of the sensory retina

Presentation:
- Exudative retinal detachment
- Nongranulomatous

Investigation:
- Lumbar puncture

Therapy:
- Steroids ineffective
- Attempts of drainage of fluid have been followed by rapid reformation of fluid
- Lamellar scleral excision leads to resolution of uveal effusion syndrome (Gass: Moorfield paper)

Prognosis:
- Variable

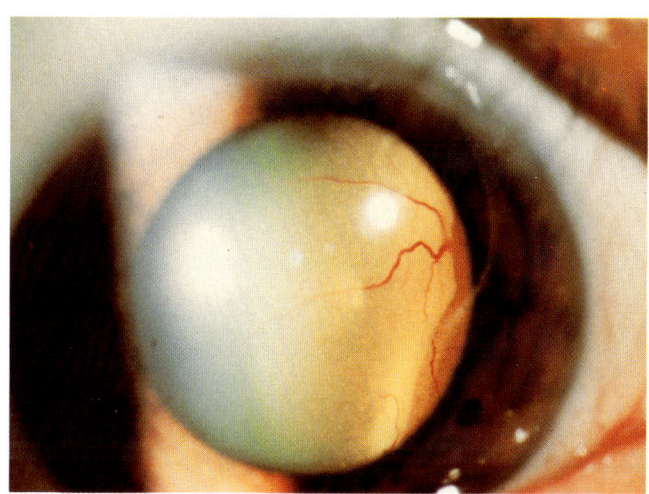

162 Uveal effusion. External photographs showing how highly elevated a uveal effusion may become where the retinal vasculature can be seen abutting the posterior lens capsule on the slit-lamp examination picture. (*Courtesy of David Fischer M.D.*)

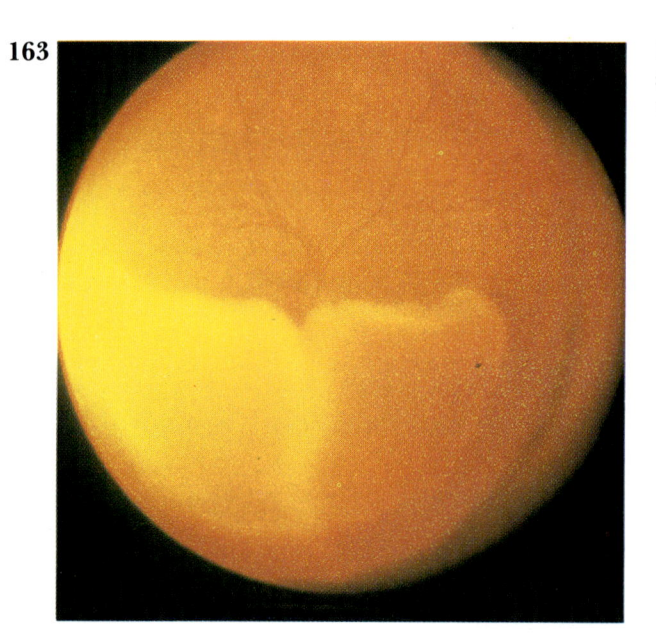

163 Wide angle fundus photograph showing uveal effusion which encompasses the entire inferior half of the retina up to the optic nerve head. (*Courtesy of David Fischer, M.D.*)

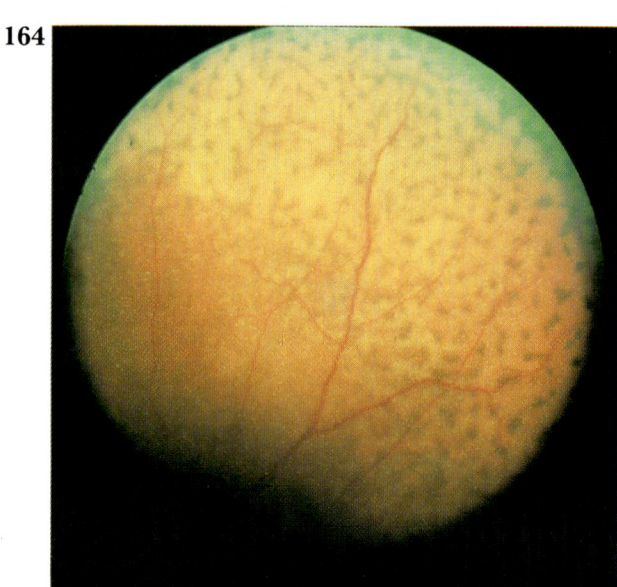

164 Resolved uveal effusion leaves behind as its 'footprints' this diffuse mottling and disruption of the retinal pigment epithelium often seen in Harada's syndrome when the serous detachment resolves in that disease entity as well.

Presumed Ocular Histoplasmosis

Presumed ocular histoplasmosis (POHS) is a disease of young adults which was originally described in the 1960s and now is very commonly diagnosed in areas where histoplasma capsulatum is endemic. It is also seen in countries where histoplasmosis is not known to occur. Currently about 3 million patients have positive histoplasma skin tests in the USA. Of these, an estimated 4% have peripheral or peripapillary scarring in the retina. Subretinal neovascular membranes that hemorrhage cause blindness in this disorder and account for a considerable proportion of young people who have a central loss of vision. The clinical features of POHS are serous and hemorrhagic detachment of the macula (**167**), peripheral and peripapillary 'punched-out' scars, (**166**), and a peripapillary depigmentation or scarring. These signs constitute the classical triad of presumed ocular histoplasmosis. It is important to observe that the anterior chamber and vitreous are clear of cells in this disease. Active disease may occur around peripapillary scarring with subretinal fluid extending underneath the macular zone. This may cause metamorphosia and reduced central vision, but the true loss of central vision occurs from subretinal neovascular membrane. Subretinal neovascular membrane may occur in the absence of the full triad of this disease and some clinicians consider these patients to have histoplasmosis until proven otherwise. However, other diseases in young people can cause subretinal neovascular membrane and these include angioid streaks, choroidal rupture, Fuchs' spot, other 'thinnings' of Bruch's membrane, Ehlers-Danlos syndrome, sickle-cell anemia, and Paget's disease.

The etiology of most cases of POHS remains unproven since many of these patients will not have documented pulmonary histoplasmosis. However, in the USA the organism is endemic in the Mississippi, Ohio, and Missouri river valleys. It is assumed that a systemic fungemia develping early may cause a mild upper respiratory infection and this may seed to the eyes and/or central nervous system. Therapy is indicated in the presumed ocular histoplasmosis syndrome for a suspected systemic fungemia, especially in the absence of pulmonary histoplasma infection. Photocoagulation appears to offer benefit in eliminating subretinal neovascular membrane, especially with krypton laser in and about the fovea. Other clinicians favour corticosteroids in addition to argon photocoagulation when subretinal neovascular membrane can be established beyond question by fluorescein angiography and if the lesion is in a treatable area outside the capillary-free zone of the fovea. When a patient has a subretinal neovascular membrane in one eye and small atrophic areas are found either by clinical examination of fluorescein angiography in the macula of the second eye, the patient has a 20–25% chance of developing macular disease from subretinal neovascular membrane in the fellow eye. Attention should be paid to early recognition of metamorphopsia and other visual complaints in the fellow eye for possible intervention with krypton or yellow dye laser photocoagulation.

PRESUMED OCULAR HISTOPLASMOSIS

Definition:
- Triad:
  Peripapillary pigment change
- Peripheral 'punched-out' lesions
- Subretinal neovascular membrane under macula

Presentation:
- Subretinal neovascular membrane in the macular region
- Peripheral 'punched-out' lesions
- Nongranulomatous choroiditis

Investigation:
- Histoplasma skin test
- Chest Xray
- HLA B7 (if macula is involved)

Therapy:
- Vigorous treatment of symptoms of metamorphosia with high-dose short course systemic steroids may be helpful. Photocoagulation of macula threatening lesions may be of benefit

Complications:
- Macular scarring
- Loss of sensual vision

Prognosis:
- Good if no lesion in or near macula
- Ominous to poor if lesion is present in macula due to recurrent activity

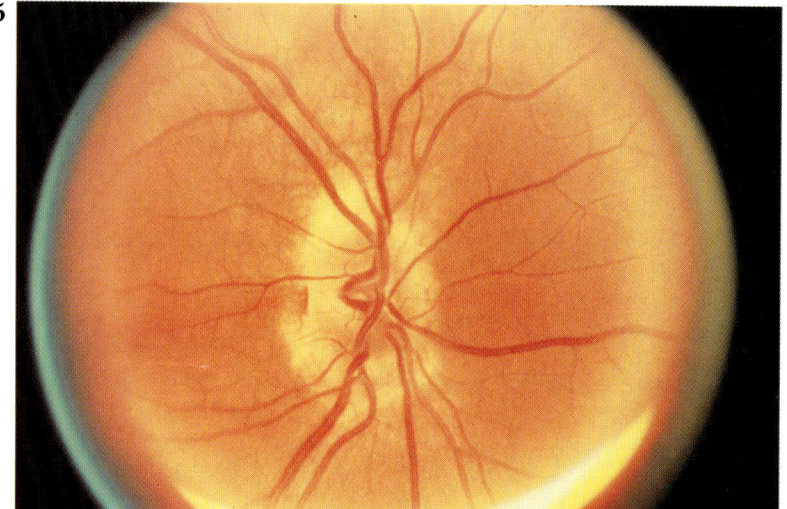

165 Peripapillary depigmentation in a 24-year-old patient with presumed ocular histoplasmosis.

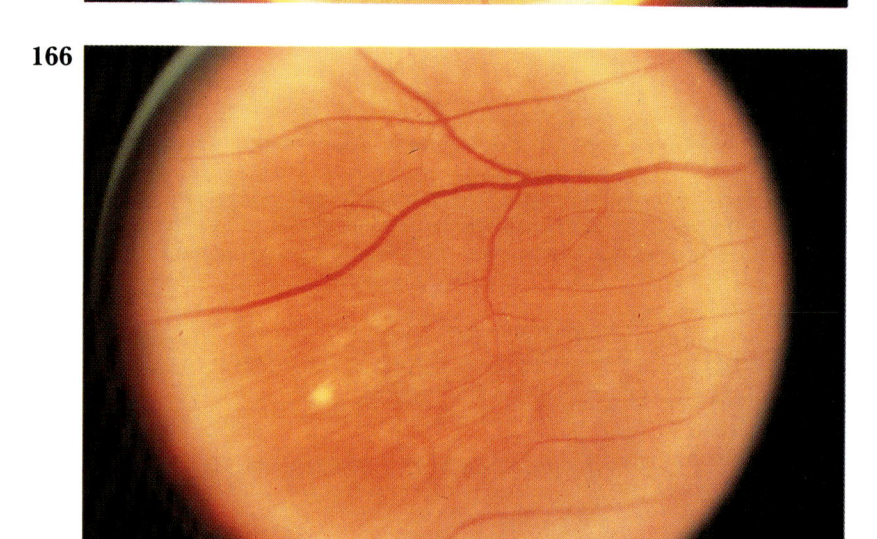

166 Peripheral 'punched-out' scar in same patient as Figure 165.

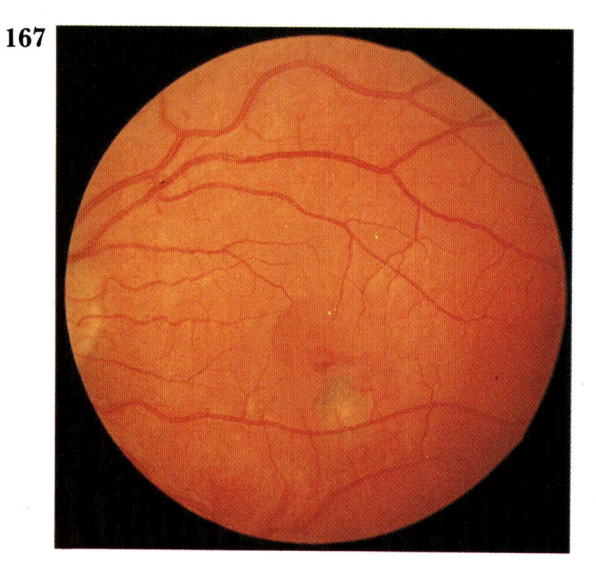

167 Subretinal neovascular membrane. A 32-year-old white woman with subretinal neovascular membrane due to presumed ocular histoplasmosis syndrome.

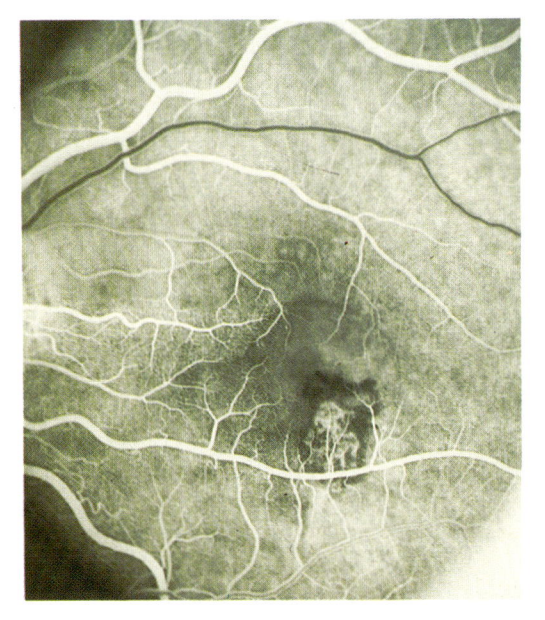

168 Early venous phase of fluorescein angiogram of the same patient showing subretinal neovascular membrane and surrounding serous detachment of the sensory retina.

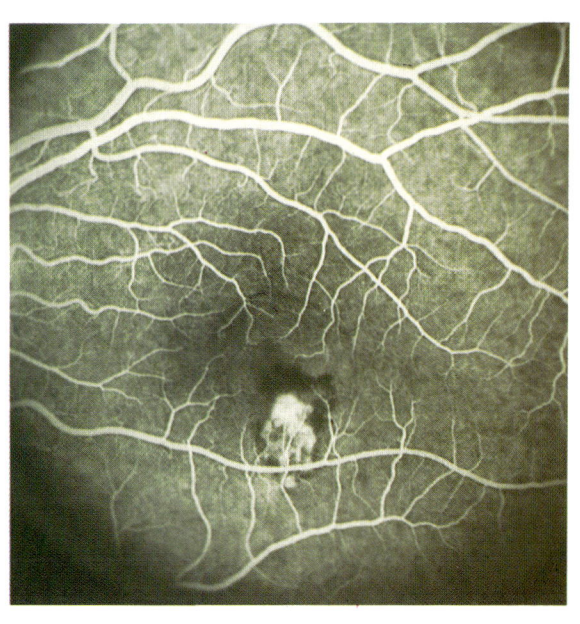

169 Late venous phase showing the accumulation of fluorescein dye in subretinal neovascular membrane now obscuring the original lacy network of the membrane seen in the previous figure.

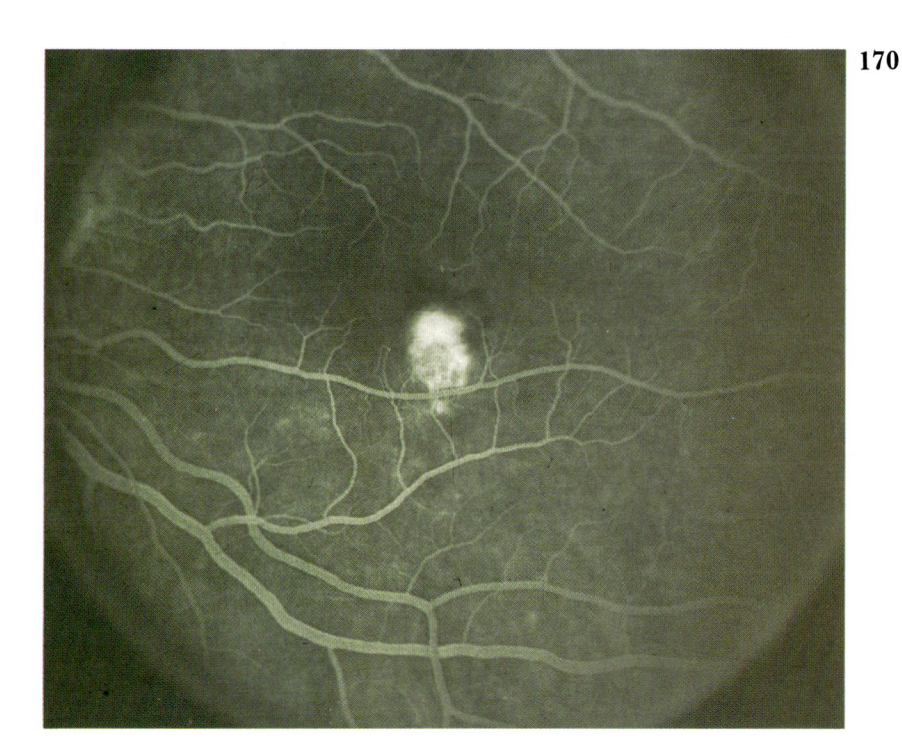

170 Late phase of accumulation of fluorescein in subretinal neovascular membrane with late staining.

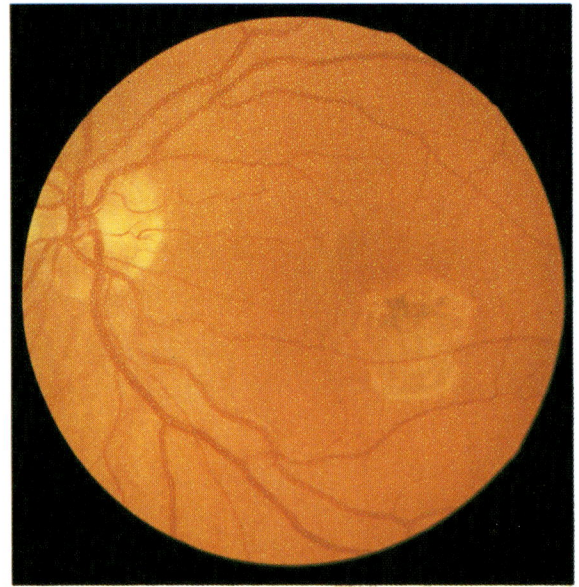

171 Argon laser photocoagulation. Same patient as in Figure 169 and Figure 168 after argon laser treatment to subretinal neovascular membrane, which occurred just outside the perifoved capillary-free zone and restored central vision of 20/25.

172 Acute macular hemorrhage in a 26-year-old Spanish woman with ocular histoplasmosis syndrome occurring acutely. Note the peripheral 'punched-out' lesion superior to the disc.

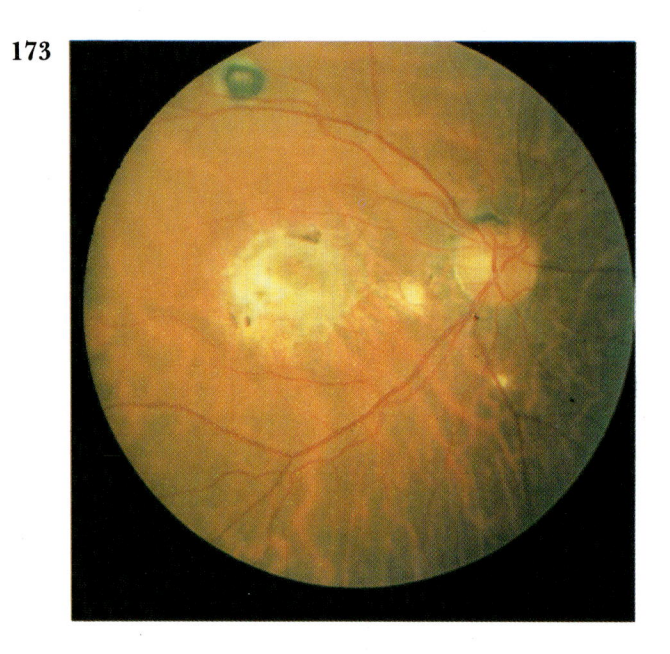

173 Old, inactive atrophic macular scar from subretinal neovascular membrane in a 32-year-old patient with presumed ocular histoplasmosis syndrome. Note two 'punched-out' lesions that are pale and devoid of retinal pigment epithelial hypertrophy inferior to the disc, and superotemporal to the disc, one hypertrophic peripheral 'punched-out' lesion with a rounded up border of retinal pigment epithelial hypertrophy.

174 Macular scarring from subretinal neovascular membrane in patient with angioid streaks noted as subtle serpiginous subretinal pigment radiating superotemporally from the disk and concentric to it. Such a condition might be mistaken for presumed ocular histoplasmosis syndrome.

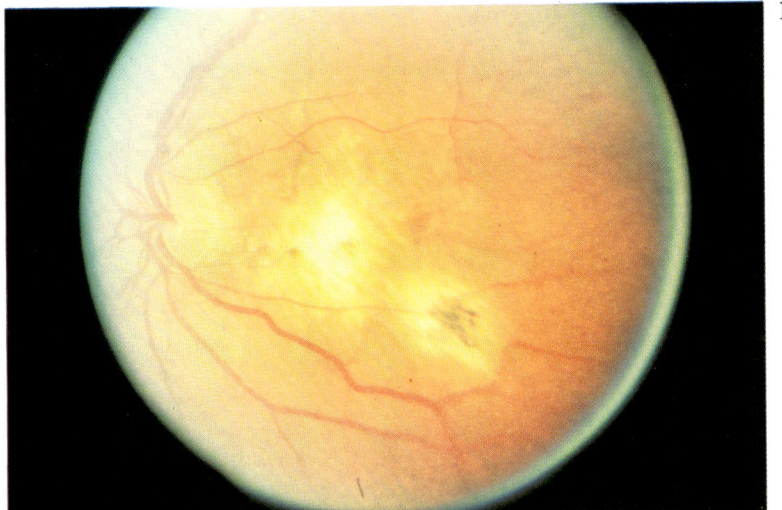

175 Fellow eye in patient with angioid streaks. Notice the streaks superotemporally, superior to the disk and concentric to it. The full extent of the subretinal darkly pigmented streaks, when carefully noted, will indicate the etiology of subretinal neovascular membrane, which is different from histoplasmosis.

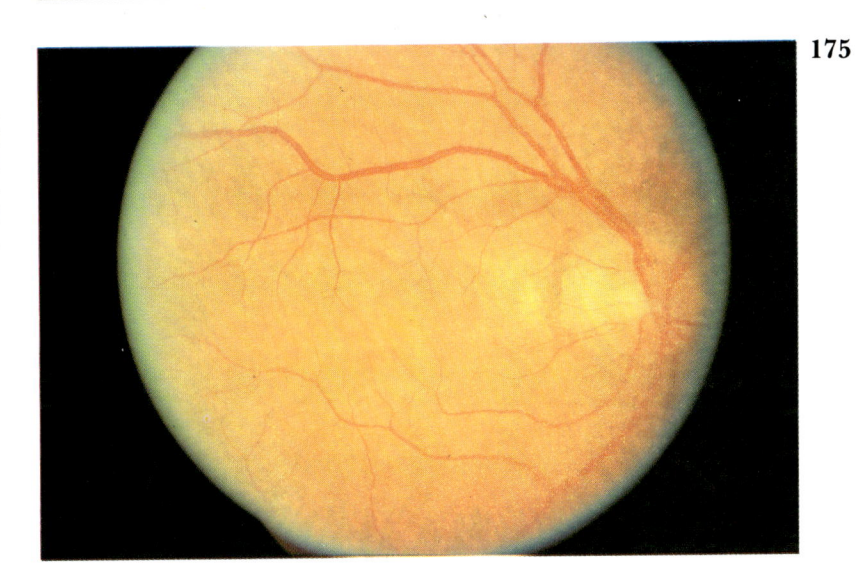

/

Coccidioidomycosis

San Joaquin Valley Fever, or desert fever, is caused by *C. immitis* and is endemic to the south western region of the USA, the north western region of Mexico, Central America, and Venezuela. Ocular involvement was first described at the turn of the century in a patient with disseminated disease with both corneal and conjunctival involvement. The infection usually begins as a pulmonary infestation and may be present without symptoms in up to 75% of cases. When manifest, a bronchial pneumonia is most common and the prognosis is good. Up to 0.5% of all patients with manifest pulmonary infection do develop disseminated disease elsewhere. The intraocular findings include iridocyclitis, often of a granulomatous nature, and multiple yellow-white corneal retinal lesions 0.1 to 0.5 disc diameter in size, often having a pigmented border and only occasionally having acute retinal exudates. Most of the retinal lesions look like 'acute' histolesions, and this is a fungal infestation, as is the organism of histoplasmosis. The usual treatment for this disease is intravenous amphotericin B. Extraocular lesions may occur as well in the lid, orbit and conjunctiva, and when these are present a phylctenular conjunctivitis and/or episcleritis may be associated with it.

COCCIDIOIDOMYCOSIS

Definition:
- San Joaquin Valley Fever
- Southwestern USA.

Presentation:
- 1° Bronchopneumonia
- Phlyctenular conjunctivitis
- Episcleral, conjunctival, lid lesions
- Multiple yellow-white chorioretinal lesions with pigmented border
- 'Punched-out' peripheral lesions

Investigation:
- Chest Xray
- Biopsy of skin, lid, conjunctival lesion
- Complement fixing antibodies
- Immunodiffusion for IgM, IgG

Therapy:
- Amphotericin B (IV; intrathecal)
- Steroids

Prognosis:
- Disease can be fatal

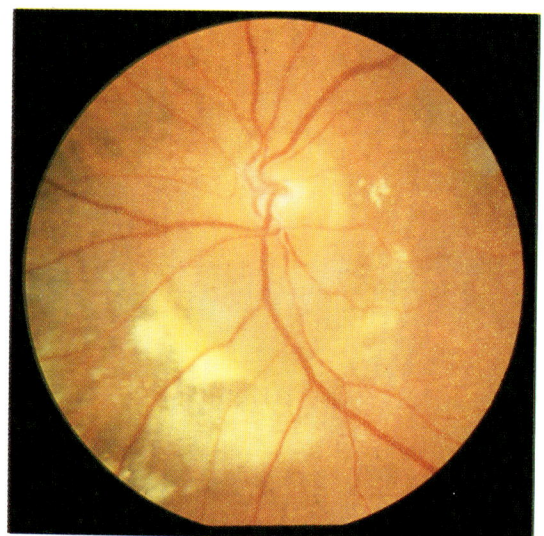

176 Coccidioidomycosis. A 54-year-old patient suffering from meningitis due to coccidioidomycosis imitis demonstrates juxtapapillary choroiditis inferior to the optic nerve head with surrounding exudate.

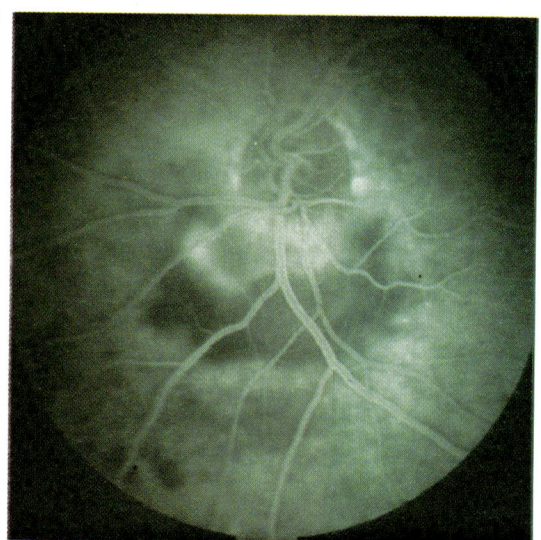

177 Fluorescein angiogram in the midvenous phase showing the blockage of the underlying choroidal fluorescence with hypofluorescence from the exudate in this abscess under the optic papilla from coccidioidomycosis. This patient was not an abuser of intravenous drugs but suffered an acquired pulmonary fungal infection endemic to the Southwest region of the USA.

Ocular Toxocariasis

Toxocara canis infection occurs in children and its clinical sign is most often leukocoria. This clinical entity may often be confused with retinoblastoma and due to the potentially profound significance of misdiagnosis, very careful attention should be paid to the clinical signs and symptoms of children who present with this entity. Toxocariasis was first described in 1950 and is now recognized in 3 forms: 1) a diffuse endophthalmitis (**183**), 2) a macular retinal choroidal granuloma (**179**) often with a scar which extends to the optic nerve head (**182**), and 3) a peripheral retinal choroidal granuloma (**181**). The *Toxocara canis* is a common ascarid (**180**) that is found in up to 50% of otherwise healthy dogs. The prevalence of human exposure as evidenced by positive serology is less than 10% of the population.

Ocular toxocariasis is almost always unilateral, although very rarely bilateral cases are reported. It is unusual to find this disease after 12 years of age. Boys are affected more frequently than girls. Frequently one can elicit a history of pica in children who become affected. It is of interest that visceral larval migrans, the systemic dermal variety of this disease, usually does not have the ocular manifestations associated with it, and vice versa. Two percent of all patients diagnosed as having ocular toxocariasis have evidence for underlying visceral larval migrans which is often characterized by fever, hepatosplenomegaly, and a high degree of eosinophilia that seldom affects the eye. However, when an acute toxocariasis affects the eye, eosinophils may be isolated from the anterior chamber by paracentesis.

ELISA, the Enzyme Linked ImmunoSorbant Assay for toxocariasis, is available through most American state laboratories or the Center for Disease Control in Atlanta. A dilution of 1 to 8 to larval antigen is considered positive and may be helpful in diagnosing over 90% of cases. An ELISA performed on the aqueous humor is even more sensitive, especially when eosinophilia may be prominent. However, skin tests are considered unreliable because there is considerable cross-reaction with other types of ascaris and many healthy persons test positively even in the absence of any larval infection.

OCULAR TOXOCARIASIS

Definition:
- Acute endophthalmitis
- Inactive usually white elevated scar on the retina with cicatrix leading to optic papilla

Presentation:
- Endophthalmitis
- Inactive uveitis
- Scar from peripheral lesion to optic papilla
- Traction retinal detachment
- Granulomatous

Investigation:
- ELISA for toxocara
- Vitreous aspiration with ELISA
- ESR CBC
- AC tap for eosinophils (B scan for calcification)

Therapy:
- Periocular steroids
- Systemic steroids during active period
- Antihelminth contraindicated

Complications:
- Cataract
- Macular scarring
- Glaucoma
- Retinal detachment

Prognosis:
- Poor if macular involved
- Poor if endophthalmitis is present
- If peripheral, prognosis is good with treatment of the severe phases of inflammation
- Once case quiet, intraocular surgery well tolerated for retinal attachment

While medical treatment of ocular toxocara is generally unsatisfactory, since antihelminth preparations release a burden of antigen which consumes the eye in immunological reaction, suppression of the reaction with steroids is preferable. Recent reports demonstrate some structural improvement with vitrectomy surgery.

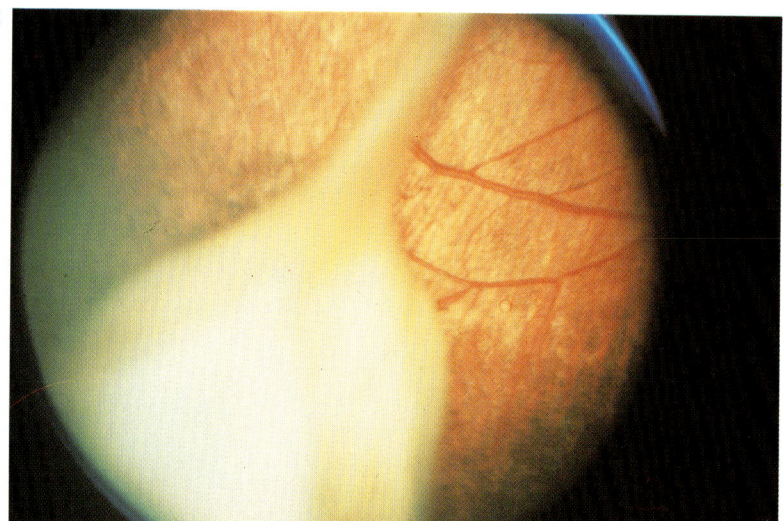

178 Peripheral retina in a 12-year-old child with ocular toxocariasis showing dense white retinal-choroidal scar in the very peripheral inferotemporal retina.

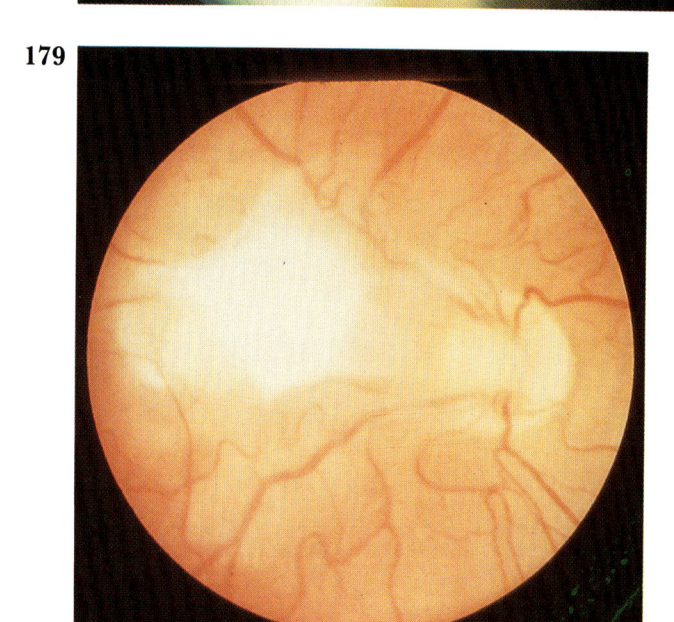

179 Presumed ocular toxocariasis in an 8-year-old child showing a white raised macular abscess with a dense fibrous band connecting to the optic papilla which is disorganizing the architecture of the retinal vasculature.

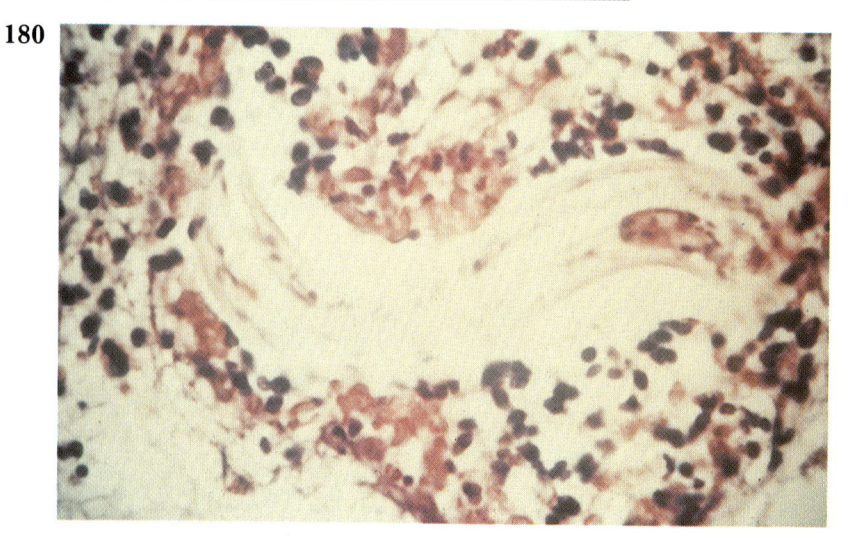

180 Toxocara abscess. Histologic demonstration of *Toxocara canis* within a retinal abscess showing a multitude of inflammatory cells surrounding the degenerating worm structure.

181 Peripheral *Toxocara canis* granuloma in retina superonasal, close to the ora serrata whose gray peak of elevation can be seen through this clear lens.

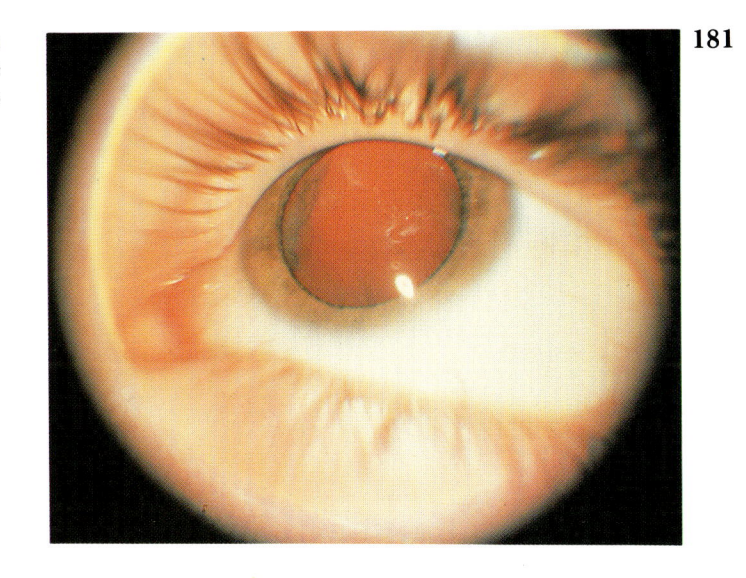

182 Dense white tensile fibrous band connected to optic papilla from peripheral abscess in an 8-year-old black child with toxocariasis.

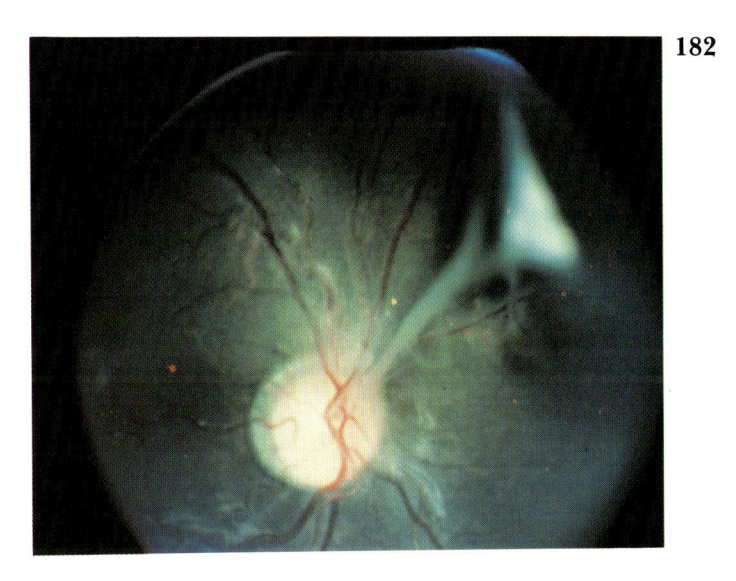

183 Diffuse endophthalmitis in a 7-year-old child with toxocariasis and visceral larval migrans showing the dense white retinal abscess in the periphery.

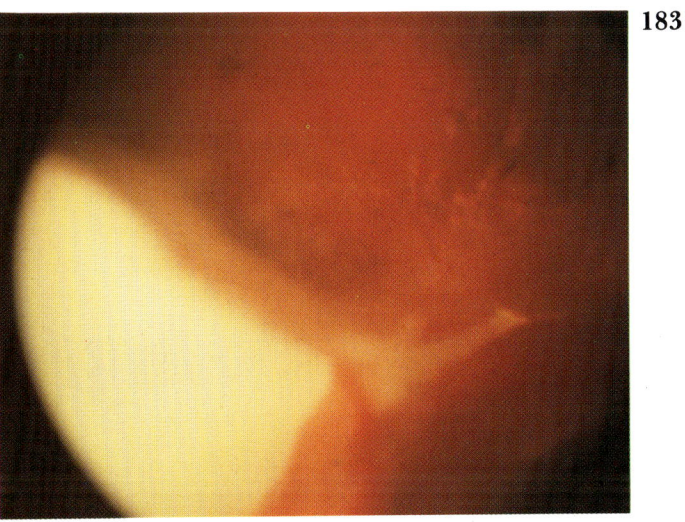

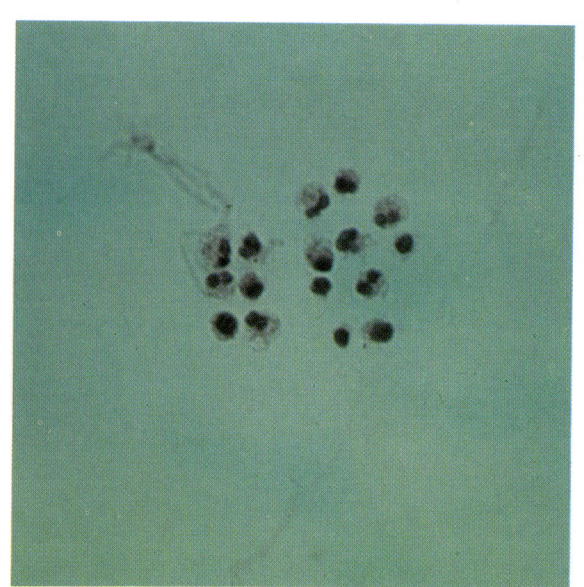

184 Multiple well-preserved eosinophils aspirated from anterior chamber in case of acute toxocariasis endophthalmitis. (*Courtesy of Jerry A. Shields, M.D.*)

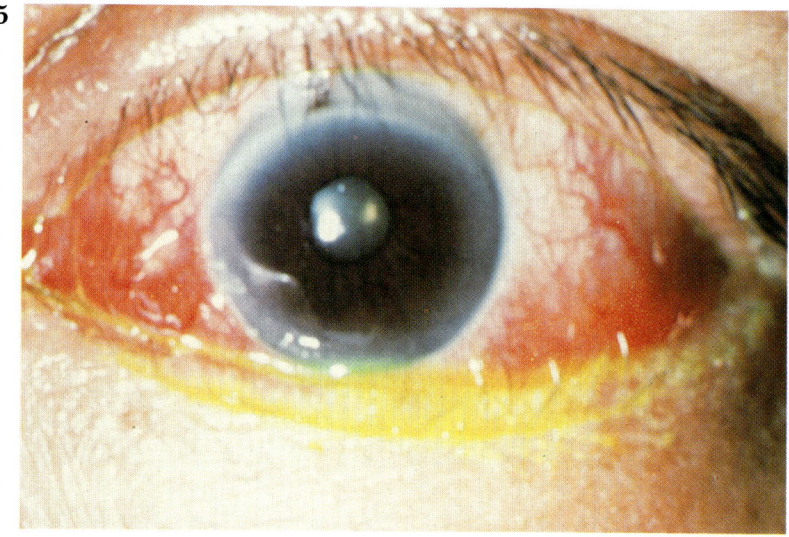

185 *Thalasia californiensis* nematode in the anterior chamber of a patient who acquired the infection from a horse in northern California.

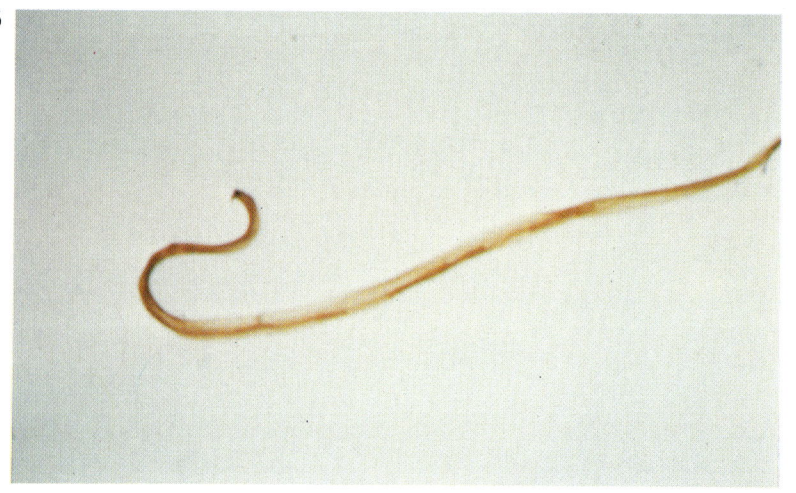

186 *Thalasia californiensis* surgically removed from the anterior segment of the patient's eye in Figure 185.

187 Loa loa worm removed from under the conjunctiva in patient with this tropical nematode infection. (*Courtesy of Jonathan Belmont, M.D.*)

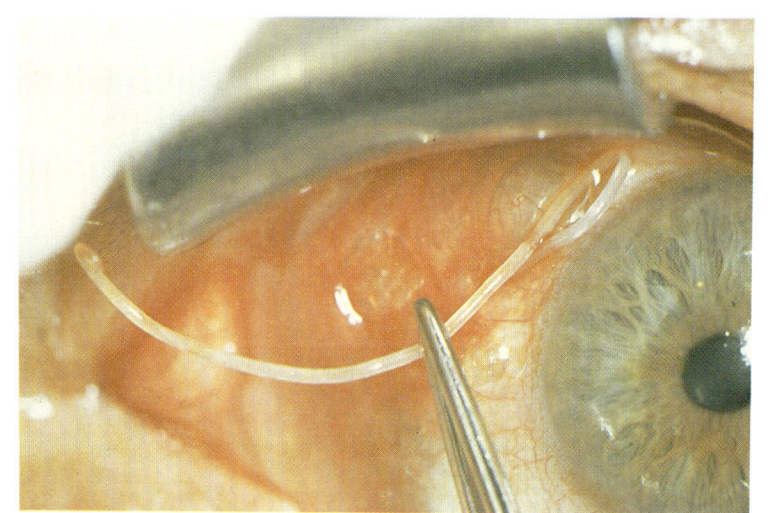

188 Bot fly larva as seen in the vitreous gel of a patient who acquired this larval infection while camping in the Sierra Nevada. (*Courtesy of Michael Goldbaum, M.D.*)

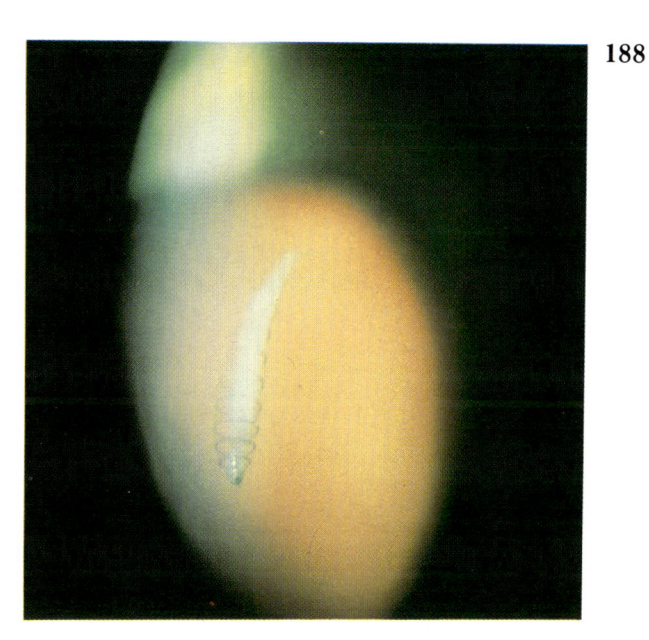

Toxoplasmosis

Toxoplasmosis is an infection by an obligate intracellular protozoan parasite and may represent the most common form of posterior uveitis in the Western world. *Toxoplasma gondii* is ubiquitous in the warm-blooded animal kingdom; the parasite undergoes the sexual stage reproduction in the intestinal mucosal epithelium in the cat, its primary host. Oocysts shed by the cat in feces are then ingested by intermediate hosts such as rodents and birds which are caught by cats again, thus perpetuating the life cycle, and who then serve as vectors to carnivorous animals and to grazing herbivorous animals. Man then eats the infected flesh of the herbivores to liberate the toxoplasma organisms (**195**). Infection may thus be acquired by the consumption of raw or improperly cooked meat. Of the systemic varieties of toxoplasmosis, approximately 1% demonstrate ocular lesions. The vast majority of patients seen by the ophthalmologist probably have congenitally acquired disease which reactivates later in life.

The organism resides in the long-term in neural tissue, and may remain dormant for long periods of time, and may reactivate in later life giving the impression of a new infection. Fetal brain and ocular tissues are especially susceptible to long-term parasitazation. Thus, affected neonates usually manifest healed scars that are susceptible to recurrent conflamation at some later time.

Systemic toxoplasmosis may manifest itself in four forms: 1) exanthematous eruption which is a skin vasculitis and resembles Rickettsial disease in appearance (this rare entity is the most fatal form of the disease) (**191**); 2) lymphadenopathic infection (**194**) which may resemble a heterophil-negative 'mononucleosis' syndrome, and includes fever, malaise, lymphadenopathy, myalgias, and perhaps a mild elevation of liver enzymes; 3) meningoencephalitic syndrome (**200**), which has a higher frequency of associated eye involvement than the more common lymphadenopathic form and usually manifests itself in seizures, fever, and profound central nervous system signs; and 4) the congenital syndrome (**189, 190**) which is the less common, most severe form of the disease, is signified by the 'Sabin' tetrad of seizures, hydrocephalus, retinochoroiditis and cerebral calcifications. Toxoplasmosis is initially a pure retinitis and forms a retinochoroiditis only secondarily. This aspect of toxoplasma infection distinguishes it from the other 'chorioretinitides.'

The clinical signs of toxoplasmic retinochoroiditis include the stigmata of 'granulomatous' uveitis. Usually mutton-fat KP (**201**) are present, an intense ant-

TOXOPLASMOSIS

Definition:
- Acute retinitis

Presentation:
- Retinitis or retinochoroiditis
- Granulomatous

Investigation:
- Toxoplasma
- Dye test (Sabin-Feldman)
- FA test for toxoplasma
- ELISA test for toxoplasma
- Aqueous antibodies (as a proportion of serum antibodies) in unusual presentation

Therapy:
- Vigorous for the lesion, if threatening: a) the macula, b) maculopapillary bundle, c) optic nerve, d) severe endophthalmitis, e) macular edema secondary to lesions superior to the macula
- Daraprim and sulfa in combination
- Can use sulfa alone
- Can use tetracycline (minocycline)
- Can use systemic or periocular clindamycin
- Concurrent systemic steroids
- Never start steroids before antimicrobials
- Avoid periocular steroids alone
- Avoid systemic steroids without antimicrobial coverage

Complications:
- Secondary anterior uveitis with posterior synechia
- Secondary cataract
- Secondary glaucoma
- Retinal scarring (macula)
- Traction retinal detachment

Prognosis:
- Fair to poor if the lesion is near the macula
- Recurrent lesions may affect the foveal region
- Excellent if peripheral lesion only (may require no treatment)

erior chamber reaction and an outpouring of cells into the vitreous, especially over the white inflammatory focus of the retina. Older lesions are usually pigmented by retinal pigment epithelium hypertrophy and may be accompanied by local retinal vasculitis. Resolution of the lesion in the retina is marked by a pigmented scar. Reactivation usually occurs in proximity to an older lesion in a so-called satellite focus (**202, 39, 57**). Vitreous membranes (198, 199) may occur when the gel is infiltrated by an intense outpouring of cells and may lead to traction retinal detachment. Retinal breaks are not uncommon in severe cases. Focal retinal necrosis may occur.

The diagnosis of toxoplasma infection is still a clinical one, but it is corroborated by the presence of antibodies in the serum of the patient. These antibodies may be assayed by immunofluorescence, Sabin-Feldman dye test, hemagglutination or the new microtiter ELISA test. A positive IgM level indicates prior exposure to the organism, but rising titers of IgG are indicative of current or recurrent infection. Patients with acquired systemic infection usually have titers over 1:256, while patients with the pure ocular form of the disease may have antibodies only to a 1:1 dilution. For this reason, it is often necessary to specify to the laboratory that the patient's serum be run undiluted, since many laboratories routinely dilute all specimens to a base level of 1:4 or 1:8.

The treatment of the infection include antiprotozoans: pyrimethamine (Daraprim©), sulfadiazine or triple sulfa and steroids. Pyrimethamine and the sulfas work synergistically, and it is appropriate to initiate these before the inclusion of steroid if either the macula or optic papilla are threatened since the local immunosuppression caused by the latter agent may cause further damage on the sensitive neural tissues. Suppression of the bone marrow may occur with the use of pyrimethamine, and the monitoring of the platelet and leukocyte count is essential. Folinic acid, a folic acid antagonist, can be given orally to prevent the marrow suppression. Clindamycin has been shown to be an effective antiprotozoan, both orally and by sub-Tenon's injection. The former method has been shown to be a very rare cause of pseudomembranous colitis which can be therapeutically avoided, (vibramycin) while the latter may be complicated by optic neuropathy. Minocycline is also advocated by some authorities as an alternative treatment. A very peripheral toxoplasmic 'hot spot' may not require treatment if the patient's immune system is intact and the essential visual structures (macula, disc) are not threatened. Toxoplasmosis is reported as an opportunistic infection in patients with AIDS.

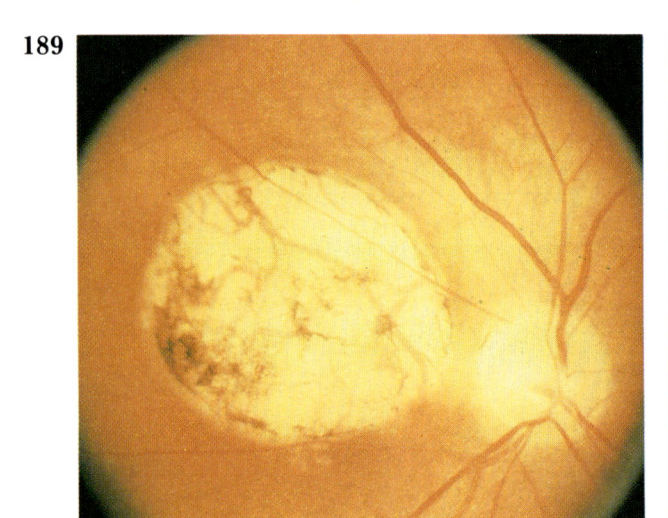

189 Large scalloped congenital toxoplasmic macular scar with retinal pigment epithelial clumping within the expanse of apparent retinal pigment epithelial absence.

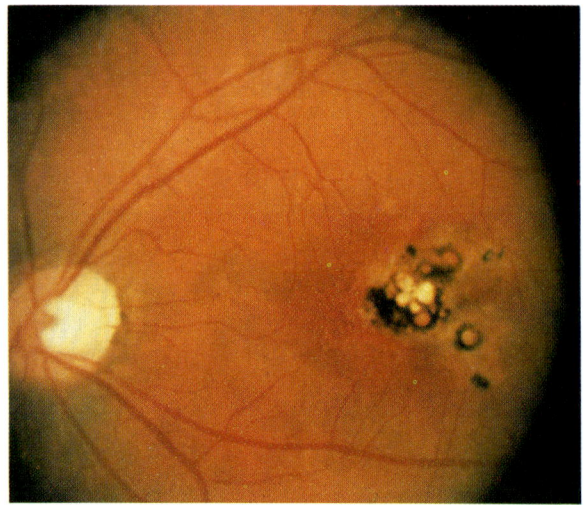

190 Inactive macular scar. Fellow eye with congenital macular scar demonstrating retinal pigment epithelial hypertrophy.

191 Exanthematous eruption of toxoplasmosis which represents vasculitis in the skin similar to Rickettsial disease.

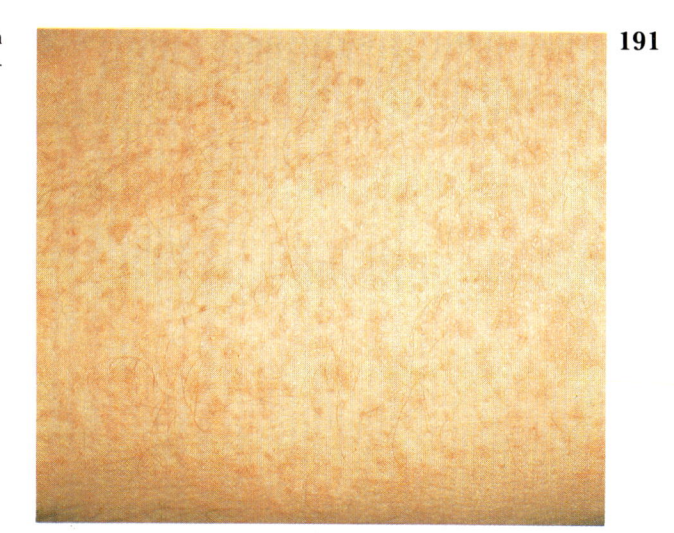

192 Classic clinical manifestation of acute retinitis with overlying vitritis, in this specific case demonstrating no associated choroiditis, resulting from a systemic acquired toxoplasmic infection with fever and lymphadenopathy.

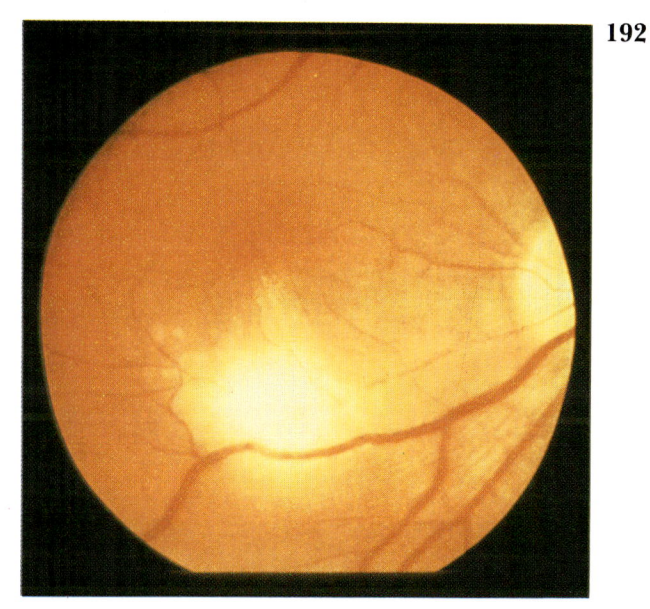

193 Fluorescein angiogram of case in Figure 192 demonstrating the hyperfluorescence of the retinal inflammation without affecting the underlying retinal pigment epithelium or the choroid. A presentation such as this with 'pure' retinitis with overlying vitritis and local vasculitis is to be considered on clinical grounds as toxoplasmosis until proven otherwise.

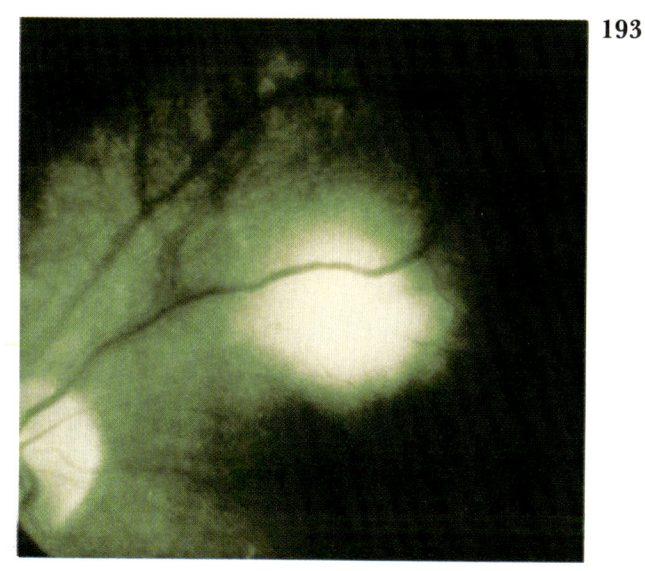

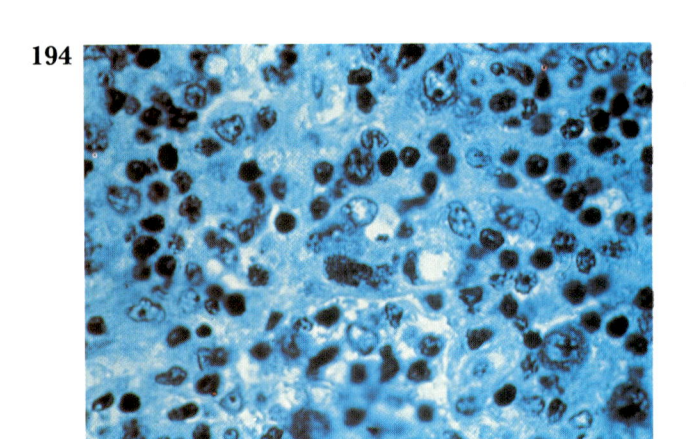

194 Lymph node biopsy of same patient in Figure 192 with systemic acquired infection, lymphadenopathy and fever demonstrates toxoplasmosis cysts.

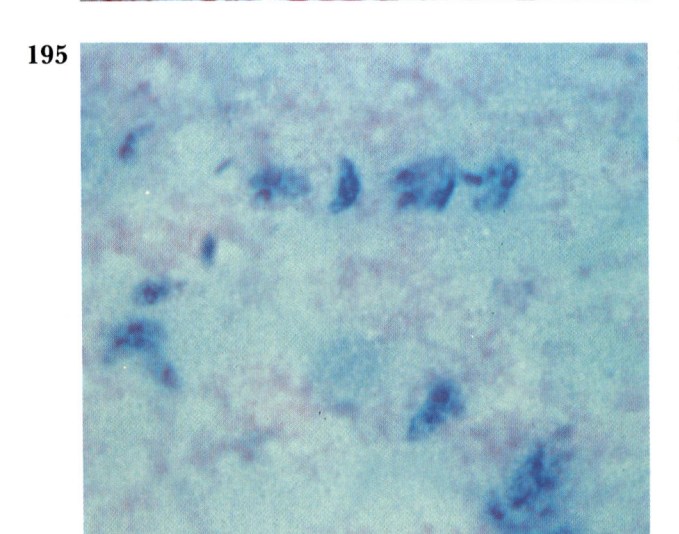

195 Typical banana-shaped protozoans (trophozoites) with central nucleus of toxoplasmosis harvested from mouse peritoneal fluid after inoculation with lymph node material to patient above.

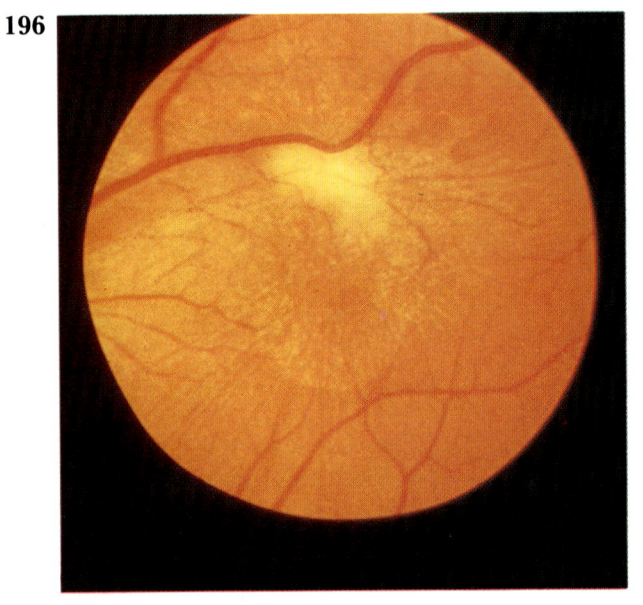

196 Healed retinal scar in foregoing patient treated with pyrimethamine, sulfa, and prednisone. The macular area demonstrates the radiating folds of the internal limiting membrane of the retina, stressed and fashioned into this pattern of 'cellophane' maculopathy.

197 Fluorescein angiogram of the healed area demonstrates the hyperfluorescence of the retinal scar and absence of pigment disruption of the retinal pigment epithelium, showing the exquisitely localized nature of this 'pure' retinal inflammation.

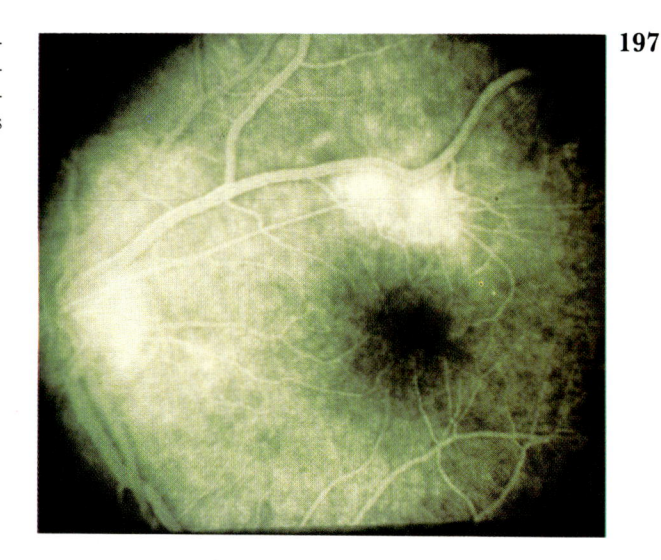

198 Toxoplasmic papillitis. Another patient with systemic acquired toxoplasmosis suffering high fever and lymphadenopathy. Intense inflammation localized over the optic nerve head indicates the neural tissue predilection of this organism.

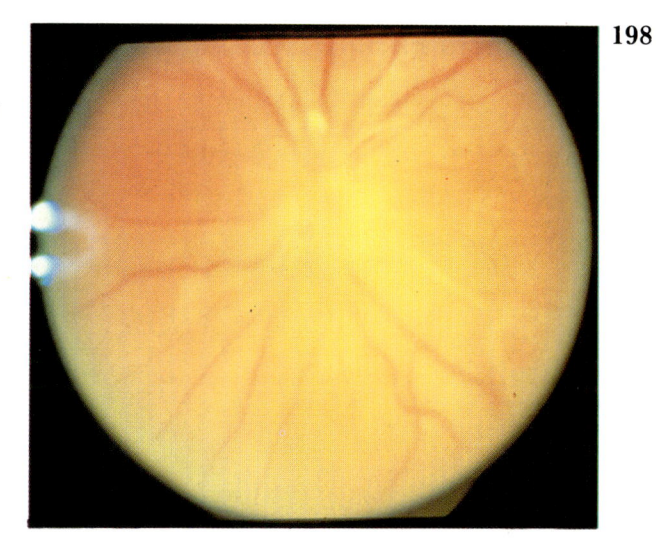

199 Vitritis and fibrous bands. Macula of same patient showing dense vitritis and diaphanous veils of inflammation forming in the vitreous gel. These fibrous bands may lead to traction retinal detachment or may cause a tear in the retina.

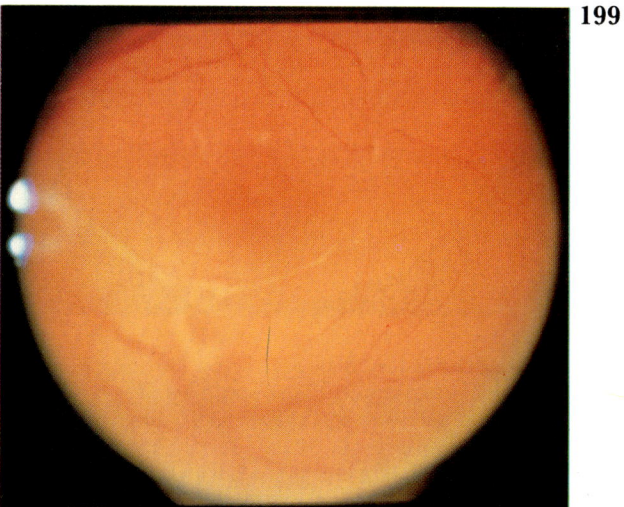

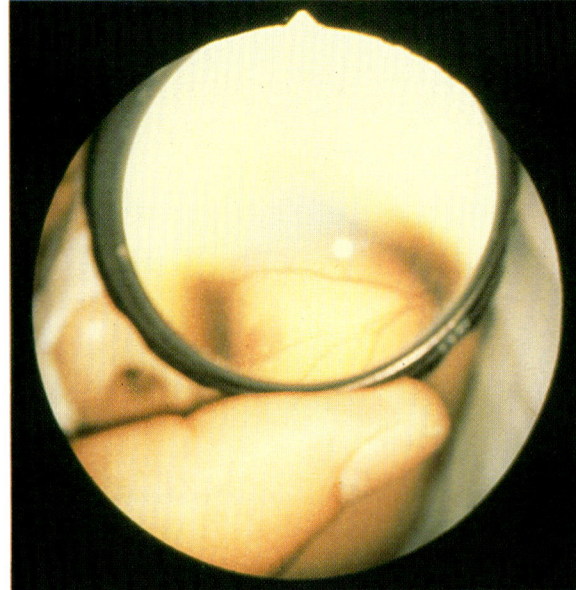

200 Roth spot. Patient with biopsy-proven meningoencephalitic toxoplasmosis, fever, seizures, and nystagmus demonstrates vitritis and a Roth spot of retinal inflammation.

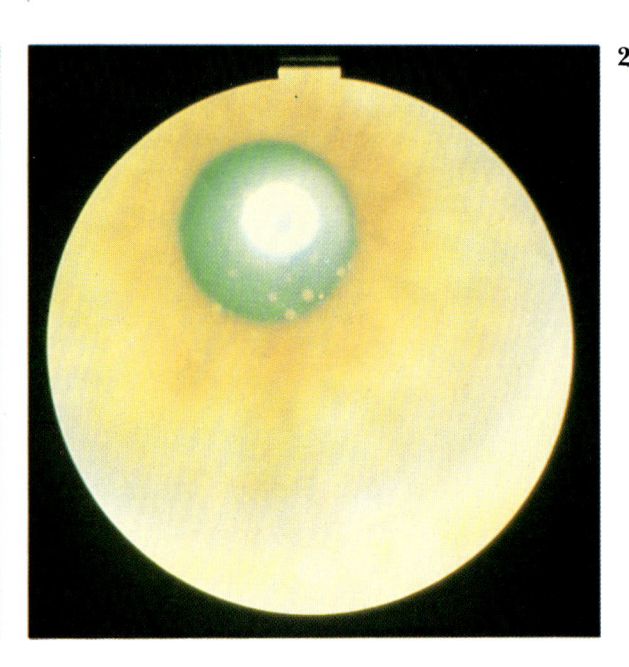

201 Mutton-fat KP. Cornea of patient with ocular toxoplasmosis demonstrates large white mutton-fat KP, usually indicative of a granulomatous process.

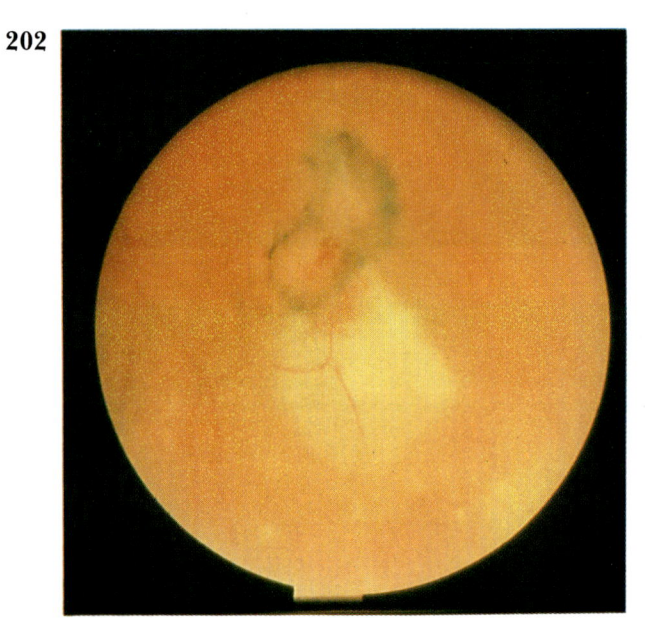

202 Satellite lesion. Retina of patient with ocular toxoplasmosis demonstrates the important diagnostic sign of recurrent inflammation occurring in a satellite lesion contiguous to the original, which is bordered by typical hypertrophic retinal pigment epithelial scarring. (See also Figure 57)

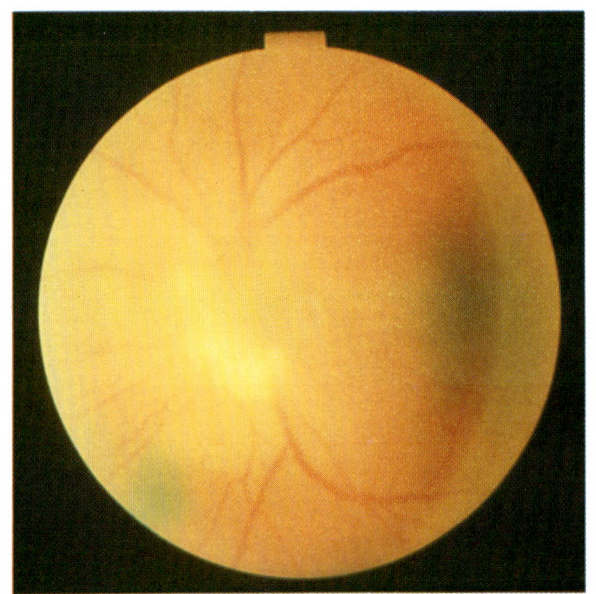

203 Recurrent active inflammatory lesions of toxoplasmosis dangerously bordering the optic papilla.

Behçet's Disease

Behçet's disease is characterized by three primary components: iridocyclitis (historically with hypopyon), aphthous lesions in the mouth (**204–207**), and ulceration of the genitalia. Erythema nodosum (**208**), arthropathy, and thrombophlebitis often accompany these manifestations, but the ocular symptoms may be the most important and serious manifestations of the disease. Central nervous system involvement, most often due to necrotizing vasculitis, may be the most protean manifestation of the disease leading to death. The frequency of ocular manifestations is 70–85% in patients with the disease; the underlying disease mechanism in all organ systems is an occlusive vasculitis. Although the most common ocular symptom is that of anterior uveitis, often with hypopyon as a not always very late sign, the presence of necrotizing peripheral occlusive vasculitis is well-known (**210, 212–214**) and often obscured by the severity of the anterior reaction. It is important to be familiar with the full spectrum of disease presentation because the ophthalmologist may be the first physician to encounter the Behçet patient. Current treatment includes steroids and immunosuppressives, chlorambucil (Imuran©), cyclosporine, Plaquenil© and colchicine.

BEHÇET'S DISEASE

Definition:
- A systemic vasculitis with multiorgan presentation

Presentation:
- Iridocyclitis
- Retinitis
- Choroiditis
- Vasculitis
- Granulomatous

Investigation:
- HLA B5, HLA-Bw51
- Antibody test with guinea pig lip
- Medical consultation
- Fluorescein angiogram
- Questionable skin puncture test (Behcetine test)

Therapy:
- Intensive local or systemic steroids
- Periocular steroids
- Low-dose chronic local or systemic steroid in chronic cases
- Immunosuppressive agents, especially chlorambucil, considered if retinal vasculitis present
- Cyclosporine

Complications:
- Cataract
- Glaucoma
- Retinal necrosis
- Optic atrophy
- Phthisis bulbi

Prognosis:
- Usually poor once eyes involved
- Blindness 3.3 yrs, after initial eye manifestations visual

204 Aphthous ulcer on tongue of patient with Behçet's disease.

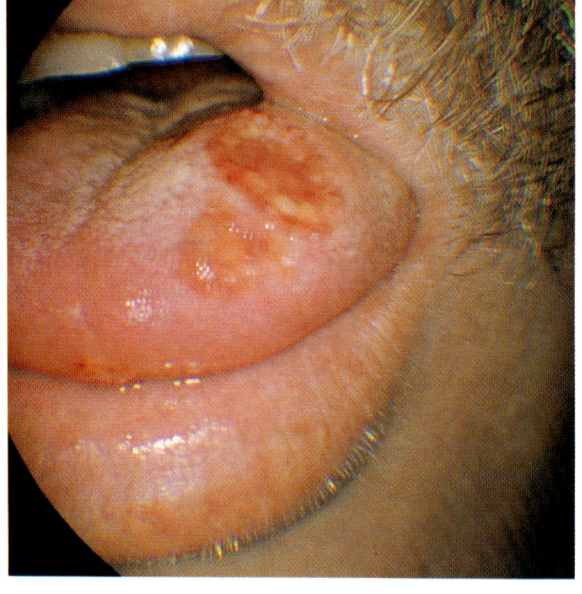

205 Recurrent necrotizing aphthous ulcer on tongue of patient with Behçet's disease.

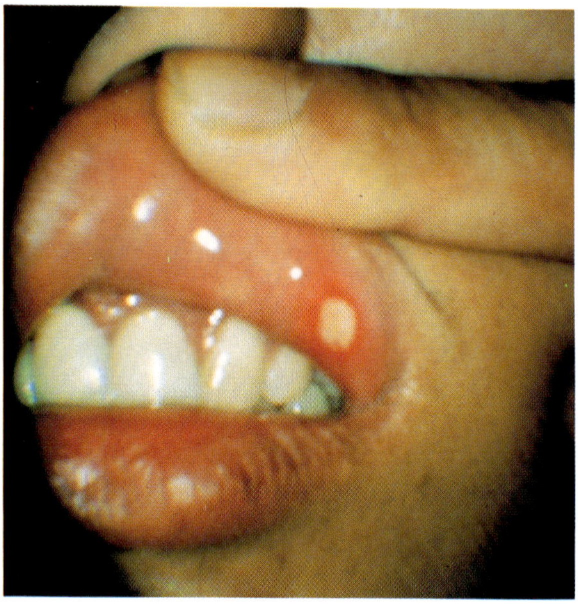

206 Aphthous ulceration on upper lip buccal mucosa.

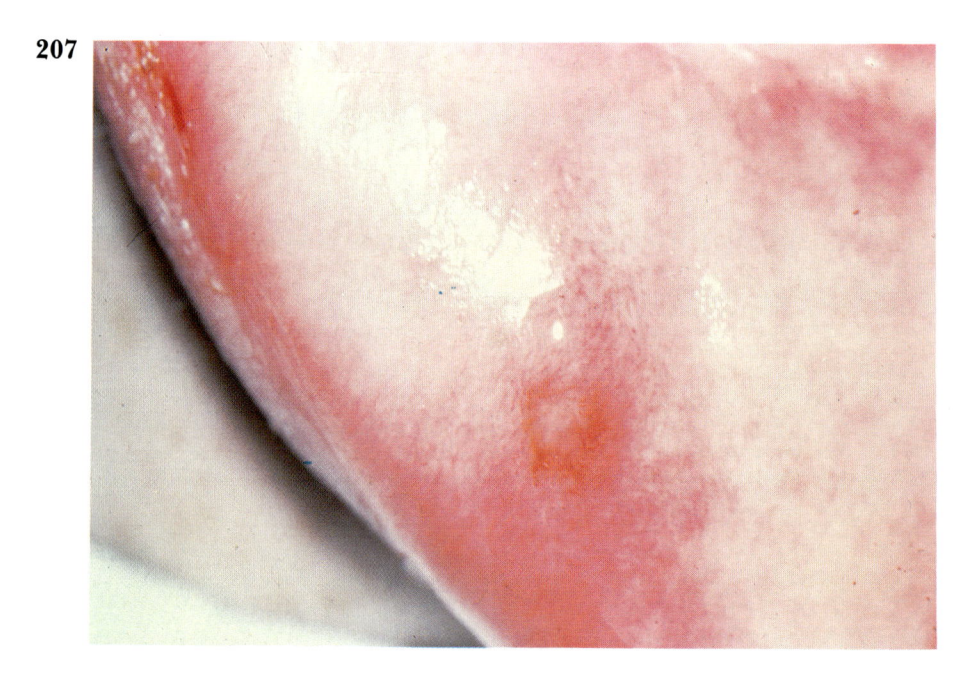

207 Healed aphthous ulcer on buccal mucosa of patient with Behçet's disease. Remaining scar is a valuable diagnostic sign in this patient with severe anterior uveitis and a history of mouth and vaginal sores.

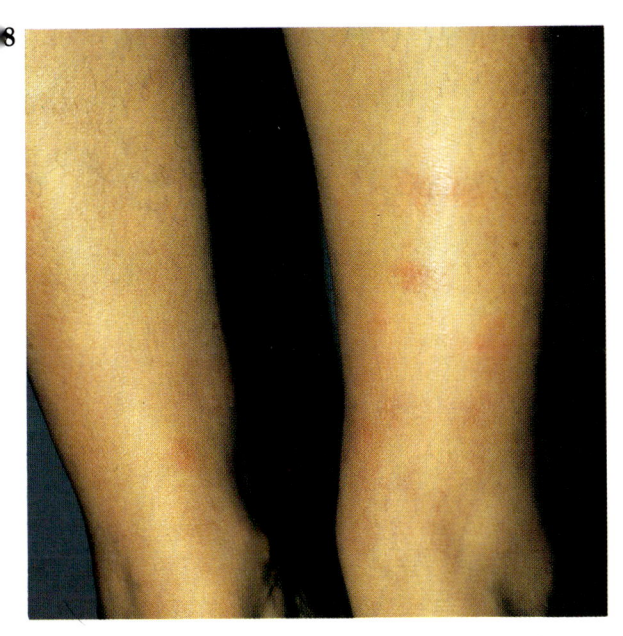

208 Classic tender maculopapular eruption of erythema nodosum.

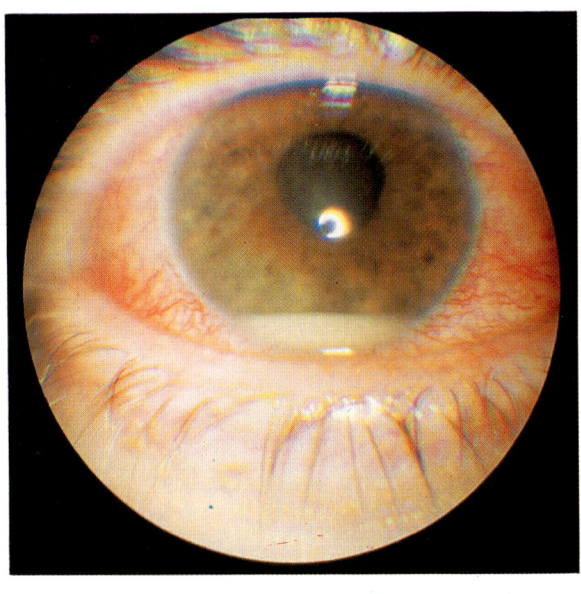

209 Classic anterior segment inflammation in a 27-year-old man with oral and genital ulceration who presents with hypopyon and intense iridocyclitis.

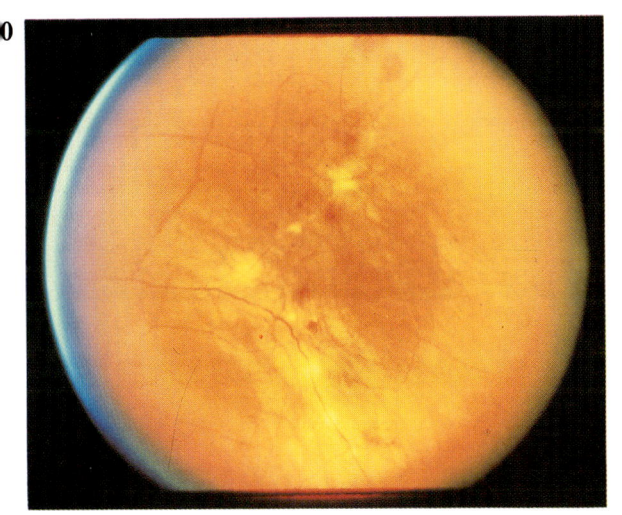

210 Areas of patchy retinal vasculitis and hemorrhage in a patient with Behçet's disease.

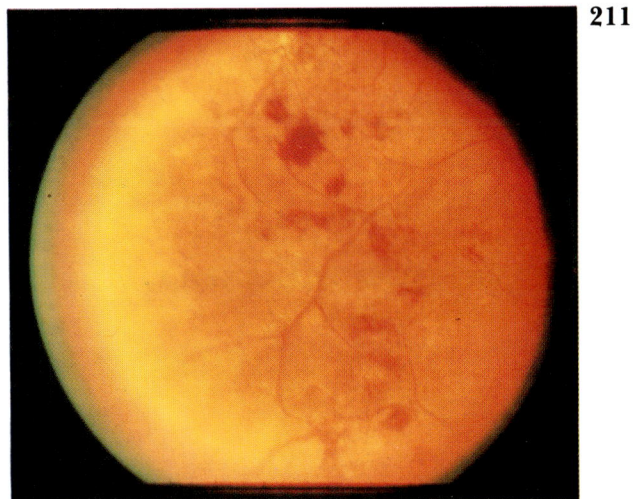

211 Focal retinal hemorrhages and vasculitis occurring concomitant with central nervous system vasculitis in patient with Behçet's disease.

99

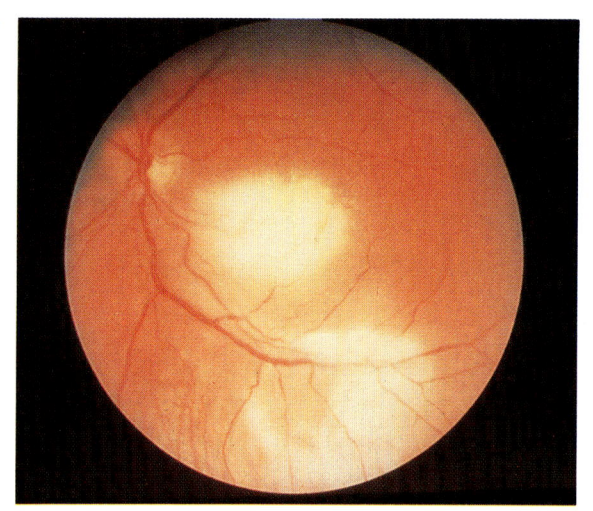

212 Necrotizing vasculitis in the retina with infarction of retina in patient with central nervous system Behçet's disease.

213 Infarction of posterior pole from necrotizing vasculitis in patient with Behçet's disease.

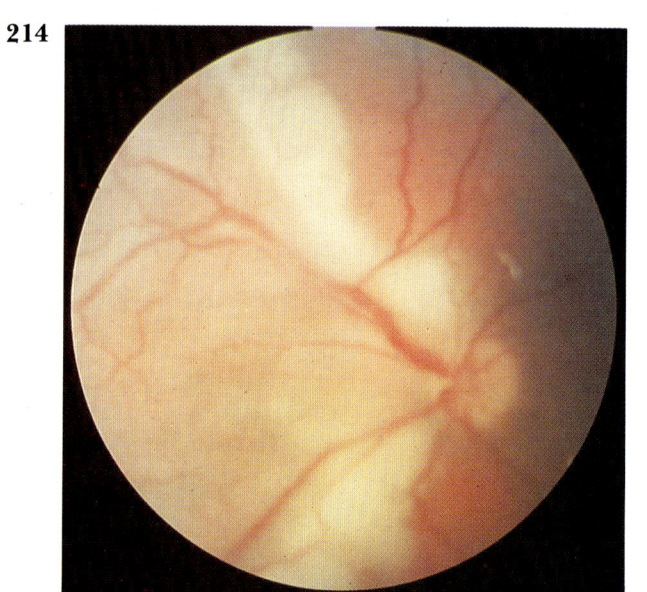

214 Retinal infarction of fellow eyeground of patient in Figure 212.

215 Actual encasement of vasculitis vessels with fibrous tissue in retina with retinal pigment epithelial changes, optic pallor and other evidence of profound episodes of retinal inflammation and vasculitis.

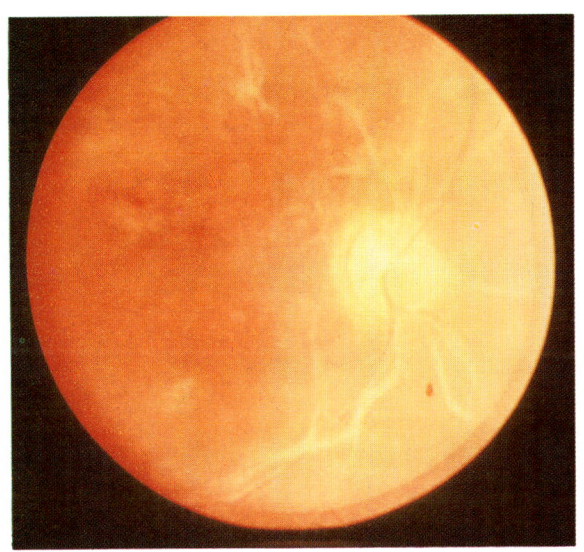

216 Almost total infarction of retina in a patient with central nervous system Behçet's disease. The patient died of vasculitic encephalitis.

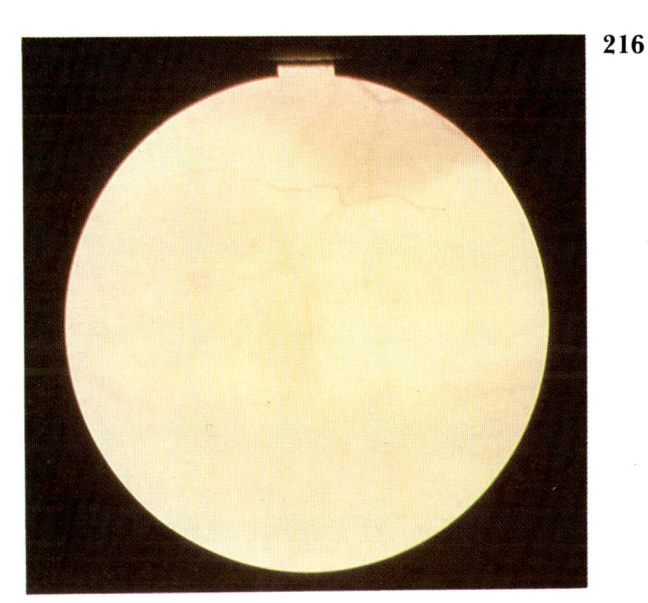

Reticulum Cell Sarcoma

Reticulum cell sarcoma is a large cell type, lymphocytic lymphoma that may occur either as a central nervous system primary malignant lymphoma (microglioma) or as an extraneural primary malignant lymphoma with accompanying infiltration in the eye. It should be classified as a large cell, non-Hodgkins', histiocytic lymphoma. The ocular form of the disease usually presents as a chronic uveitis with a vitreous cell infiltrate (**217**) accompanied by subretinal and choroidal infiltrates, with or without papillary hyperemia. Reticulum cell sarcoma is an important vitritis in the 40–65 years and over age group. It may masquerade as chronic uveitis and frequently lacks systemic involvement (less than 25% of patients), as it is confined to the central nervous system and the eye.

Unlike its uveitis counterparts, reticulum cell sarcoma responds poorly to therapy with steroids or immunosuppressant drugs. Radiation therapy is the treatment of choice. However, its possible derivation from B-lymphocytes would theoretically suggest a susceptibility to chemotherapy to supplement irradiation if necessary. Therefore, it is essential to identify this disorder properly. A vitreous biopsy is suggested for older patients, in whom a comprehensive uveitis evaluation is otherwise negative, in order to rule out this perplexing and potentially fatal entity. It usually presents as an externally white, seemingly quiet eye, until slit-lamp examination and ophthalmoscopy reveal apparent intraocular inflammation.

RETICULUM CELL SARCOMA
(Large Cell Lymphoma, B-Cell Lymphoma)

Definition:
- Masquerade inflammation; malignant infiltration of B-cell histiocyte

Presentation:
- Vitreous cells
- Subretinal infiltrate
- Iridocyclitis
- Nongranulomatous

Investigation:
- Vitreous biopsy
- Morphology of cells
- Stains of light chains on vitreous cells for monoclonal derivation
- Systemic evaluation for lymphoma
- Lumbar puncture for cells
- CT scan, MRI of brain for microgliomatosis

Therapy:
- Radiation therapy to orbit and CNS
- Adjunctive chemotherapy

Complications:
- Central nervous system disease
- Panophthalmitis complications
- Cataracts
- Glaucoma
- Retinal detachment

Prognosis:
- Poor (90% of patients die within 1 year of CNS disease if untreated)

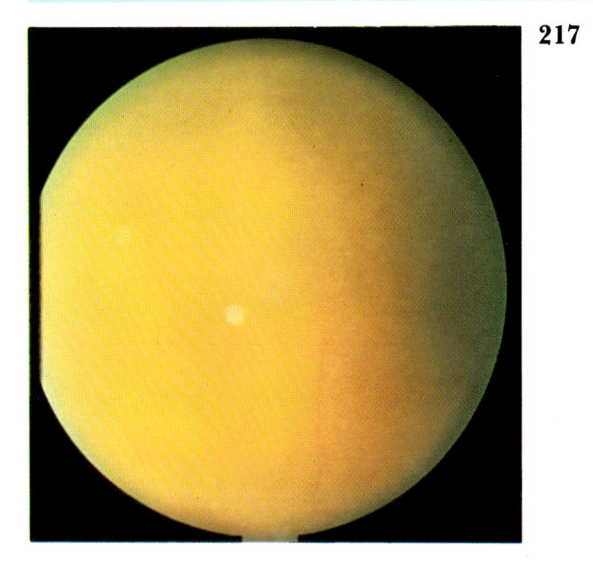

217 Dense vitritis overlying areas of white subretinal infiltration in patient with large cell malignant lymphoma (reticulum cell sarcoma).

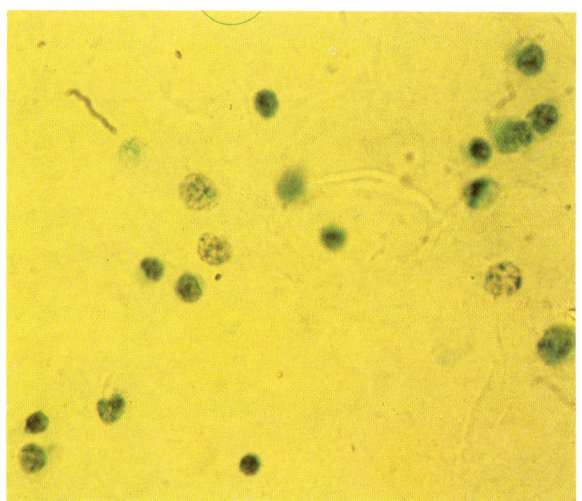

218 Vitreous specimen from patient demonstrating infiltration with large cell malignant lymphoma (lymphocytic lymphoma, reticulum cell sarcoma).

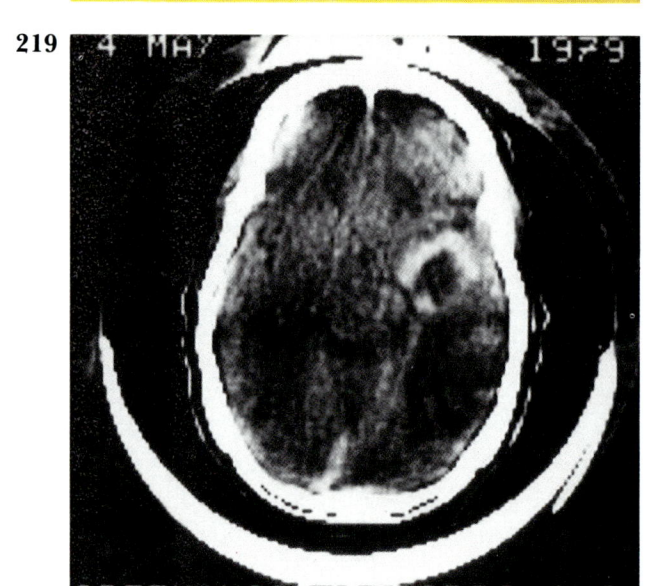

219 Computerized axial tomogram of brain with contrast to demonstrate a large temporal lobe infiltrate of large cell malignant lymphoma (reticulum cell sarcoma).

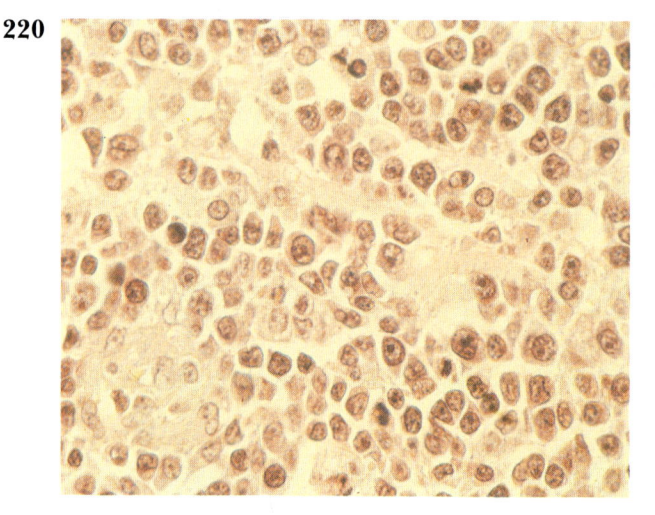

220 Brain biopsy specimen of large cell malignant lymphoma in temporal lobe with characteristic large, noncleaved nuclei with multiple large nucleoli, chromatin clumping, and thickened nuclear membrane. An occasional plasma cell and malignant small lymphocyte are present. (Original magnification times 400.)

221 Vitritis and subretinal infiltration. Another patient with dense vitritis, demonstrating multiple large areas of subretinal infiltration in the posterior pole.

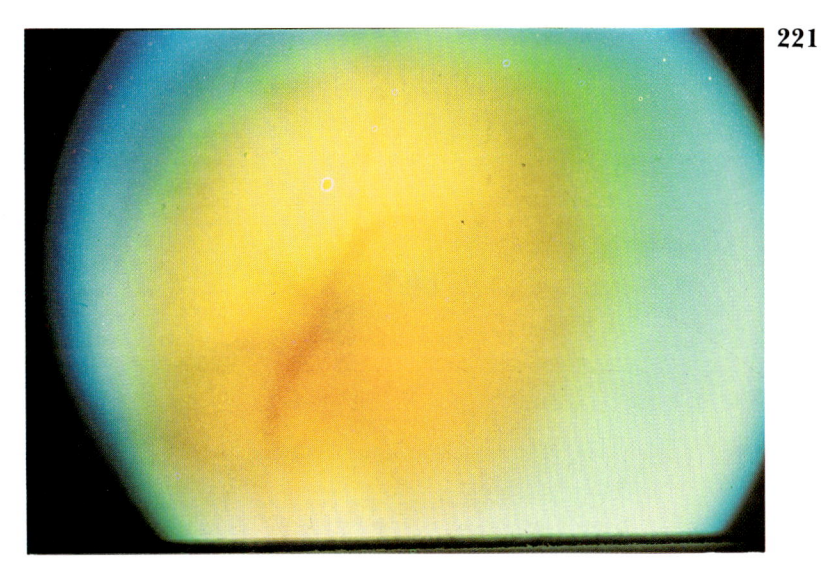

222 Immunoglobulin molecule. Schematic diagram of antibody demonstrating its central paired heavy chains and the outer light chains.

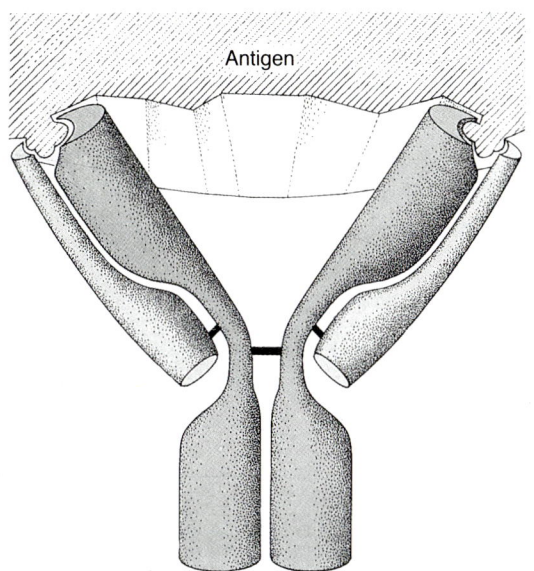

223 Particulate intracytoplasmic deposits of only lambda light chains stained for immunofluorescence on vitreous cells from a biopsy specimen to demonstrate the monoclonal basis of the B-cell infiltrate in the vitreous gel. (Original magnification times 400.)

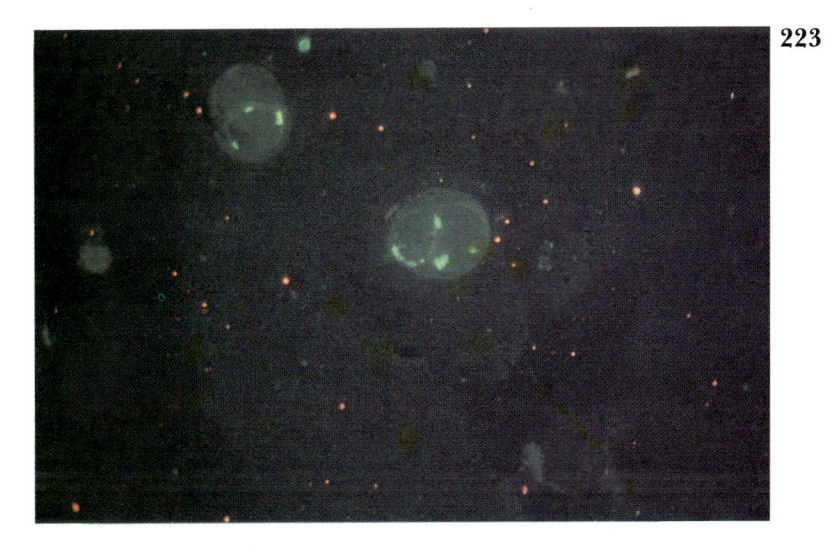

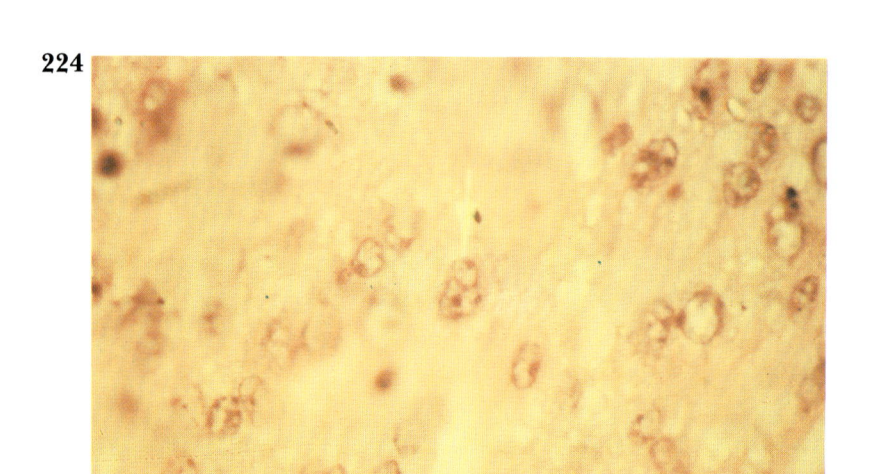

224 Brain biopsy of patient with parietal lobe large cell malignant lymphoma in whom vitreous cell infiltrate was presenting sign. The patient later developed this brain tumor after an unrevealing initial central nervous system evaluation.

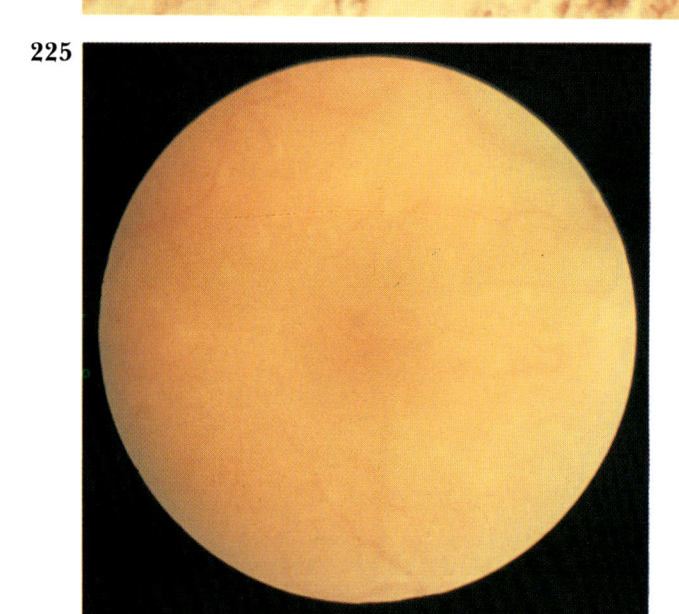

225 Dense vitritis in an 80-year-old man in whom an extraneural large cell malignant lymphoma was present. Vitreous biopsy disclosed infiltrate of malignant lymphocytes, and diagnostic vitrectomy restored vision in this eye from 20/200 to 20/30 for the remaining 19 months of this patient's life. His other eye had a macular hole with vision of 20/400 and no evidence of malignant infiltration.

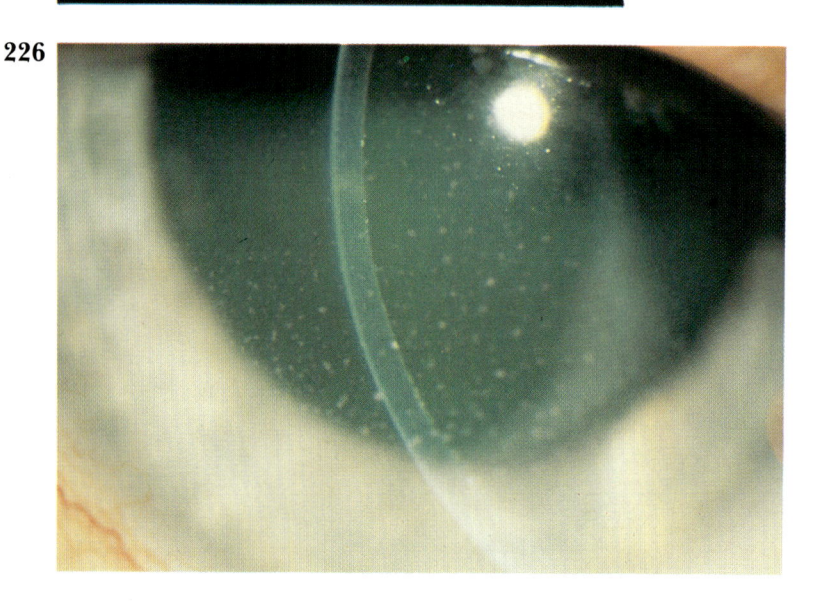

226 'Masquerade' mutton-fat KP. Dramatic array of large, greasy, white KP on endothelium of cornea in patient who died from large cell malignant lymphoma (reticulum cell sarcoma). These precipitates are usually seen in the inflammations associated with histologically granulomatous processes, but in this patient underscore the 'masquerade' nature of this disease, which portrays all of the clinical stigmata of an intraocular inflammation or infection.

227 Richter syndrome. A 60-year-old man presents with such dense vitritis, his slit-lamp appearance simulates a cataract. His eye is white, quiet, with a clear lens; this presentation suggests a large cell lymphoma (reticulum cell sarcoma).

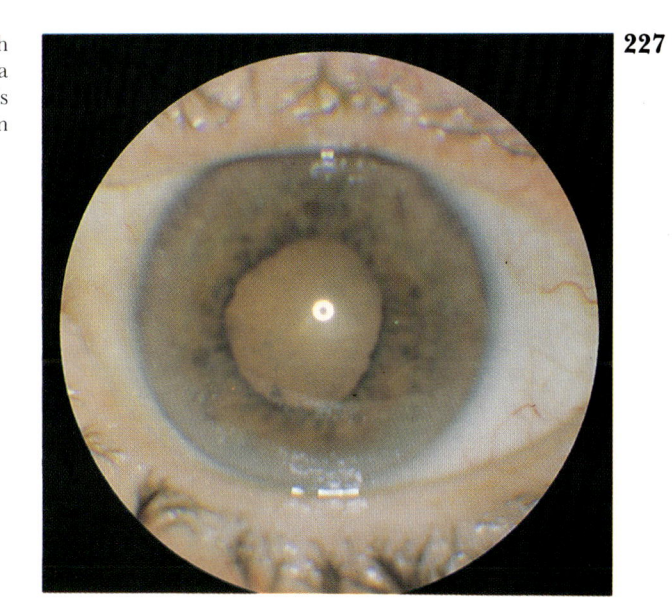

228 Large pigmented mutton-fat KP are seen in inferior cornea of same patient.

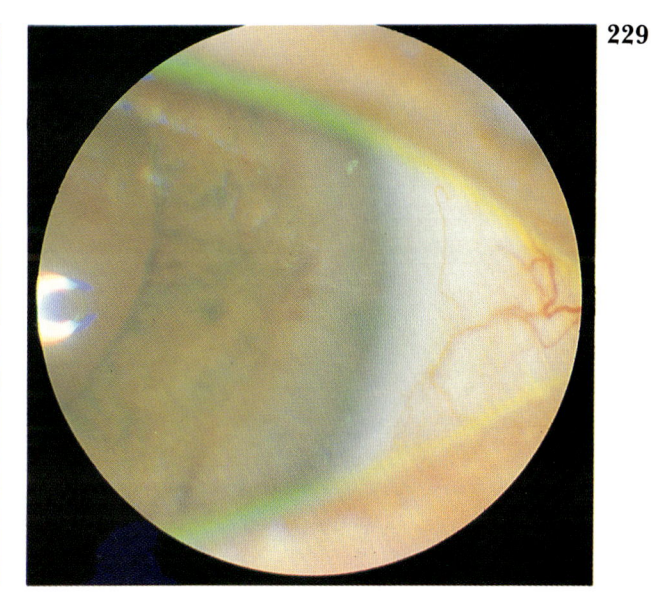

229 Peripheral iris of a patient demonstrates grayish white infiltrate uncommon for reticulum cell sarcoma.

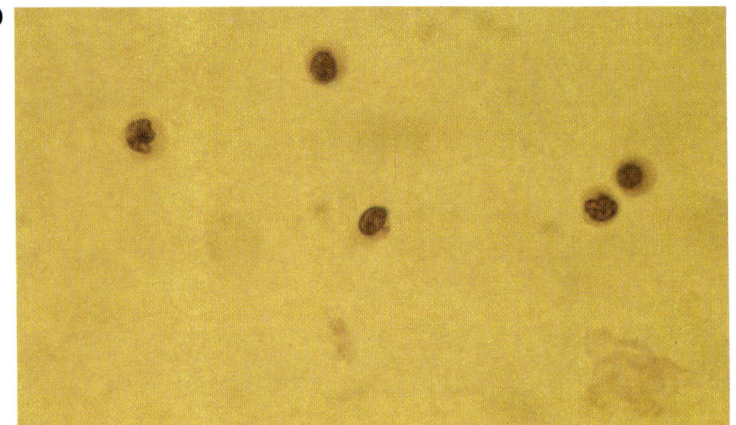

230 Vitreous biopsy reveals cells with irregular hyperchromatic nuclei and nucleoli suggestive of chronic lymphocytic leukemia infiltration of vitreous, not reticulum cell sarcoma (Fundus exam is normal).

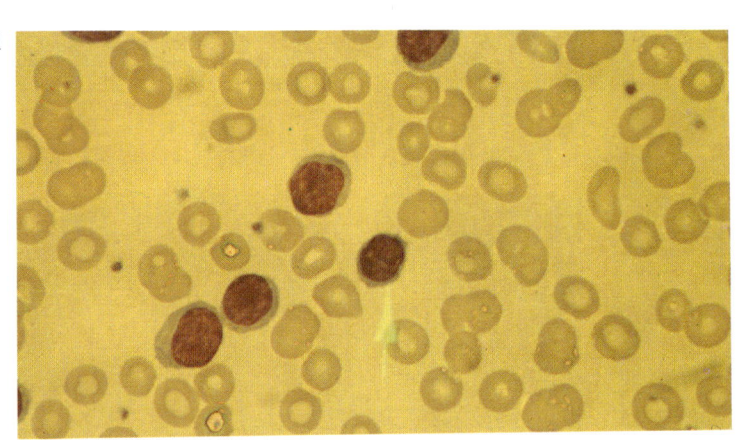

231 Peripheral smear demonstrates chronic lymphocytic leukemia which is responsible for this 'pseudo-reticulum cell sarcoma' picture in the eye. (Richter syndrome.)

Mycobacteria

Mycobacterium leprae, an unusual and exotic infection in the USA, should nevertheless be considered a cause of uveitis for patients in America. Native populations from China, Samoa, Hawaii, the Philippines, and the Sonoran province of Mexico may bring endemic leprosy with them. A prolonged period of contact is necessary in order to acquire the infection. The clinical manifestations of lepromatous uveitis differ considerably from the other mycobacteria, tuberculosis, in that *M. leprae* exclusively affects the anterior segment of the eye, preferring the cooler temperatures for its survival and multiplication.

Leprosy occurs in two distinct forms, lepromatous and tuberculoid, with intermediate varieties between them. The basic difference between these two forms depends upon the patient's intact or absent cell-mediated immunity. In the lepromatous form of the disease, which is diffuse and can involve many organs, profuse numbers of organisms are seen, due to the lack of the patient's cell-mediated immunity. When this immunity is intact in the tuberculoid form, there is a localized form of the disease affecting one organ or one organ system only. Its predilection is for neural tissue, and only isolated organisms can be identified in histologic specimens. Patients who have leprosy may no longer feel the need to confine themselves to leprasaria and may be found in the general population. A high index of suspicion for this type of infection must now be engendered in physicians in the USA, because of the recent influx of Indochinese who were susceptible to leprosy and tuberculosis.

MYCOBACTERIA

1. Tuberculosis

Definition:
- Iridocyclitis, choroiditis, retinitis with vitreous

Presentation:
- Usually choroiditis first
- Granulomatous

Investigation:
- Sputum/bronchial lavage culture
- Tuberculin skin test
- Chest Xray
- ESR
- Medical consultation
- Serum lysozyme
- HIV test

Therapy:
- Treat acute recurrent iridocyclitis with steroids
- Treat chronic iridocyclitis and choroiditis lesions with systemic steroids covered by antituberculous therapy (INH and Rifampin)

Complications:
- Variable

Prognosis:
- Variable

2. Leprosy (Hansen's Disease)

Definition:
- Anatomic iridocyclitis only (predilection of organisms for cooler parts of the body)

Presentation:
- Acute or chronic iridocyclitis
- Granulomatous or nongranulomatous

Investigation:
- Anterior chamber tap (FITE stain or Ziehl-Neelsen stain)

Therapy:
- Dapsone
- Rifampicin
- Treat iridocyclitis with steroids after covering with antimicrobial

Complications:
- Secluded pupil
- Corneal decompensation
- Cataract

Prognosis:
- Variable

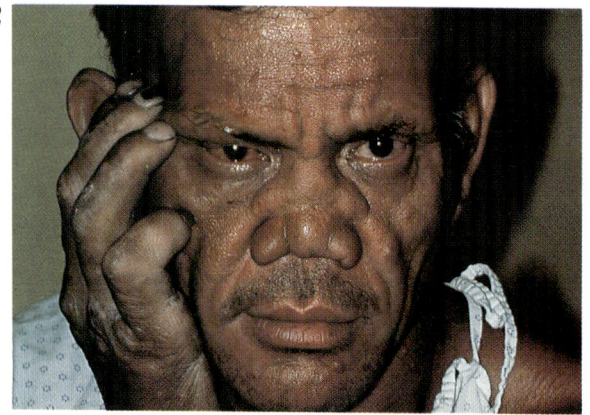

232 Typical leonine facies of lepromatous leprosy. Patient has resorbed nasal cartilage and multiple anesthetic skin lesions on the face.

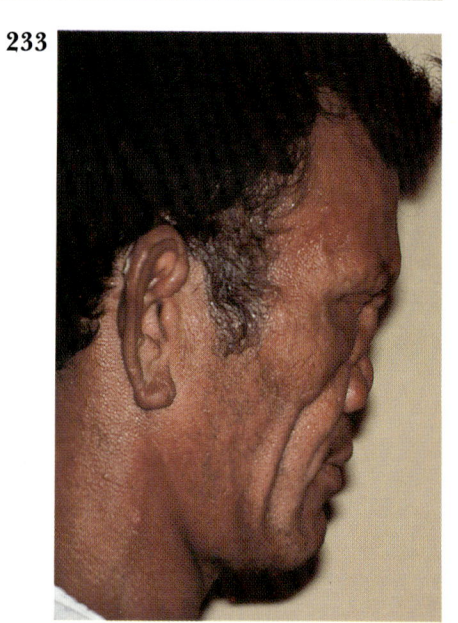

233 Profile of patient in Figure 232 showing the resorbed nasal cartilage and its striking effect on the profile.

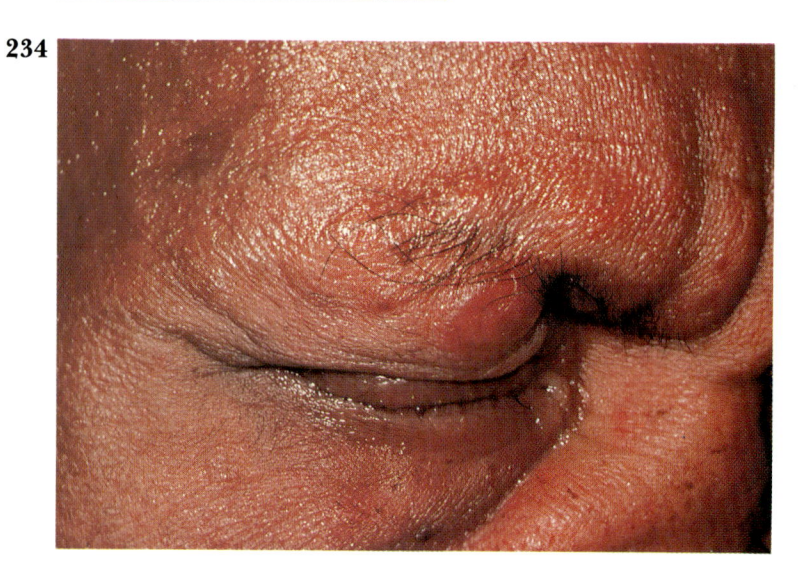

234 Anesthetic nodular lepromata on the skin of upper lid.

235 Scleral inflammation over an anesthetic nodule in patient with lepromatous leprosy.

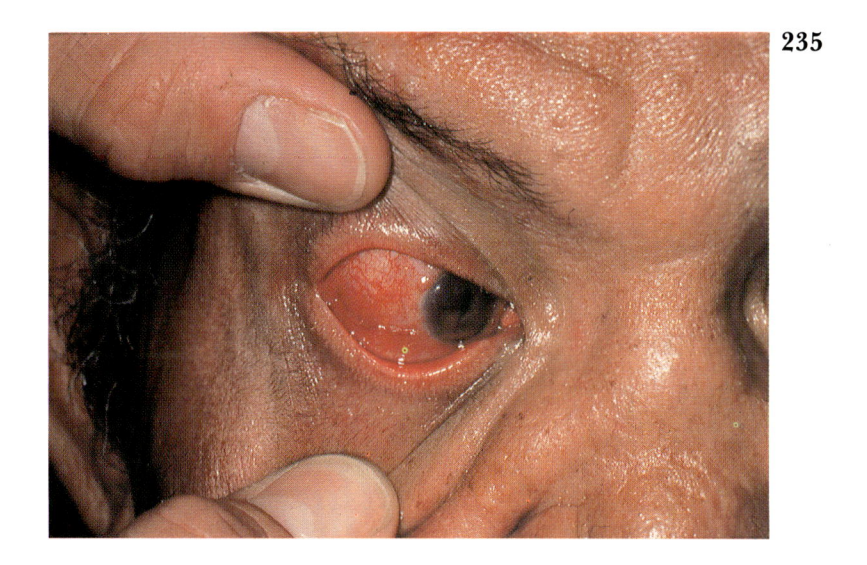

236 Scleral nodule. Higher power of inflamed scleral nodule.

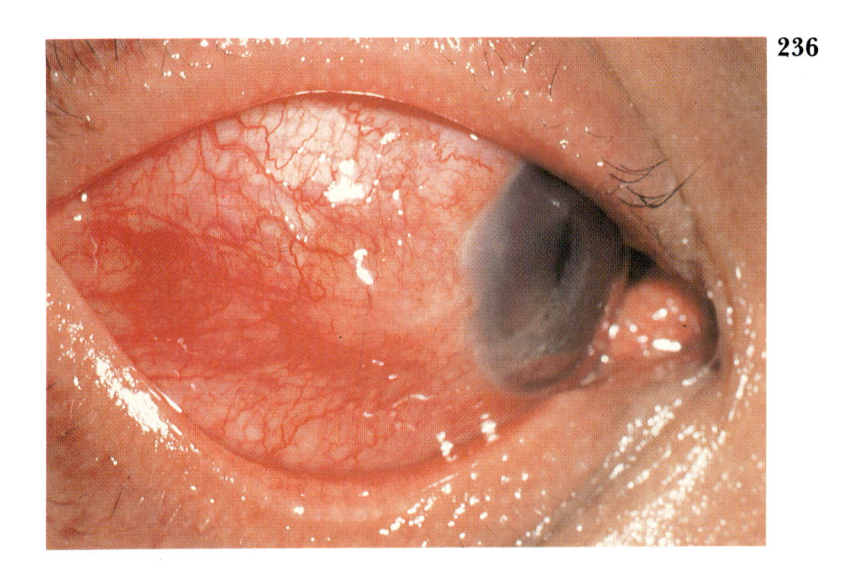

237 Profound anterior segment inflammation in patient with acute plastic iridocyclitis.

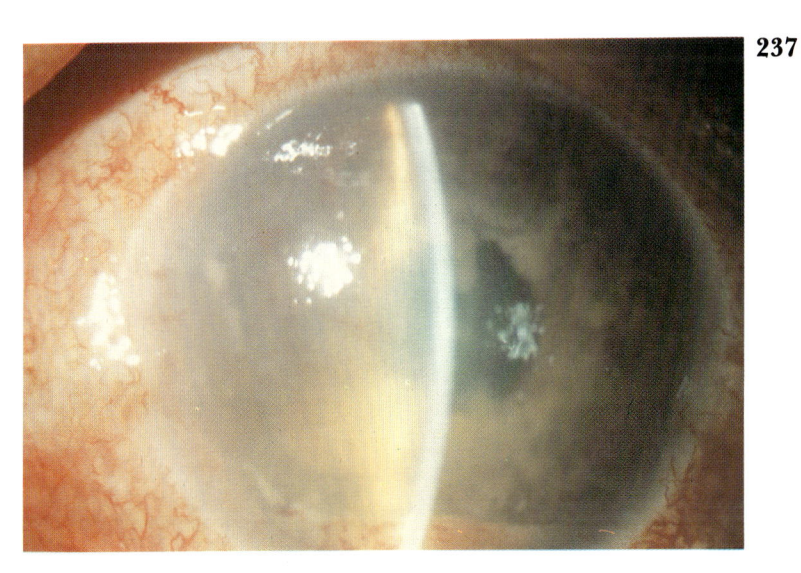

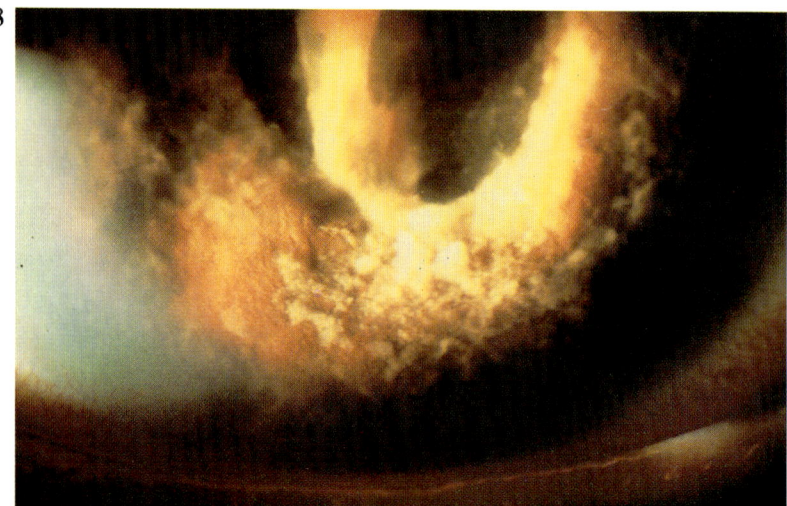

238 Nodular lepromata noted as cheesy, white superficial exudative accumulations of inflammatory material on the surface of the iris.

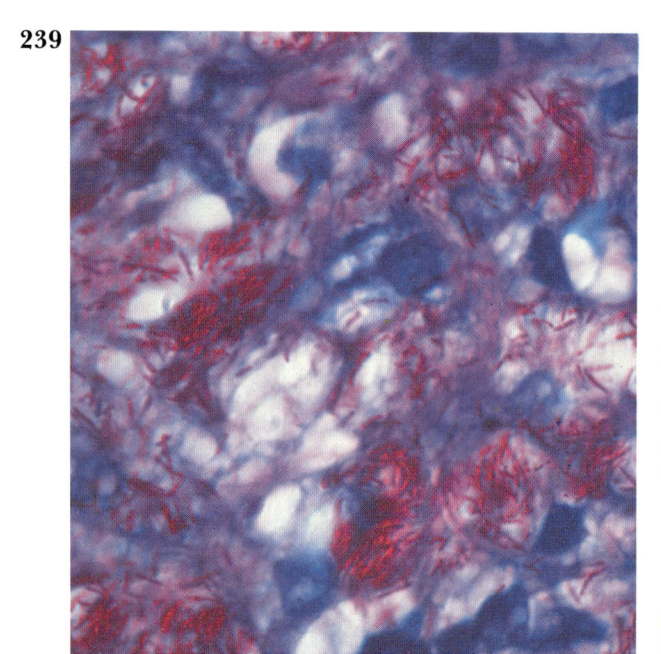

239 Clumps of acid-fast bacilli demonstrated in the scleral nodule patient with acute plastic iridocyclitis noted in Figure 237.

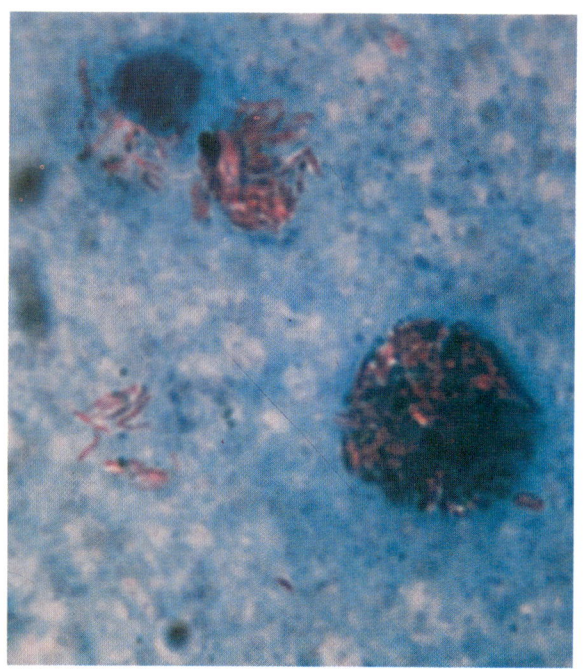

240 Clumps of acid-fast bacilli are isolated from the aqueous of the patient.

Mycobacterium tuberculosis can manifest itself in many types of ocular inflammations. Tuberculous conjunctival granulomas are a cause of Parinaud's ocular glandular syndrome, phlyctenular keratitis and conjunctivitis are supposed hypersensitivity reactions to tubercular proteins, and tuberculous iridocyclitis occurs with and without associated corneal lesions. Panuveitis may be the most profound manifestation of the ocular-acquired form of the disease. Vasculitis may occur in the retina along with choroiditis either as focal choroidal tubercles (**241**) or more diffuse inflammatory material under the retina. Tuberculous nodules may range in size from ¼ to ½ in disc diameter, may have either distinct or indistinct borders, and in Caucasian patients may simulate a malignant melanoma of the choroid. Nodules, whether located in the conjunctiva, iris, choroid, retina or optic nerve head, consist of the characteristic caseating necrosis: tubercles surrounded by mononuclear infiltrate of cells. Inflammation may be diffuse and may affect all coats of the eye. In contradistinction to sarcoidosis, which is a noncaseating granuloma, tuberculosis usually occurs as the necrotizing variety. Historically, it may be identified with acid-fast stains such as Ziehl-Neelsen or Fite stain and found in lesions of the retina, choroid, ciliary body, iris, cornea, conjunctiva, and orbit.

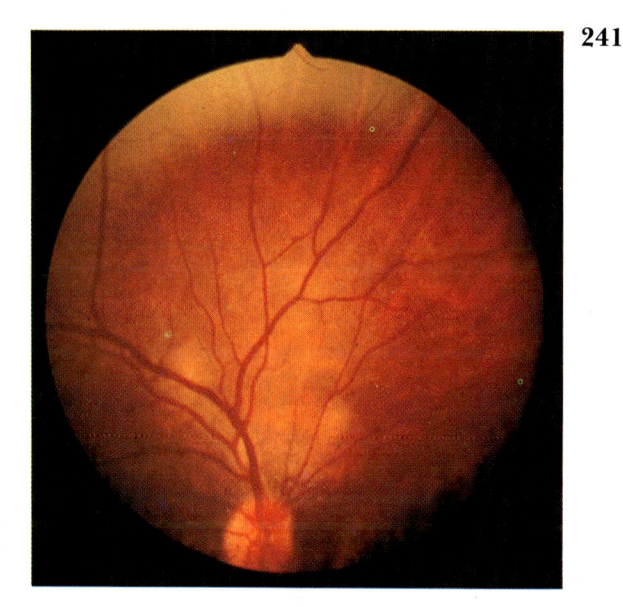

241 Focal choroidal infiltration. Note prominent discrete focal choroidal infiltration superior to the optic papilla in a 28-year-old female with choroidal tuberculosis.

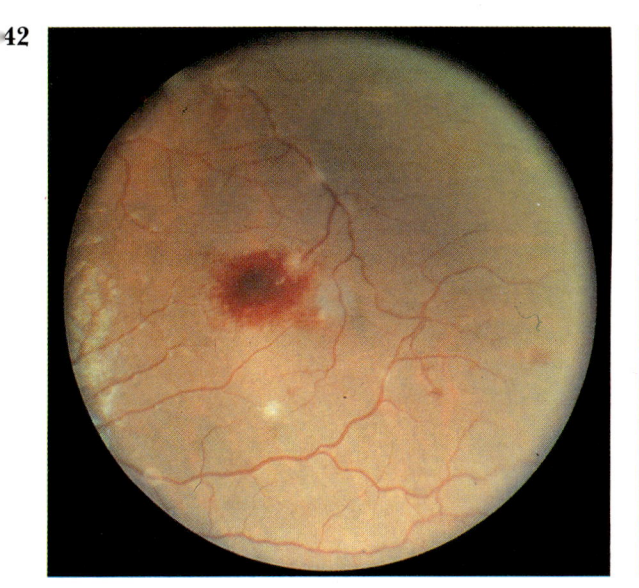

242 Patchy vasculitis and hemorrhage in an 11-year-old patient with acquired ocular tuberculosis.

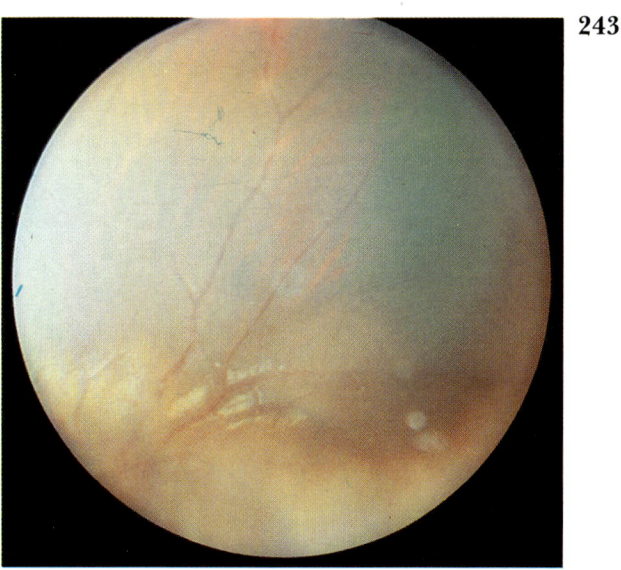

243 Diffuse vasculitis may be seen along each of the vessels encasing the vessel wall.

113

244 Red-free photograph to demonstrate fully both the hemorrhagic and exudative vasculitis as seen in this patient with acquired tuberculosis.

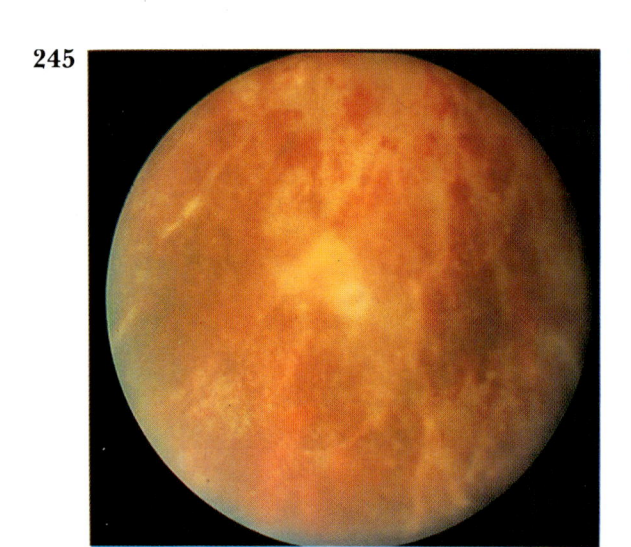

245 Extreme hemorrhagic vasculitis in macula of patient with acquired tuberculosis.

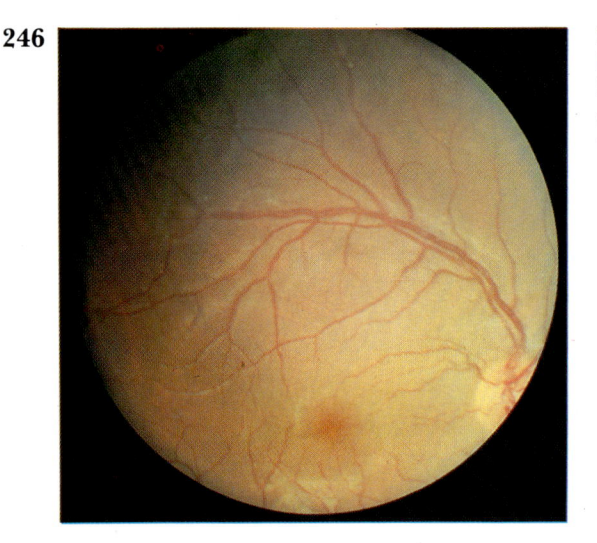

246 Resolved tuberculosis vasculitis. Patient noted in Figure 245 after successful treatment with INH, rifampicin, and prednisone. Note the absence of perivascular sheathing and perivascular exudate compared to the pretreatment photo.

Herpes Virus

The herpes virus family consists of DNA viruses which are attracting increasing attention from clinicians and researchers because of their prevalence in the population both as a venereal infection and otherwise. The herpes family includes herpes simplex virus (HSV) sometimes referred to as herpes hominis, herpes zoster virus, cytomegalovirus and Epstein-Barr virus. All cause ocular inflammation but have varying manifestations of disease. Herpes simplex most commonly causes keratitis both with stromal and disciform lesions (**252, 254**) that may have an accompanying anterior segment inflammation with chronic precipitates. This may sometimes initiate a recurring iridocyclitis that may occur in the absence of active keratitis. Acute or chronic glaucoma may complicate the iridocyclitis. Herpes simplex virus has been isolated from the aqueous humor and has been noted by electron microscopy to be present in the iris and stroma. Antibody titers to the herpes viruses are usually of little diagnostic significance because of the ubiquitous nature of the virus. Routine studies done both in infants and adults show that there is over 90% positivity in patients who have no known herpes infection. Herpes simplex may rarely cause a retinal inflammation in the newborn or in immunodepressed patients who are debilitated.

Herpes zoster ophthalmicus may often be accompanied by iridocyclitis and vitritis. There may be hyphema, hypopyon, and vitreous involvement in very severe cases; optic nerve infection may also occur. The iridocyclitis may be profound (**249, 253, 254**), but the virus has only rarely been recovered from the aqueous in patients with this infection. Often patients with diabetes or lymphoma are more prone to this infection (**258, 259**), but a person need not be immunocompromised to acquire it. Zoster virus has a predilection for neural tissue and may cause an intense perineuritis and perivasculitis in and around the optic nerve head.

HERPES VIRUS

1. Cytomegalic Inclusion Disease

Definition:
- Retinitis

Presentation:
- Acute
- Granulomatous

Investigation:
- Laboratory workup
- Viral studies of urine, serum and titers
- Pediatric consultation
- Complement-fixing antibodies
- HIV test

Therapy:
- DHPG. Gancyclovir is a new effective, antiviral agent. Recurrences may occur after the drug is stopped or tapered
- Foscarnet. Recent collaborative study demonstrates efficiency to lengthen patient's life
- High doses of systemic steroids and immunosuppressants unless contraindicated

Complications:
- Usually the complication of AIDS
- Drug abuse, organ transplantation, exogenous or endogenous immunosuppression

Prognosis:
- Poor, especially in AIDS patients

2. Herpes 1 Simplex, Herpes 2 Genital, Zoster

Definition:
- Iritis
- Iridocyclitis
- Keratouveitis chronology, can be either acute or chronic
- Granulomatous

Investigation:
- Diagnosis based on previous history of herpetic corneal disease
- Test for corneal sensation
- Skin lesion in zoster or look for previous keratitis

Therapy:
- Topical antivirals
- Systemic acyclovir
- Topical steroids may be necessary with antiviral coverage
- Glaucoma therapy, if necessary

Complications:
- Glaucoma
- Cataract
- Corneal scarring and vascularization

Prognosis:
- Fair in absence of glaucoma or scarring
- Poor, if glaucoma or frequent recurrences and poor response to treatment
- These may be exquisitely sensitive to steroid treatment and, therefore, steroid reduction

3. Epstein-Barr Virus

Definition:
- Iritis
- Iridocyclitis
- Can be keratitis
- Can be choroiditis
- Acute and chronic

Presentation:
- Granulomatous

Investigation:
- Titers of anticapsidigms and early antigen demonstration

Therapy:
- Acyclovir, prednisolone, topical steroids and mydriatics

Complications:
- Synechiae
- Cataract
- Glaucoma
- Cystoid macular edema
- Possible subretinal neovascular membrane

Prognosis:
- Poor if posterior pole is involved

4. Acute Retinal Necrosis

Definition:
- Retinitis
- Vitreoretinitis

Presentation:
- Acute
- Granulomatous/NA

Investigation:
- Herpes simplex, herpes zoster titers (serum/vitreous)
- Corneal/retinal biopsy (demonstrated virus)

Therapy:
- Systemic acyclovir
- ?Intravitreal acyclovir
- Photocoagulation posterior to area of necrosis if visibility allows (to prevent RD from necrotic, thin retina)
- Retinoscopy with broad posterior sclerobuckle if RD develops, or if photocoagulation deemed necessary

Complications:
- Retinal detachment occurs in >75% of patients
- Optic atrophy
- Retinal pucker

Prognosis:
- Poor. (See pages 131–132)

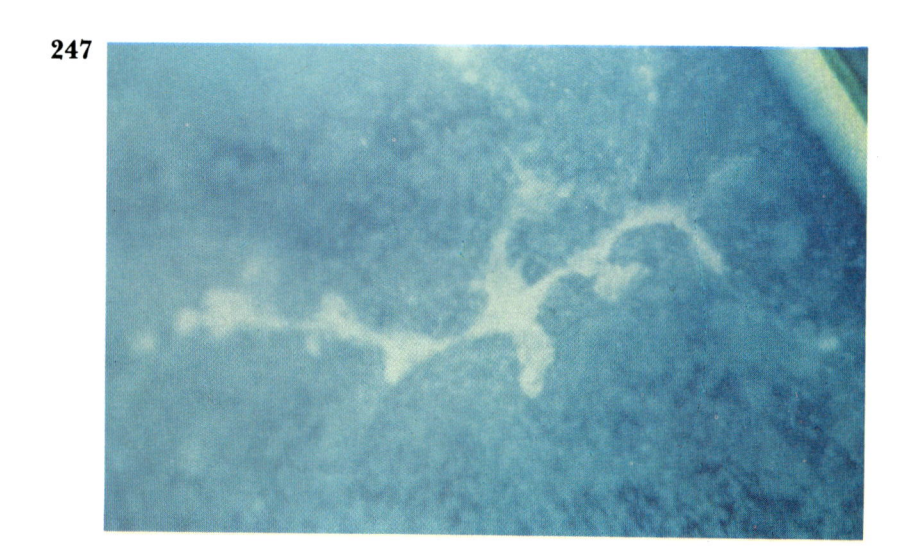

247 Herpes dendrite. Large fluorescein staining dendrite in patient with acute keratitis from herpes simplex hominis (HSH) disease.

248 Profound iris atrophy in a 30-year-old male with herpes zoster uveitis.

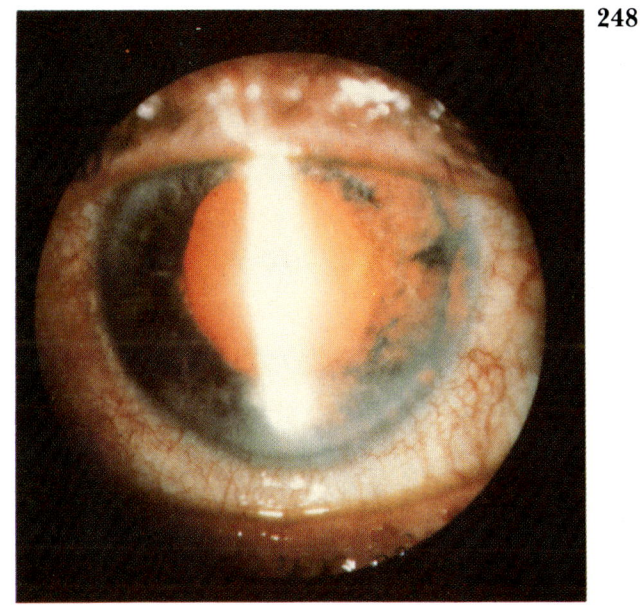

249 Large dendritic inflammation in patient covering almost entire cornea with an acute herpetic keratitis.

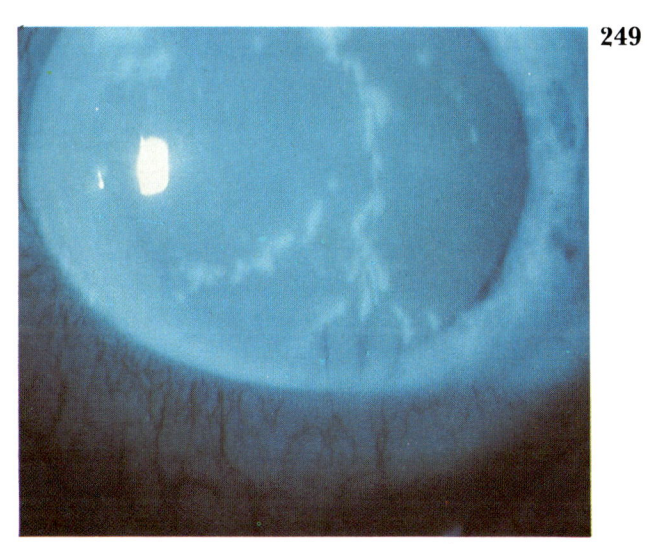

250 Stromal scar in disciform keratitis from herpes simplex disease.

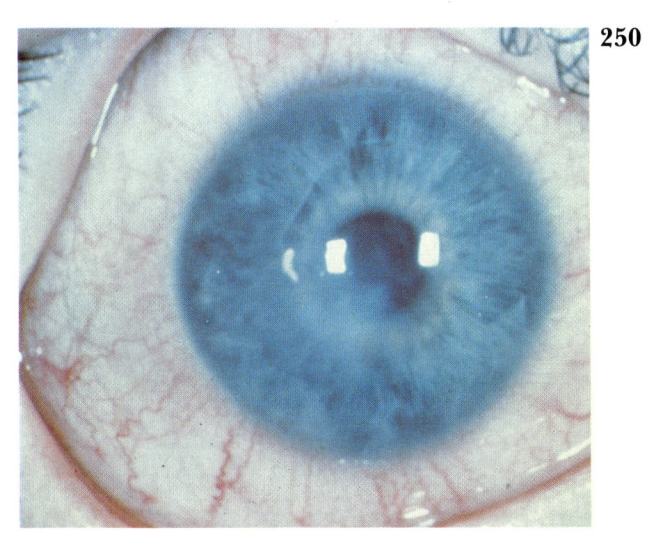

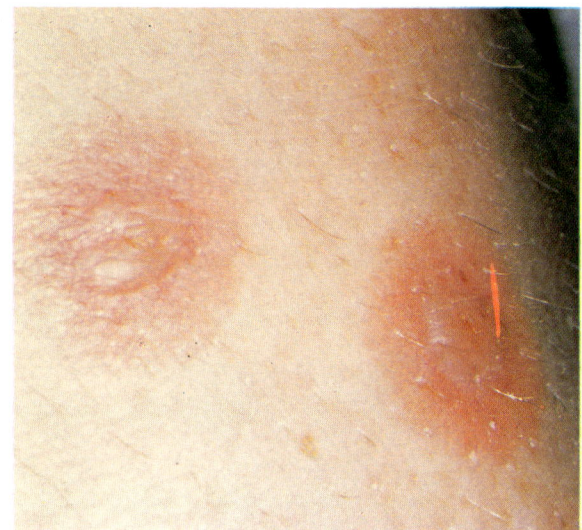

251 Dermal vesicles from acute herpetic skin infection which has spread to eye in patient with herpes simplex disease.

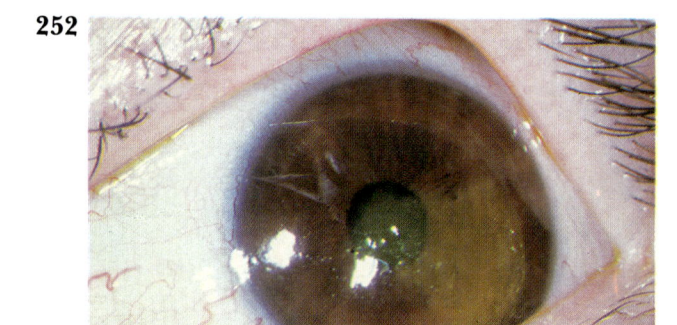

252 Fluorescein staining geographic ulcer in a patient with herpes simplex keratitis.

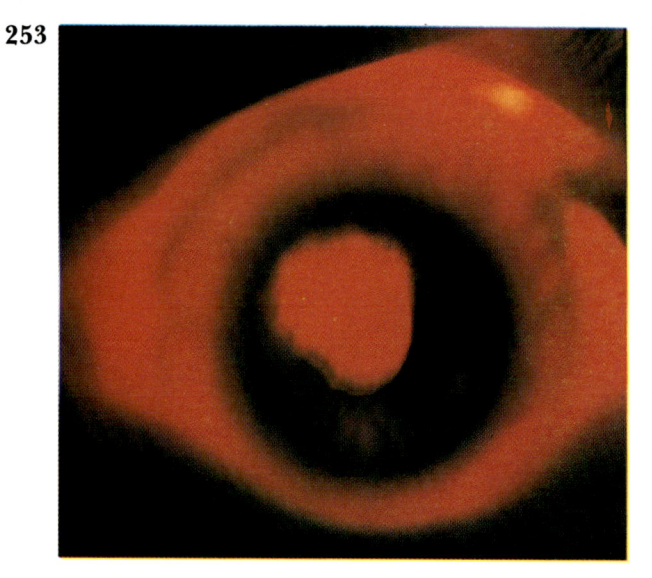

253 Transillumination of the globe to demonstrate resultant iris atrophy in a patient who has recovered from severe herpetic zoster ophthalmicus iridocyclitis.

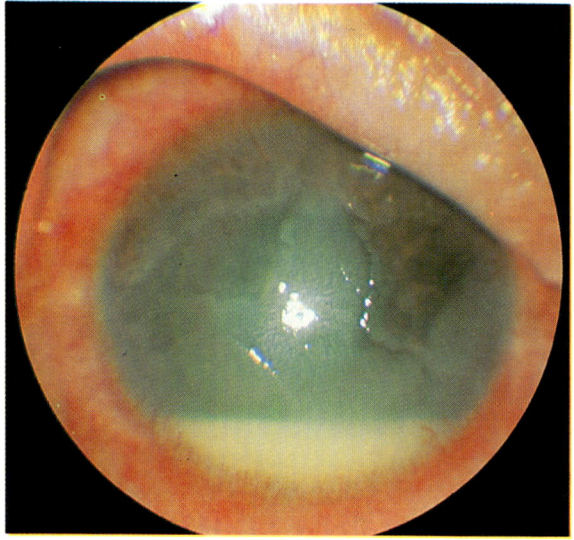

254 Hypopyon with profound anterior segment inflammation in a patient with recurrent herpes simplex geographic infection of cornea.

Cytomegalic Virus Inclusion Disease (CID)

Cytomegalovirus causes a distinctive retinitis in newborns, infants, and immunocompromised adults who are usually undergoing organ transplant surgery or cancer therapy, or suffer from AIDS. There is an exudative retinitis with occlusive necrotizing vasculitis and retinal hemorrhage which has been described as 'pizza pie' retinopathy (**130, 255, 256, 257**). Serological assessment has revealed that a high percentage of the normal population has been exposed to this virus. However, very rarely, some seemingly healthy patients may have the ARN or BARN syndrome as a consequence of CID in the retina.

This organism is an opportunist that causes significant ocular disease in infants and small children or in compromised adult hosts. The iridocyclitis that occurs is usually secondary to the necrotizing occlusive vasculitis seen in the retina. There is often a moderate number of cells in the vitreous and vitreous precipitates, which appear on the posterior vitreous face of the internal limiting membrane of the retina. Large areas of confluent retinal necrosis are caused by the neural cell-to-cell transmission of this virus. The retina may take on a gray-brown totally necrotic appearance. Vessels become sheathed with perivascular accumulations of monoclear inflammatory cell infiltrations. The typical clinical appearance of CID when manifested in an adult who has had either organ transplantation (kidney or heart) or is otherwise immunosuppressed (i.e., cancer chemotherapy) may be enough to substantiate a clinical diagnosis. The presentation is the most common infectious manifestation of ocular AIDS. The disease usually occurs bilaterally but can be more pronounced in one eye. CID increasingly has been found to be responsive to AZT, gancyclovir and foscarnet.

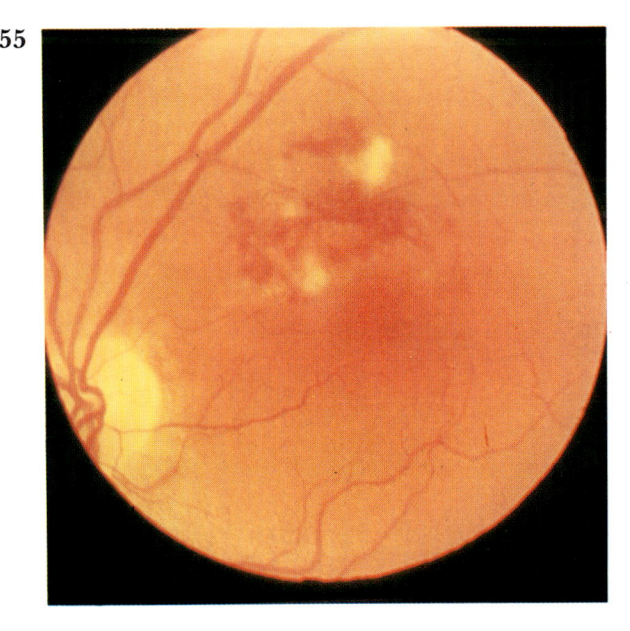

255 Cytomegalic retinitis. Fundus photograph of the typical 'pizza pie' picture of cytomegalic inclusion retinitis in a patient treated with prednisone and cytoxan as cancer chemotherapy for metastic breast disease.

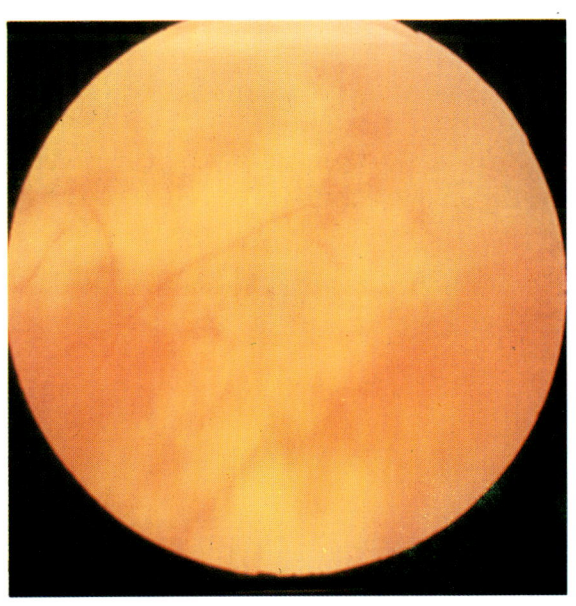

256 Peripheral retina showing accumulation of white exudate in a patient with cytomegalic inclusion retinitis secondary to immunosuppression from metastic breast cancer treatment.

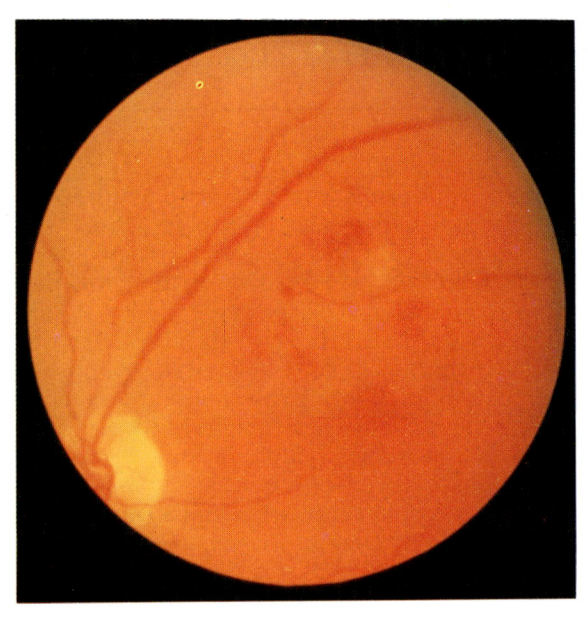

257 Fundus of same patient in Figure 255 showing improvement of inflammation and hemorrhage in macula after reduction of immunosuppression drugs.

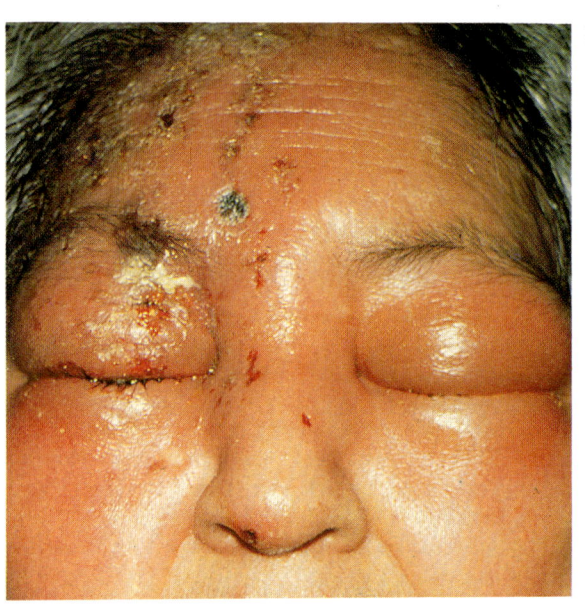

258 Facial nerve dermitome distribution of herpes zoster ophthalmicus in patient with lymphoma. (*Courtesy of James Gealy, M.D.*)

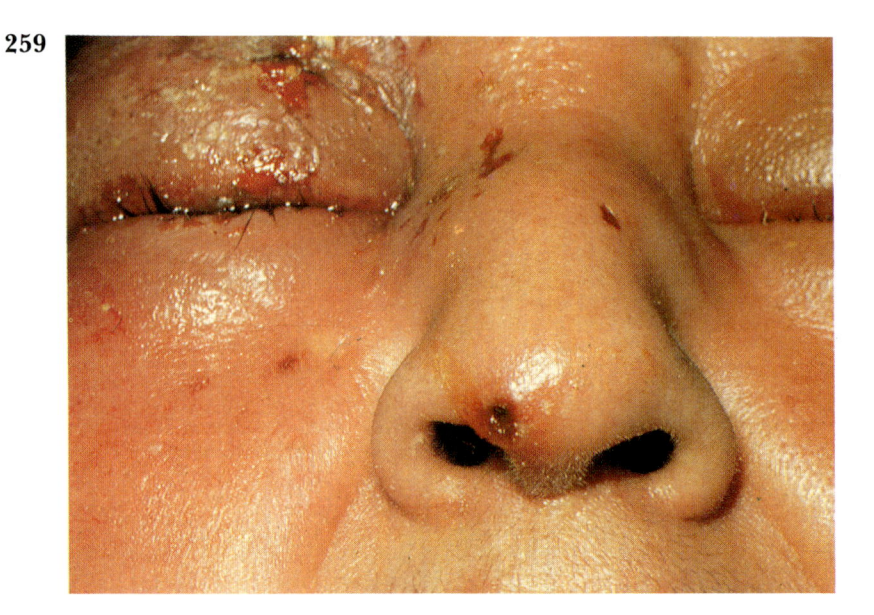

259 Zoster vesicle. Enlargement of Figure 258 showing distribution of herpes zoster ophthalmicus noting its course along the naso-lacrimal nerve, manifesting an acute herpetic vesicle on the tip of the nose. Such a location of a vesicle in a patient whose lids cannot be opened due to swelling almost certainly would indicate the cornea is involved in this infection. (*Courtesy of James Gealy, M.D.*)

Serpiginous Choroidopathy *(Geographic Choroiditis, Helicoid Choroiditis)*

This very rare intraocular inflammation is usually classified as one of the uveitides. It occurs in both eyes and usually begins in the fourth or fifth decades, although it may be seen in the thirties. Patchy inflammation begins concentrically around the nerve head (**265**), entails the retinal pigment epithelium, the choriocapillaris, and outer layers of the retina and spreads peripherally (**264**) from the papilla in all directions. It is called either serpiginous or geographic choroiditis because of this serpentine crawling of the inflammatory process with its profound retinal pigment epithelial affection. There is often evidence of retinal edema and inflammatory cells overlying the retina at the advancing edges of the lesion (**263, 264**) and there may be, on occasion, hemorrhage within or at the edge of the advancing inflammation. There may be areas that heal entirely, the only sequela being an alteration in the retinal pigment epithelium with scarring and windowed scarring or just window defects. In other areas the advancing margins of the inflammation are quite active, as noted with focal cellularity in the vitreous overlying it. There is often the rapid and abrupt diminution of vision with loss of acuity. However, occasionally some lesions may remain limited to the posterior segment but spread unevenly around the macula, leaving the macula spared. Nothing is known about the pathology or etiology of this syndrome and there are no laboratory tests for it. Corticosteroids have been tried therapeutically, but there is no evidence that they effectively suppress the inflammation, which may run a limited course over a period of several months to years in most patients. Because there is no proven treatment, it would seem reasonable that a trial of high dose systemic or periocular steroids is indicated in the acute phase of this disease when central acuity is threatened. Recently, a combination of cyclosporine, azathioprine (Imuran©) and prednisone has been suggested.

SERPIGINOUS CHOROIDOPATHY OR GEOGRAPHIC CHOROIDOPATHY (Also Helicoid Choroidopathy)

Definition:
- A choroiditis involving retinal pigment epithelium (iridocyclitis)

Presentation:
- Acute or chronic

Investigation:
- Fluorescein angiography

Therapy:
- None known
- Proposed combination chlorambucil, cyclosporine, prednisone

Complications:
- Macular scarring

Prognosis:
- Fair to poor (good if macula spared)

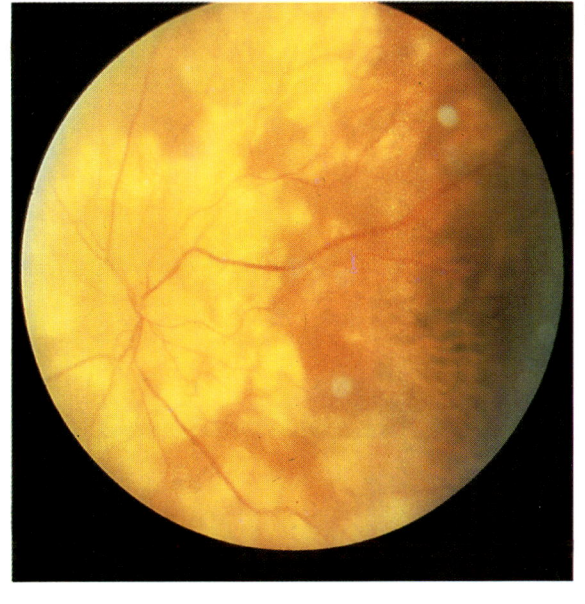

260 Geographic choroiditis. A 40-year-old man demonstrating a profound alteration of the retinal pigment epithelium. An advancing margin of inflammation radiates out from the optic papilla and extends over the entire posterior pole.

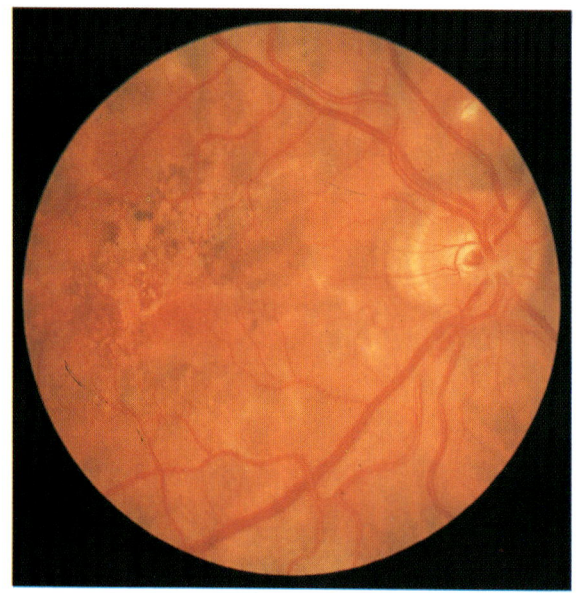

261 Macular scarring at the level of the retinal pigment epithelium from inactive inflammation of serpiginous choroiditis.

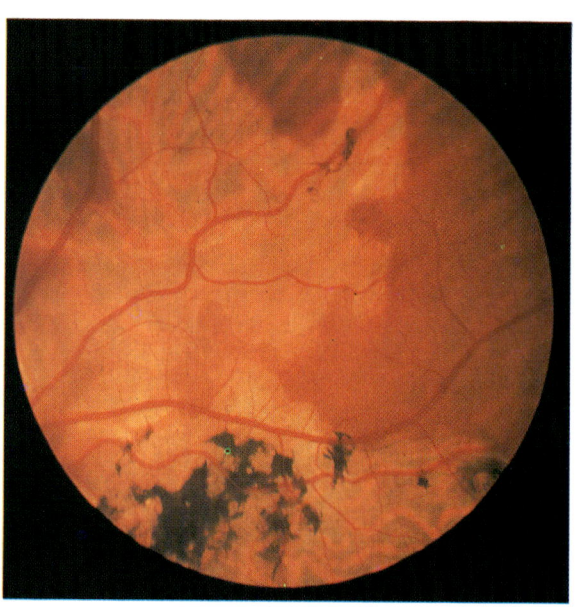

262 Serpiginous borders. Fellow eye of a patient showing inactive scarring superior to macula with its characteristic serpiginous border or edges.

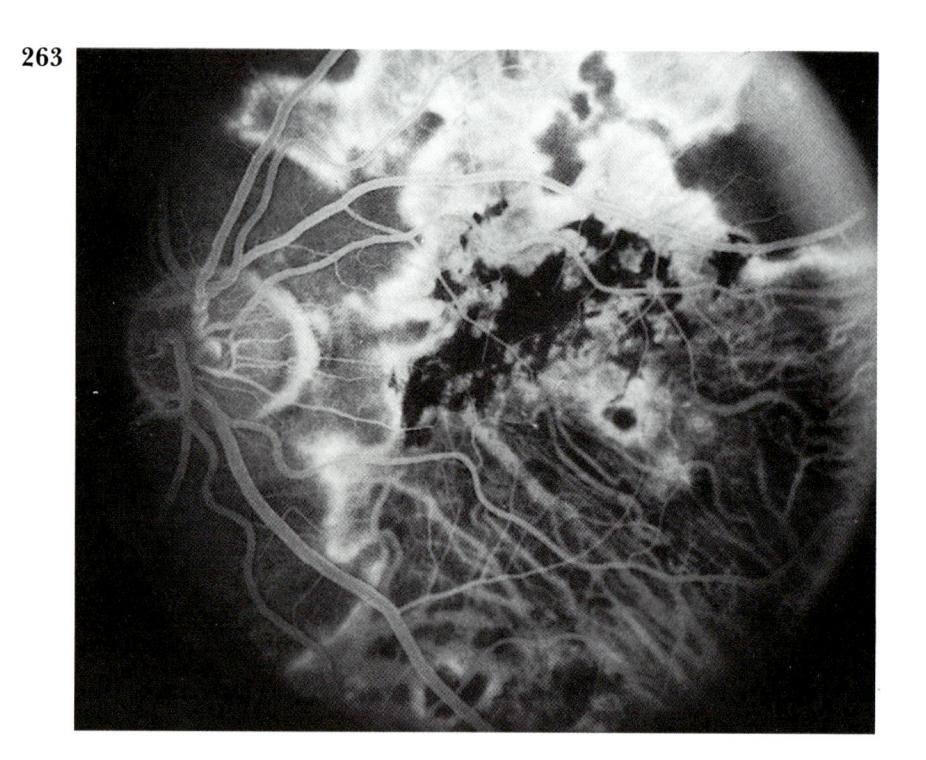

263 Fluorescein angiogram demonstrating profound alteration and focal areas with complete absence of retinal pigment epithelium.

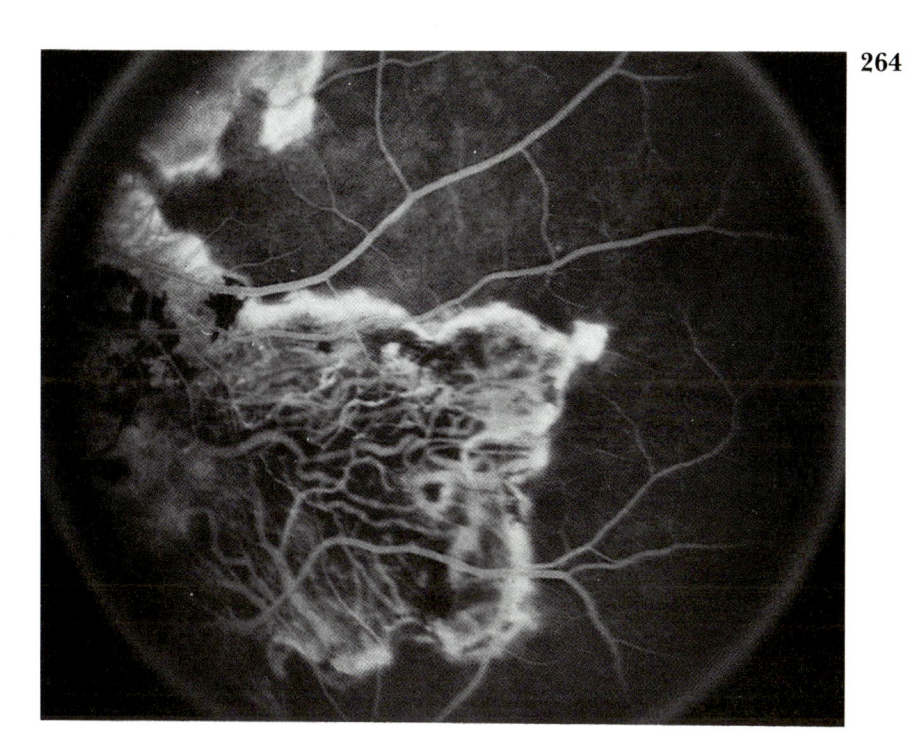

264 Fluorescein angiogram in late phase showing the active, advancing edge of this inflammation as a distinct border of persistent hyperfluorescence.

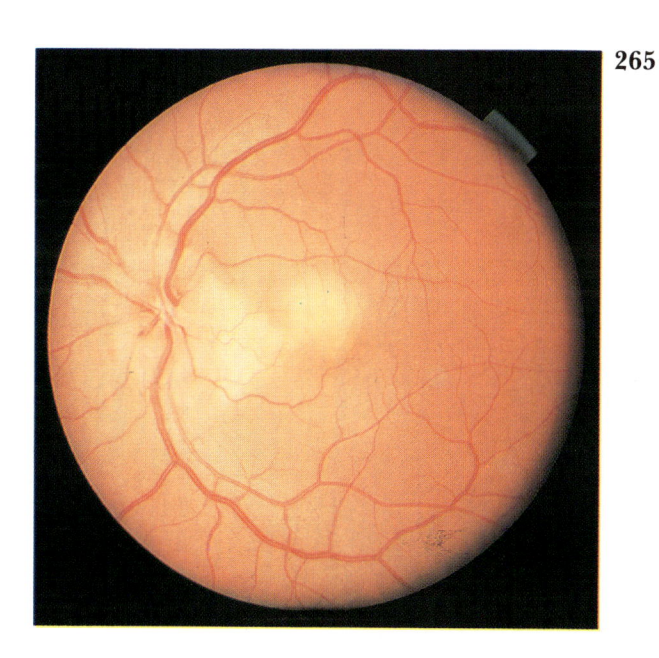

265 Very early involvement of peripapillary inflammation in the eye of a young patient with serpiginous choroiditis. (*Courtesy of Jonathan Belmont, M.D.*)

Subacute Sclerosing Panencephalitis (SSPE)

Inflammatory retinopathy occurs in association with SSPE, which may be due to a slow measles virus infection. Clinically, the disease occurs mainly in children and young adults, showing up months or years after apparent recovery from a rubeola infection. There may be concomitant neurologic signs noted, such as acute personality changes, lethargy, muscle weakness, and seizure activity. The disease is frequently fatal. The ocular changes seen in the fundus include a focal retinitis with edema, hemorrhages and folds in the retina in corresponding areas where acute retinal necrosis had occurred and left pigmented scars. Although the etiology of this disease is still questioned, laboratory evidence suggests that a slow measles virus infection may be the cause.

SUBACUTE SCLEROSING PANENCEPHALITIS

Definition:
- Acute retinitis

Presentation:
- Acute

Investigation:
- Antibodies to measles virus

Therapy:
- None

Complications:
- Severe central nervous system effects, death

Prognosis:
- Poor

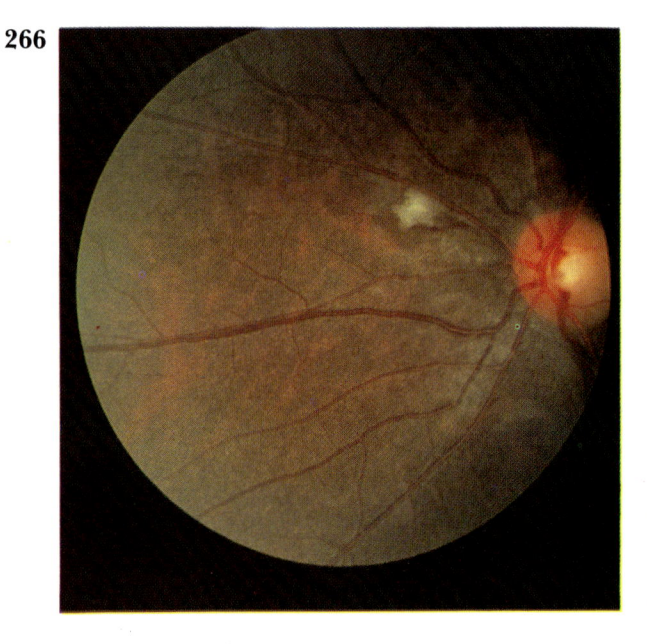

266 Focal lesion of inflammatory retinitis in an eight-year-old black child, who died from subacute sclerosing panencephalitis two years after having had a clinical diagnosis of measles infection.

Pars Planitis *(Peripheral Uveitis, Chronic Cyclitis)*

Pars planitis is a common inflammatory disease of children and young adults in their 20s and 30s. It accounts for a large number of the cases of intraocular inflammation seen in our panorama of uveitis syndromes and shares with its two fellow uveitides, juvenile rheumatoid arthritis and reticulum cell sarcoma, the fact that it is often seen in a quiet white eye.

The incidence of this entity has a peak in teenage years and a second peak in young adults in their 20s and 30s. Although the disease is most often bilateral and is usually more active in one eye than the other, it can be unilateral for many years in some patients. The symptoms consist of floaters and poor vision, especially if the macula is affected with cystoid edema. There is almost always no pain, erythema or photophobia, and rarely any external sign of iridocyclitis, such as limbal flush or injection. Synechiae are almost never seen.

The principal finding in pars planitis is an organization of exudation over the pars plana (**268**) which forms a 'snowbank' over the pars and snowballs also may be seen in the vitreous just over or posterior to the pars plana (**267**). The eye is usually externally quiet, although the initial attack may be accompanied by some redness and iridocyclitis. In some few cases, few fine, white KP may be noted on the endothelium of the cornea, but the anterior chamber reaction is usually minor in proportion to the anterior and posterior vitreous, especially over the pars plana.

Hence, the designation cyclitis is used because the vitreous is usually most affected anteriorly. Posterior vitreous attachments are often present in young people with this disorder. The snowball opacities are for the most part preretinal and concentrated inferiorly, although they may be elaborated at the pars plana superiorly. They are almost always inferior in location when observed clinically.

The retina may have a concomitant patchy peripheral vasculitis, which involves the venules rather than the arterioles. For this reason this disease entity may be confused with sarcoid in some young patients. There may be peripapillary retinal edema and cystoid macular edema as a common concomitant side effect, which may be found angiographically without obvious evidence for it being present clinically.

The complications of pars planitis include cataract, usually the posterior subcapsular type, either from iatrogenic corticosteroid administration or from inflammation, secondary glaucoma, vitreous hemorrhage from vascularization of the snowbanks, dragging of the vascular architecture off the nerve head toward the inferior exudate, cystoid macular edema, and subsequent chronic cystoid macular edema and degeneration, retinal vasculitis and, of course, detachment. Other complications include band keratopathy, cyclitic membrane, and retinoschisis. (Band keratopathy is very rare and would suggest either the entity of juvenile rheumatoid arthritis, or toxocara canis in a young patient.) But in spite of the many potential complications of this disease, more than 80% of the patients have a visual acuity of 20/40 or better after 10 years. Long-term studies show that this mysterious inflammatory disorder with no apparent etiology tends to 'burn out' after the duration of unexplained intraocular inflammation.

PARS PLANITIS (Intermediate Uveitis)

Definition:
- Chronic cyclitis

Presentation:
- Chronic cyclitis
- Nongranulomatous

Investigation:
- Fluorescein angiogram for cystoid macular edema

Therapy:
- Periocular (posterior, subtenon) steroid injection for secondary macular edema or disk edema only
- Occasionally short-course systemic steroids for exacerbations
- Immunosuppressive agents or cyclocryotherapy may be considered for severe recalcitrant cases
- Retinal detachment surgery for traction retinal detachment

Complications:
- Cystoid macular edema
- Cataract
- Secondary steroid glaucoma
- Traction retinal detachment

Prognosis:
- Good if case is treated vigorously for CME. Cases do well with cataract surgery
- Poor if patient goes on to retinal detachment changes and/or neovascularization of the ora

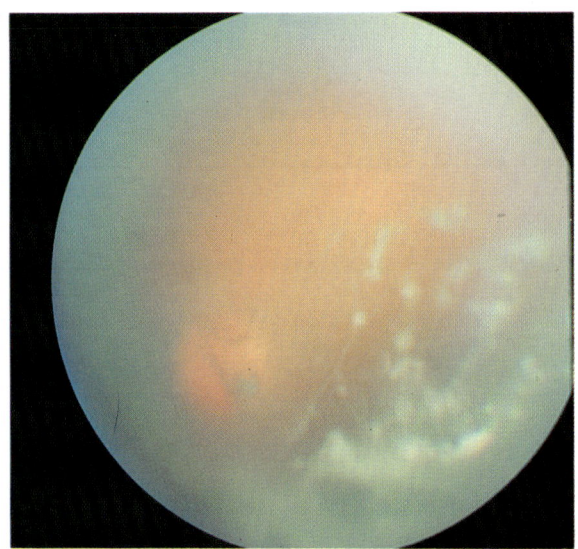

267 Snowballs and intense vitreal inflammation behind the lens of this 14-year-old patient with pars planitis.

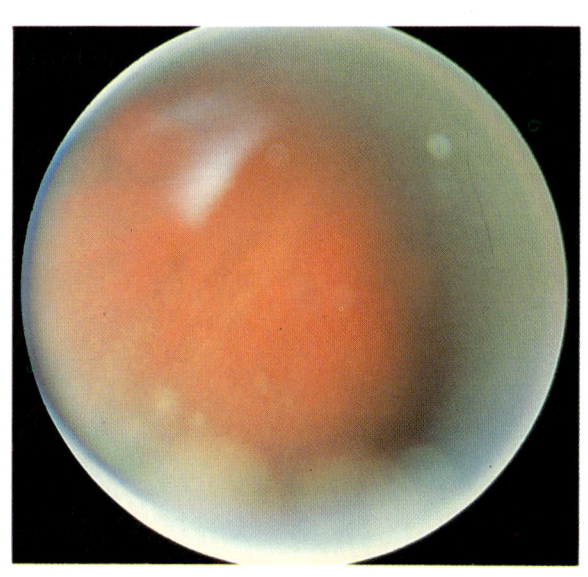

268 Dense exudation over pars plana in a 24-year-old patient with pars planitis.

Acute Multifocal Placoid Pigment Epitheliopathy (AMPPE)

This postdromal viral illness usually effects an intraocular inflammation limited to retinal pigment epithelium and follows on the heels of an upper respiratory viral illness, sometimes manifesting itself with headache and erythema nodosum. There is usually an abrupt drop in vision in an otherwise symptom-free eye. While the disease is usually bilateral, one eye is often affected before and sometimes more severely than the other. In many instances, it may be difficult to elicit the previous viral symptoms, but it is usually several days to several weeks before.

Clinically, gray-white deep retinal lesions are found in the level of the retinal pigment epithelium (**269, 271**) or in the choriocapillaris and frequently affect the macula. There are paracentral or central scotomas and reduced central vision. The degree of visual reduction depends upon the location of the inflammatory lesions. There are usually cells in the vitreous gel overlying this posterior inflammation and only occasionally a mild iridocyclitis present with it. Serous detachment of the retina is rare but has been reported.

This inflammatory disorder usually resolves over a period of several weeks, often with scarring and alterations in the appearance of the retinal pigment epithelium and the choriocapillaris. However, the vision frequently returns to normal.

ACUTE MULTIFOCAL PLACOID PIGMENT EPITHELIOPATHY (AMPPE)

Definition:
- Retinal pigment epithelial inflammation with secondary iridocyclitis

Presentation:
- Acute
- Nongranulomatous

Investigation:
- Fluorescein angiogram
- Rule out systemic viral infection

Therapy:
- None

Complications:
- Macular pigment alteration
- Macular scarring

Prognosis:
- Good

269 AMPPE. Obvious and profound inflammatory alterations in the retinal pigment epithelium in this 23-year-old woman, who suffered from an upper respiratory infection one week prior to the onset of abrupt loss in vision in both eyes.

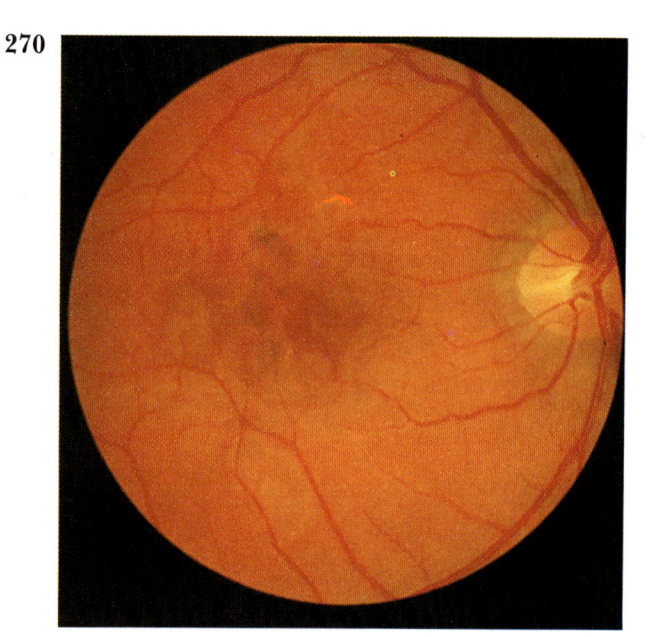

270 More subtle changes in the retinal pigment epithelium in a case of AMPPE. The AMPPE is resolving; however, the central vision was still 20/100 at the time of this photograph, but two weeks later returned to 20/20 with an unchanged fundus picture.

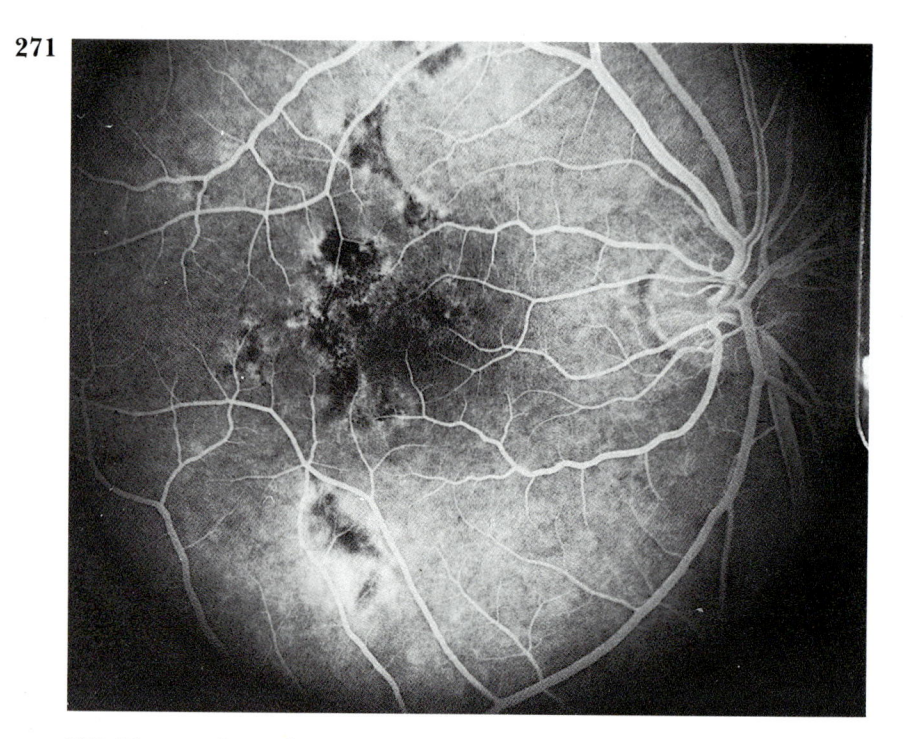

271 Fluorescein study of patient in Figure 270, showing how much more profound the retinal pigment epithelial alterations are demonstrated by the contrast of an angiogram.

Multiple Evanescent White Dot Syndrome (MEWDS)

Multiple evanescent white dot syndrome, or MEWDS, is an inflammation of the retinal pigment epithelium, choriocapillaris, Bruch's membrane and overlaps into the neurosensory retina. It is an entity with an unknown etiology that has a profound but short-lasting effect upon the vision and electrophysiologic function of the eye. Its anatomic presentation may only be mild to moderate, while visual changes may be quite severe. Symptoms usually consist of a blurring of vision, flashing lights or black spots, which are described as fixed in position in contrast to the floating or moveable spots ascribed to vitreous floaters. The visual acuity is often in the 20/50 to 20/70 range. It unusually falls to a poor level such as 20/200 or 20/400. A mild afferent pupillary defect may be present and the vision usually recovers to normal within two to 12 weeks.

Observable yellow-white lesions are seen deep to the retina at the level of the retinal pigment epithelium. Ranging from 100 to 200 microns in diameter, these spots can rarely become as large as 1 disc diameter; they may be confused with AMPPE. They are usually discrete lesions and do not become confluent such as AMPPE. They usually appear to be clusters of small discrete dots at the level of the RPE. Most cases descrive a sparing of the macula, with the largest focus of these small spots being in the peripapillary area and the mid-periphery. Vasculitis is not a prominent finding in this disorder. There is also a curious absence of anterior chamber inflammation. At most, a 1 plus cell and flare is described, as well as an 1 to 2 plus vitreous cellular reaction. Keratic precipitates are not described. A fine granularity is noticed in the foveal area which is described as a reddish excavation somewhat similar to that seen in solar retinopathy measuring between 50 to 75 micra. This granularity may be a disturbance of the retinal pigment epithelium and in the early fluorescein angiographic stages, these lesions show focal hyperfluorescence in the RPE and may again be composed of smaller clusters of tiny dots or specs. They later may demonstrate as window defects in the retinal pigment epithelium due to alteration or death of the cells in that layer. In late-phase angiograms, diffuse staining of the RPE and staining of the optic disc may be noted. Mild leakage of dye from the retinal and disc capillaries is observed. Interestingly, fluorescein angiographic changes may persist long after the white dots are no longer clinically apparent, either by ophthalmoscopy or slit-lamp examination with a 60 or 90 diopter lens. In the late resolution stages of this disease, a fluorescein angiogram usually reverts to normal, although a few focal punctate defects may be seen in the RPE as transmission lesions.

Electroretinographic studies performed in several of the patients have shown that MEWDS has a profound effect on the retinal physiology. The photopic a-wave and b-wave amplitudes are decreased as well as the scotopic a-wave and b-waves. These ERG findings indicate a widespread retinal physiologic involvement out of proportion to the seemingly small anatomic involvement of the retina and RPE with the clusters of tiny white dots. As the disease resolves, the ERG responses are noted to return to normal. In the acute phase of the disease the electro-oculogram also shows moderately light-dark ratios that appear to correspond with the severity of the disease, reflecting a more severe RPE and photoreceptor abnormality then is often observed clinically. Once again, as with the ERG, as the disease resolves the EOG also returns to normal.

MULTIPLE EVANESCENT WHITE DOT SYNDROME (MEWDS)

Definition:
- Discrete, small, focal, multiple exudate of the retinal pigment epithelium combined with choriocapillaris, Bruch's membrane, overlapping into neurosensory retina.

Presentation:
- Yellow-white lesions deep to the retina, at level of RPE
- Occasional minimal iritis
- Occasional minimal vitritis

Investigation:
- ERG
- EOG

Therapy:
- Unknown etiology
- Non-specific, sympathomatic treatment

Complications:
- RPE pigment changes may persist
- Usually vision returns to normal
- Usually ERG/EOG returns to normal

Prognosis:
- Excellent

The etiology of MEWDS is obscure. Because its clinical course appears to resolve as well as the seemingly profound ERG and EOG findings out of proportion to the clinical signs, it is presumed that this may be a consequence of virus infection, similar to AMPPE. Several patients have been described as having a preceding flu-like illness. Chorioretinitis observed in this disorder appears to be self-limited, which would reflect the development of antibodies to a virus or some other inflammatory agent. While the function of the RPE appears to be profoundly disturbed during the course of the disease, these cells apparently do survive intact and resume normal function, as reflected by the ERG and EOG. Residual scars and defects of the RPE are rare. The differential diagnosis for MEWDS would include AMPPE, serpiginous choroidopathy, multifocal choroiditis, bird-shot retinopathy, and a nonspecific retinal pigment epitheliitis. All of these entities have in common an unknown etiology and all have a profound effect on the electrophydiologic function of the eye in excess of the apparent clinical signs that are involved. Most or all of these are suggested to have a viral etiology.

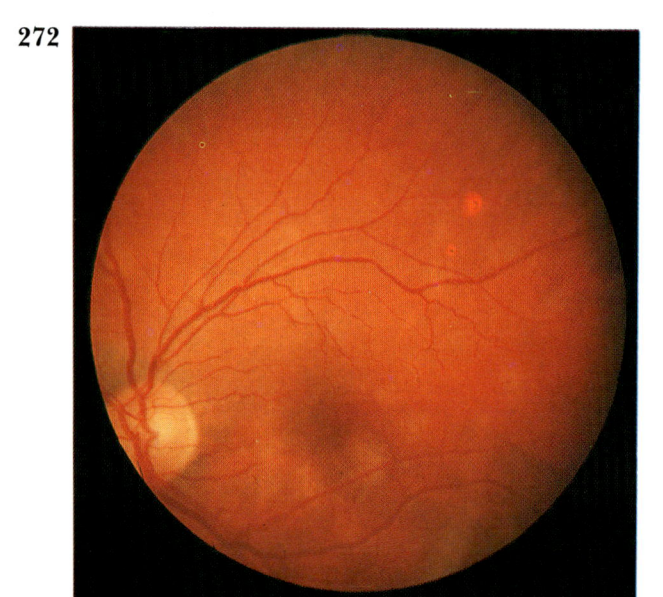

272 MEWDS. A 24-year-old white female with 20/20 (6/6) vision, but dense paracentral scotoma, who demonstrates discrete yellow-white lesions deep to the retina at the level of the RPE.

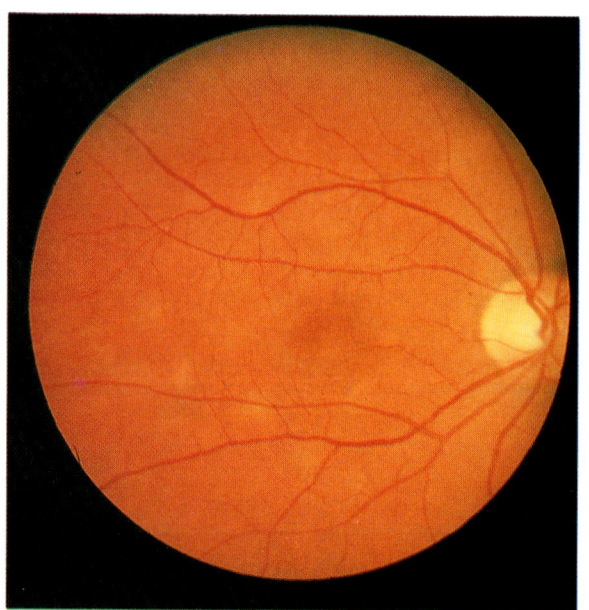

273 MEWDS. Other eye of same patient shows more white lesions, but temporal to the macula.

Bilateral Acute Retinal Necrosis (BARN Syndrome or ARN Syndrome)

This very severe manifestation of ocular inflammation, only recently described, occurs in men and women of almost any age. These patients are seemingly otherwise healthy and have no systemic prodromal complaints. There is increasing evidence that this syndrome may be related to a cytomegalovirus or herpes simplex infection. Interestingly, patients who have cytomegalovirus retinitis in the usual sense are infants or immunoincompetent patients who are compromised either by steroids as part of cancer treatment or by organ transplantation.

The onset of this syndrome is abrupt. Vision usually drops rapidly in the first eye and quite significantly in the second eye. Although usually affected sometime after, the second eye may remain symptomless for a year or more after the onset of the disease. Only occasionally is one eye alone affected.

The major fundus picture includes severe retina necrosis with occlusive vasculitis and generalized edema of the whole retina, with a peripheral whitening spreading to the macular region (**274, 275**). As this disease progresses, there is hemorrhage into and in front of the retina and the formation of retinal tears and holes, marked vitreous traction, and often inoperable retinal detachment with phthisis. Laser photocoagulation to the peripheral necrotic retina may prevent or stall retinal detachment. Most recently, herpes virus (H. Zoster, 1982; H. Simplex, CMV, Epstein-Barr) are thought to mediate this disease. Treatment with acyclovir is advocated by most authorities. All of this may happen rapidly, in a matter of days to weeks. There is usually an associated mild to moderate inflammation, often with minimal KP formation. Usually, the final and catastrophic visual outcome is no light perception.

ACUTE RETINAL NECROSIS (ARN)

Definition:
- Acute inflammatory necrosis of the retina of unknown etiology

Presentation:
- Retinitis, retinal vasculitis with vitreous cells
- Nongranulomatous

Investigation:
- Titers:
  - Herpes simplex
  - Herpes zoster (serum/vitreous)
  - Corneal/retinal biopsy (to demonstrate CMV-like particles)

Therapy:
- Systemic acyclovir
- Intravitreal acyclovir
- Photocoagulation posterior to area of necrosis if visibility allows
- Retinopexy with broad posterior scleral if TRD develops or if threatens

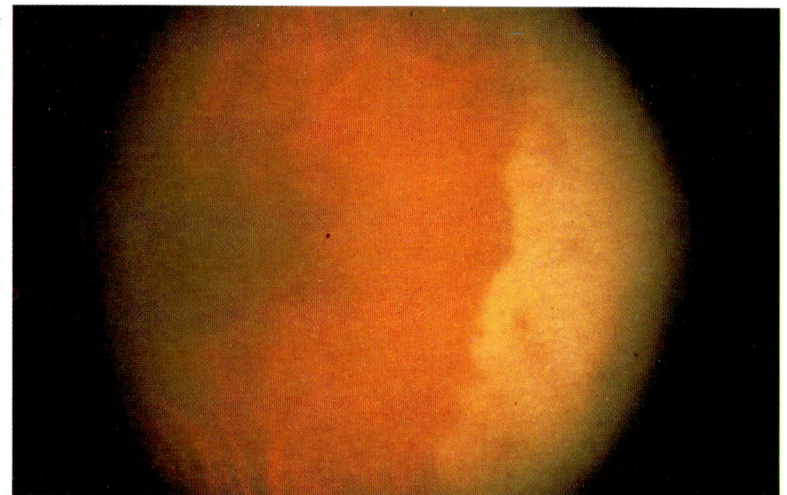

274 Acute peripheral retinal necrosis in an otherwise healthy 38-year-old male.

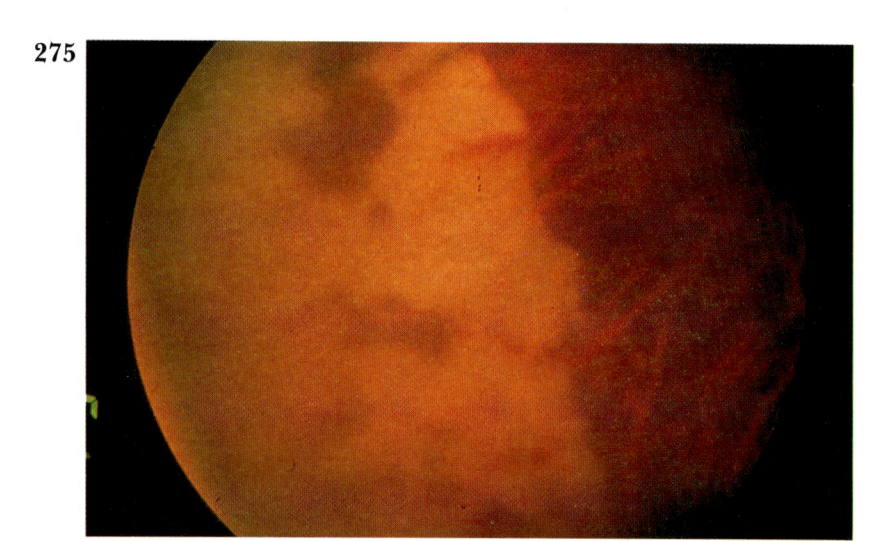

275 Acute retinal necrosis now progressing with white exudation covering the retina in a necrotic fashion directing toward the posterior pole.

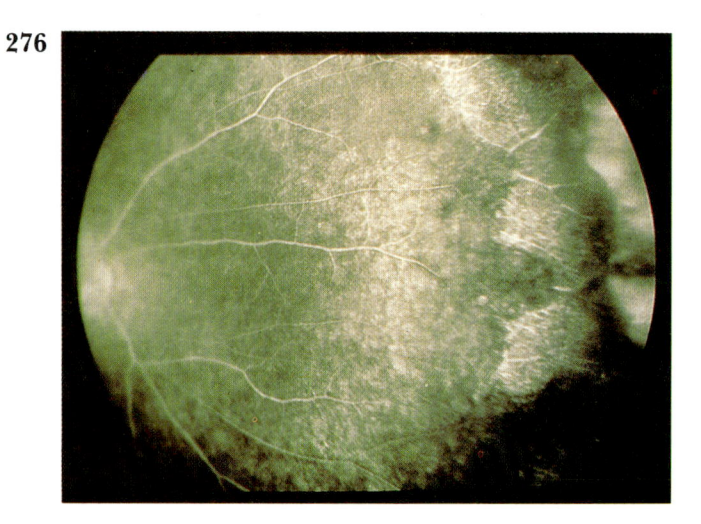

276 Fluorescein angiogram demonstrates the profound retinal pigment epithelial alteration in a patient with acute retinal necrosis.

Birdshot Choroidopathy

This rare ocular inflammatory disorder has only recently been described by Ryan and Maumenee. It usually affects middle-aged patients and occurs in both sexes. Multiple patches of what appear to be a dropout of the retinal pigment epithelium or multifocal choroiditis occur in both eyes abruptly (**278**). There is usually an associated mild iridocyclitis with a more abundant cellular infiltration into the vitreous cavity. This disorder resembles pars planitis in some respects, except there are no exudates over the pars plana. There is involvement of the choroid or choriocapillaris, and there may be subtle discoloration or patchy areas waving in the choroid on examination with a contact lens. The disease progresses bilaterally with late arteriolar sheathing, and optic atrophy may ensure. The etiology of birdshot choriopathy is unknown and there are no reports of its histopathology. Some of the early patients first described had a prodromal viral illness, suggestive of an acute multifocal placoid pigment epitheliopathy-type picture. It is not clear whether this disease is a true inflammation or a degenerative condition that mimics uveitis.

BIRDSHOT CHOROIDOPATHY

Definition:
- Retinal choroiditis with retinal pigment epithelium inflammation
- Secondary iridocyclitis

Presentation:
- Chorioretinitis
- Nongranulomatous

Investigation:
- Fluorescein angiogram
- HLA-A29 (highly specific)

Therapy:
- Systemic or periocular steroids (often with poor results)

Complications:
- Cystoid macular edema
- Retinal scarring

Prognosis:
- Fair to poor

277 Birdshot choroidopathy. Patient with patchy focal macular inflammation at the level of the retinal pigment epithelium following an abrupt onset of minimal anterior segment intraocular inflammation with posterior vasculitis, thought to be 'birdshot'.

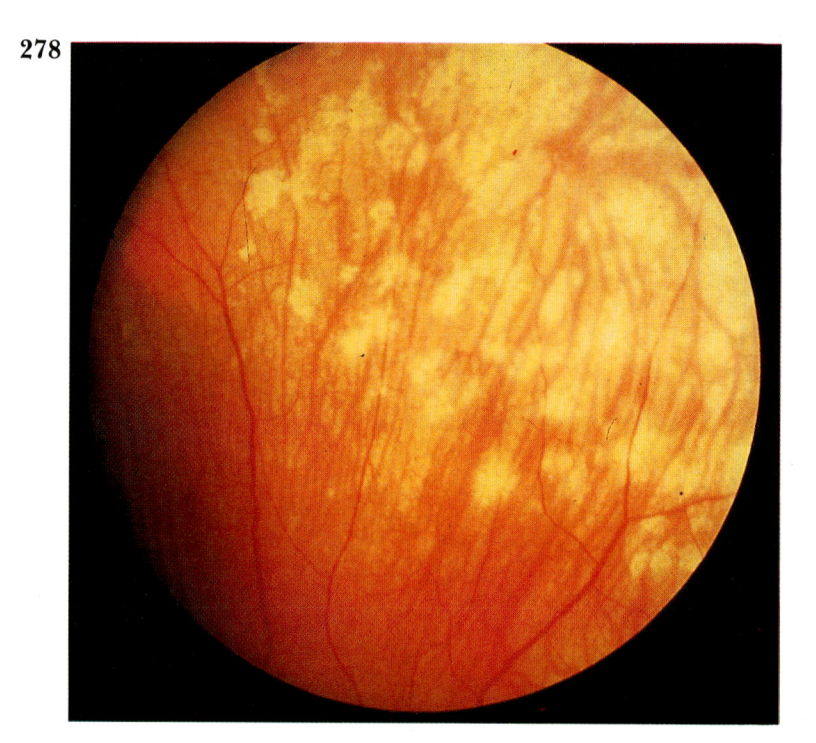

278 Peripheral retina of the same patient showing diffuse focal spots of retinal pigment epithelial inflammation, then depigmentation as if the retinal periphery were showered with 'birdshot'.

Fuchs' Heterochromic Iridocyclitis

Fuchs' iridocyclitis is an unusual unilateral uveitis and is often the most misdiagnosed of all the uveitides. It occurs in men and women in the third and fourth decades and accounts for two percent of all cases of uveitis. Fuchs' iridocyclitis is often unrecognized. When it is recognized, it may be overtreated and cause iatrogenic or natural cataract and glaucoma. Rare bilateral cases have been reported. Occasionally there is erythema and photophobia with the onset of Fuchs' cyclitis. A mild inflammation is discovered in many patients on a routine eye examination, either because of mild iridocyclitis or because of heterochromia that the patient called to the attention of an eye doctor.

It is often best to examine the two irides in sunlight, rather than in the usual dark examining room. Sunlight may highlight the very subtle differences in iris pigmentation. In almost all cases, the fellow eye is entirely normal. The usual situation is for the lighter eye, which is depigmented, to be the eye affected by Fuchs' (**279**); however, if there is hypertrophy of the iris pigment epithelium, the darker eye may be the one affected.

There is usually no pain, and the major complication is reduced vision due to cataract. This is another uveitic situation where the affected eye is usually white and quiet with only a mild limbal ciliary flush. It may thus simulate the same 'quiet uveitis' as in juvenile rheumatoid arthritis, peripheral uveitis (where usually there are no synechiae formed) and in the pseudo-inflammations, such as reticulum cell sarcoma.

Clinically, there are usually small, diffuse, fine KP that are not pigmented and that disappear and reappear spontaneously. KP are not concentrated in the inferior triangle of the cornea as they are in almost all other uveitides, but rather are usually evenly distributed throughout the back and at the center of the cornea, much as with a Krukenberg spindle. In most cases, there are no large mutton-fat-type KP. There is usually a mild anterior chamber reaction and 1–2+1 cells with a similar amount of flare. Transillumination should reveal the irregular defects in the iris pigment epithelium with thinning of the stroma (**280**). There are usually no synechiae at the pupil and the pupils dilate well. The vitreous cavity usually possesses a small amount of cellularity with strands, but the posterior pole and retinal vessels are usually normal. Cystoid edema is not a feature of Fuchs' iridocyclitis.

Abnormal blood vessels in the chamber angle have been reported and may be a feature of this disease, but they are not usually found. The vessels of the angle usually become more prominent as a result of a contrast caused by an atrophied iris. The clinical course of Fuchs' iridocyclitis in up to 50% of the cases is usually that of a slowly progressive cataract, and anywhere from 20% to 50% of the patients develop chronic open angle glaucoma. The mild iridocyclitis is usually not a problem in this disorder.

FUCHS' HETEROCHROMIC IRIDOCYCLITIS

Definition:
- Iridocyclitis

Presentation:
- Acute or chronic iridocyclitis
- Nongranulomatous

Investigation:
- None

Therapy:
- No treatment needed in vast majority of cases
- Night-time dilatation with short-acting mydriatic cycloplegic agents (if Koeppe nodules present)
- Periocular steroids for posterior pole edema
- Therapy for glaucoma which may be refractory

Complications:
- Cataract
- Glaucoma

Prognosis:
- Often good with no treatment
- Cases do well with cataract surgery
- One of the rare uveitides amenable to posterior chamber intraocular lens
- Glaucoma may be refractory to treatment requiring seton surgery

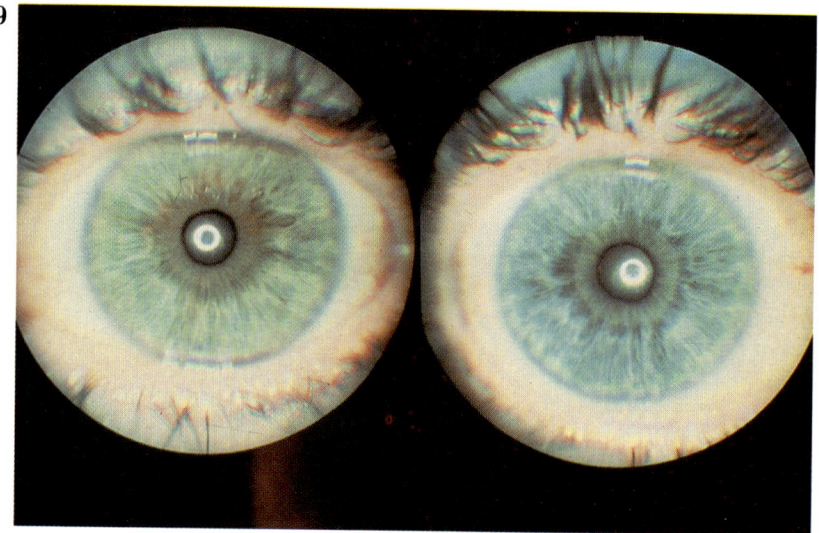

279 Fuchs' heterochromia. Irides of patient with Fuchs' heterochromic iridocyclitis, demonstrating the contrast in color of the two eyes (hazel versus blue).

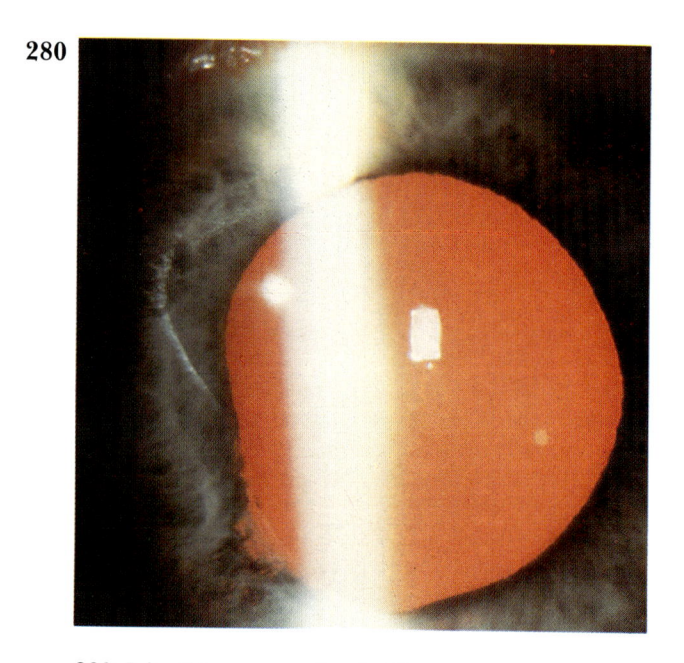

280 Iris of the same patient in Figure 279, demonstrating pigment atrophy at 7:00 o'clock on the pupillary margin and posterior subcapsular cataract changes can be noted.

Relapsing Polychondritis

Relapsing polychondritis (chronic atrophic polychondritis) is an uncommon arthritic disorder characterized by the development of recurrent inflammation in cartilaginous tissues throughout the body. It occurs in both sexes and usually has its onset between the ages of 20 to 60 years. Its pathogenesis is unkown but is often classified with the other collagen vascular and connective tissue diseases.

Inflammation of the pinnae of the ears is the most common feature of this disorder (**283**), when one or both become red, swollen, and painful. Repeated attacks lead to resorption of ear cartilage and floppy, drooping ears. Arthralgias and arthritis are often seen. Inflammation and resorption of the nasal cartilage (**282**) is another frequent finding, sometimes resulting in a saddle nose deformity. A number of systemic diseases have been found in association with this disorder, including vasculitis, rheumatoid arthritis, systemic and discoid lupus erythematosus, ankylosing spondylitis, ulcerative colitis, and sarcoidosis. There may be considerable overlap in the types of uveitis etiology in patients who present with these unusual connective tissue manifestations. Episcleritis (**281, 284**) is probably the most common complication but conjunctivitis and keratitis occur as well. Scleritis may involve primarily the anterior portions of the eye and many patients often have an associated keratoconjunctivitis sicca. Involvement of the retina and optic nerve is seen far less often than the anterior ocular complications. However, there are several reports of active and inactive chorioretinopathy associated with this disorder, and there is one case in which the clinical picture was similar to that of a juvenile Coats' disease. Optic neuritis has also been reported in this connective tissue disorder.

RELAPSING POLYCHONDRITIS

Definition:
- Iridocyclitis

Presentation:
- Iridocyclitis, keratitis, keratouveitis
- Episcleritis scleritis
- Nongranulomatous

Investigation:
- Physical exam (cartilage absent, floppy ears, decreased nasal cartilage)

Therapy:
- Topical steroids
- Immunosuppressives (especially chlorambucil)
- Cyclosporine

Complications:
- Corneal scarring

Prognosis:
- Good

281 Corneal inflammation. Left eye of a 24-year-old white woman with relapsing polychondritis, showing limbal conjunctival and episcleral injection with peripheral corneal infiltrates involving the stroma, as well as superficial cornea.

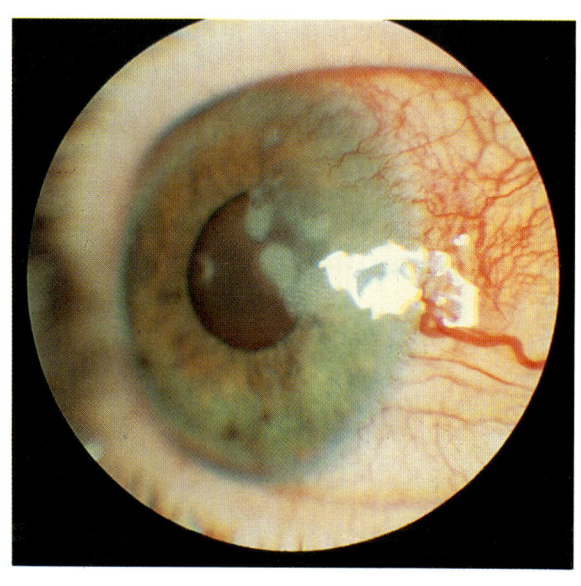

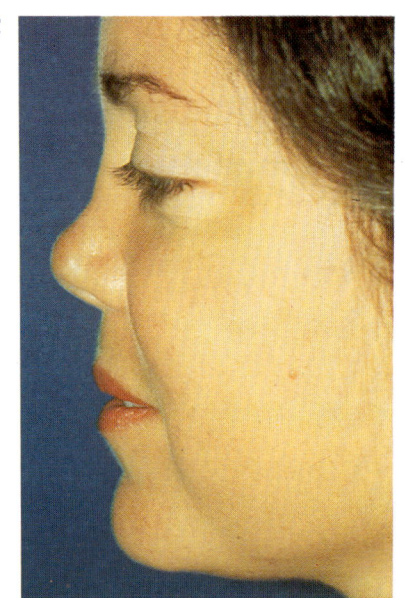

282 Typical saddle nose appearance in the same patient as in Figure 281, with relapsing polychondritis.

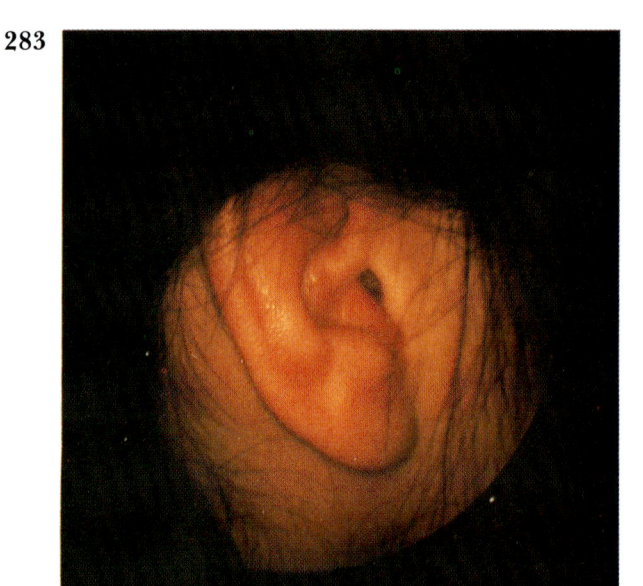

283 Swollen pinna with pain, erythema, and heat in patient with relapsing polychondritis.

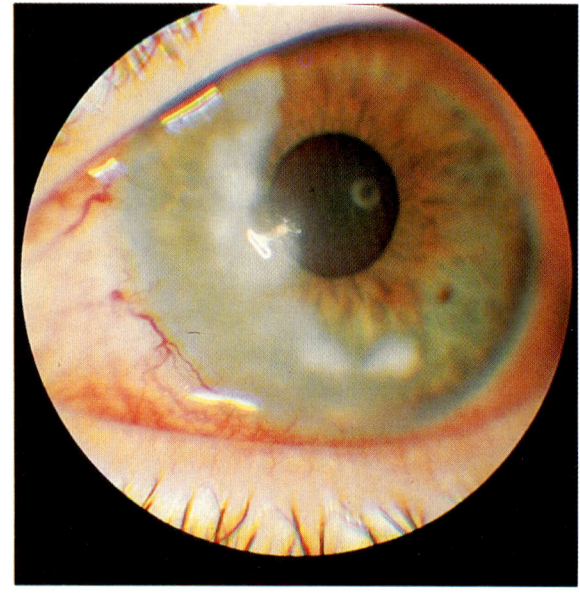

284 Polychondritis episcleritis. Fellow eye of a patient with an acute episcleritis and adjacent keratitis.

Drug Abuse

Fungal endophthalmitis and particulate matter emboli to the eye. Drug abuse is a growing problem worldwide as well as in the USA where it ushers in a host of new considerations in the medical management of patients with mysterious complaints and illnesses. A young person not having undergone ocular surgery who presents with what appears to be a metastatic endophthalmitis (**289, 291, 295**) should be suspect of intravenous drug use until proven otherwise. Patients who suffer metastatic endophthalmitis caused by either intravenous drug abuse or metastatic emboli due to drug treatment can have devastating damage done to their ocular structures before the etiology of this phenomenon is recognized and treated. Particulate matter may embolize to the eye (**285**), particularly in intravenous drug abuse patients who 'cut' and dilute their intravenous substances with talc, cornstarch, and other particulates, which may embolize to the eye either in a shower or as a single focus of inflammation or infection.

DRUG ABUSE

Definition:
- Vitritis
- Retinitis secondary to hematogenous embolization

Presentation:
- Usually vitritis
- Secondary retinitis
- Secondary choroiditis
- Granulomatous

Investigation:
- Ultrasonography of globe
- Paracentesis with centrifugation of anterior and posterior chamber for fungal or bacterial elements
- Directed biopsy of vitreous for candida
- Systemic evaluation of patient

Therapy:
- Specific treatment for fungal or bacterial etiology

Complications:
- Panuveitis
- Cataract
- Retinal detachment
- Glaucoma

Prognosis:
- Usually poor (good if caught and treated early, especially candida endophthalmitis)

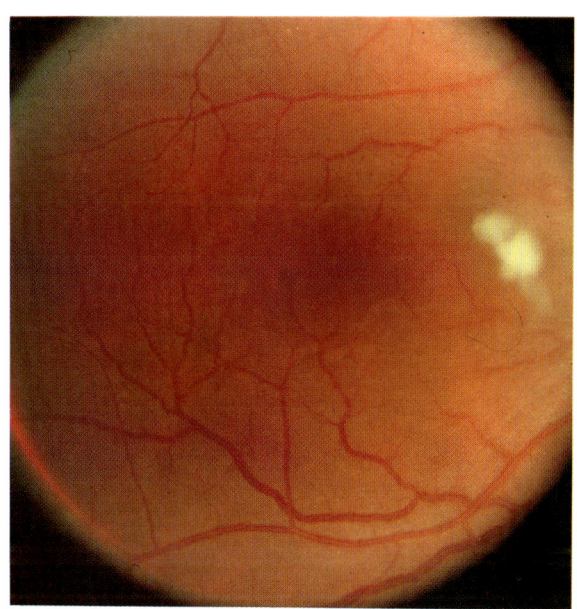

285 Particulate embolus of refractile talc in a patient abusing intravenous cocaine.

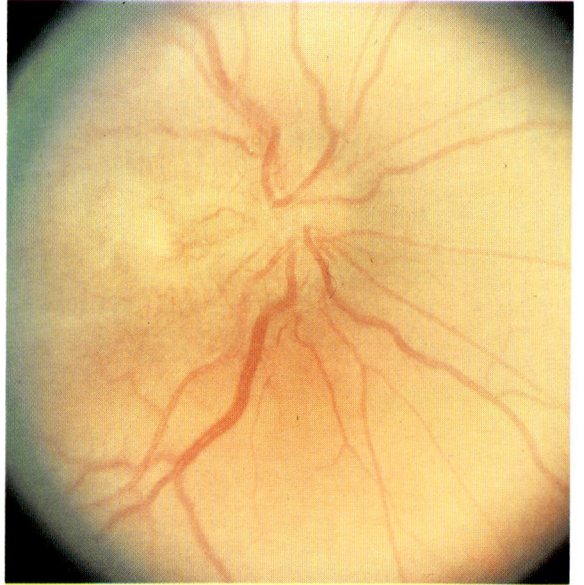

286 Talc embolus in Figure 285 is seen developing into a retinal granuloma where the fractile particle of talc crystal can no longer be recognized.

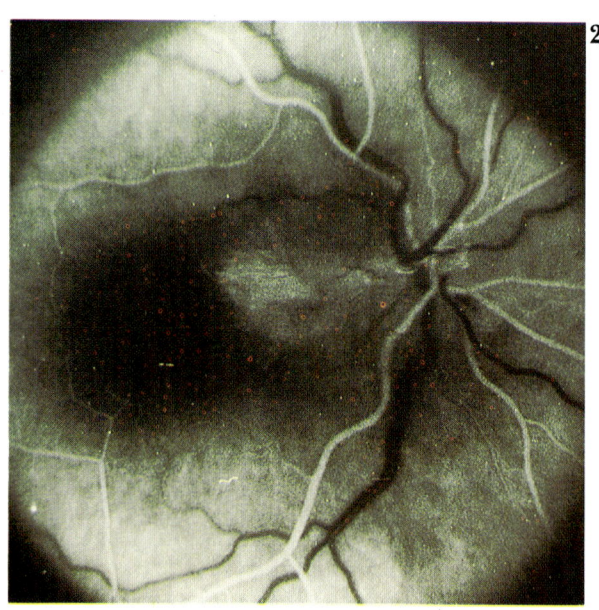

287 Fluorescein angiogram in the early venous phase showing the accumulation of fluorescein beginning in this talc granuloma.

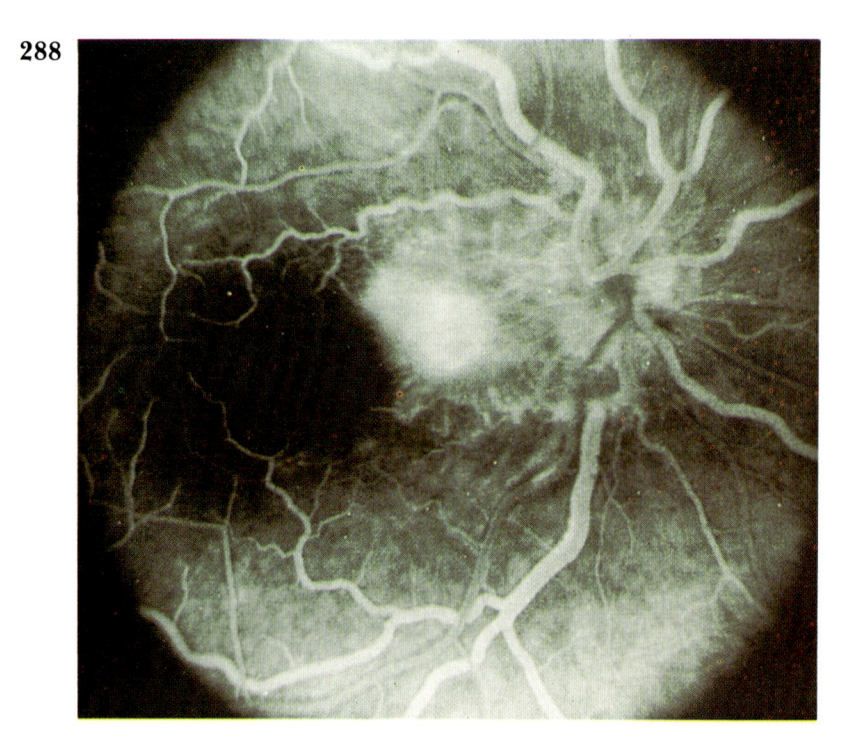

288 Late venous phase of fluorescein angiogram showing that the talc granuloma encompasses almost the entire papillomacular bundle.

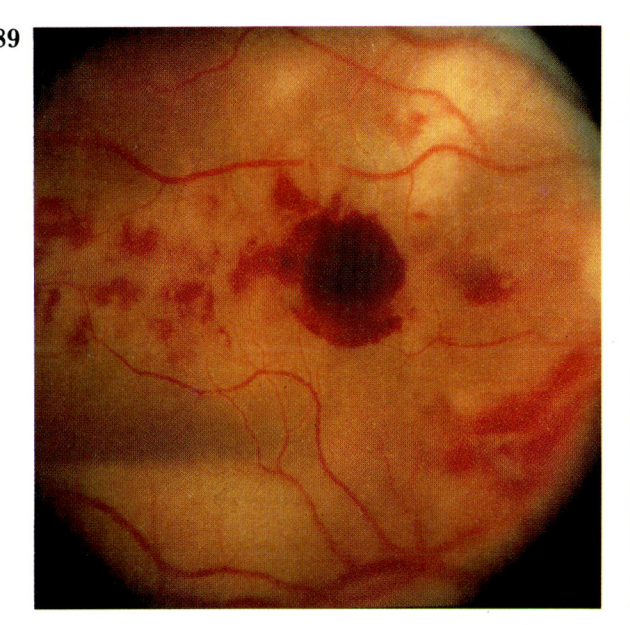

289 Macula showing meniscus of exudate lying deep to the retina with patient in upright position.

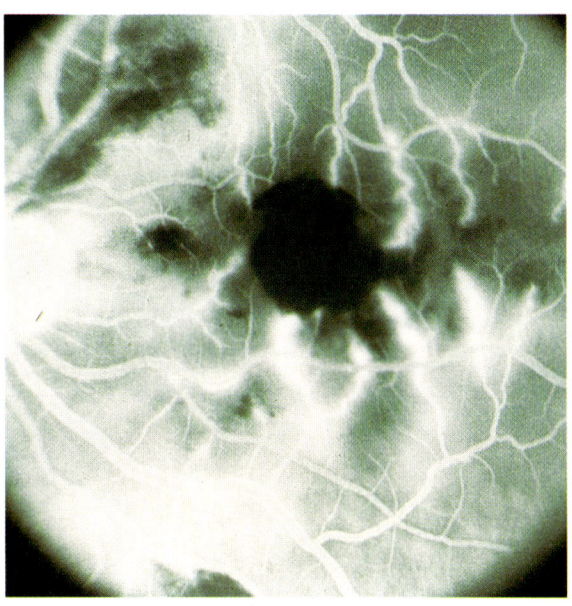

290 Fluorescein angiogram showing a profound leakage due to vasculitis of all vessels in the posterior pole in the same patient with aspergillus endophthalmitis.

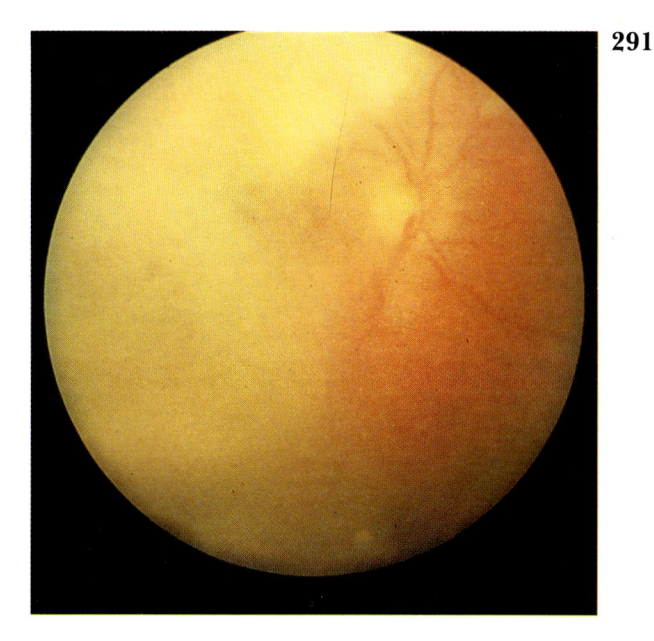

291 Vitreous fluff balls. Another patient suffering aspergillus endophthalmitis from intravenous drug abuse. Almost the entire vitreous body is filled with 'fluff balls' which are coalescing to allow only a peek through to the posterior pole from a central opening

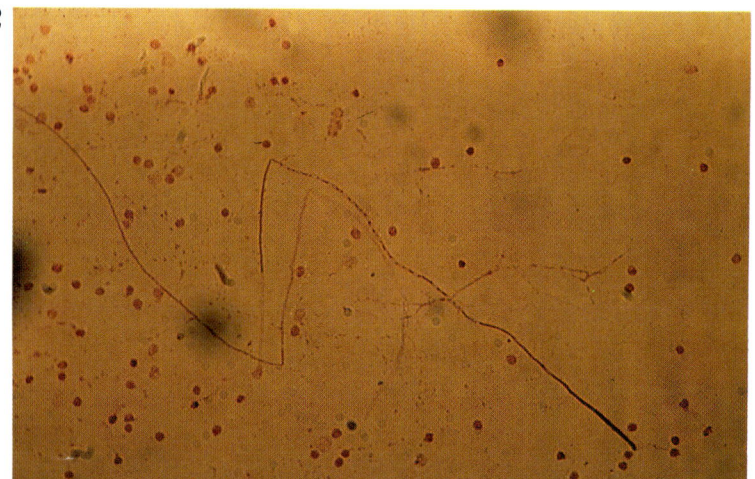

292 Hypha of aspergillosis recovered from fluffy vitreous exudate of previous patient with aspergillus endophthalmitis.

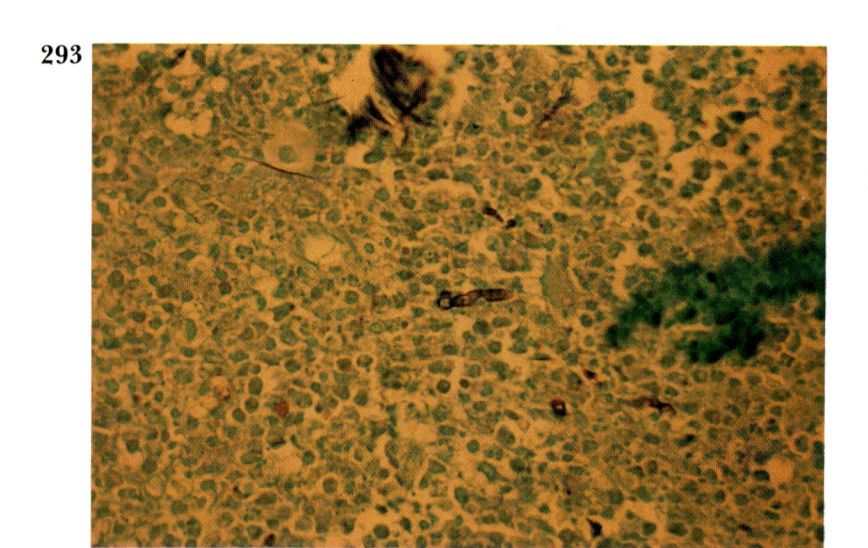

293 Hypha of aspergillosis recovered from inflamed rib in patient with metastatic osteomyelitis whose overall condition of systemic fungemia was called to attention by endophthalmitis from intravenous drug abuse.

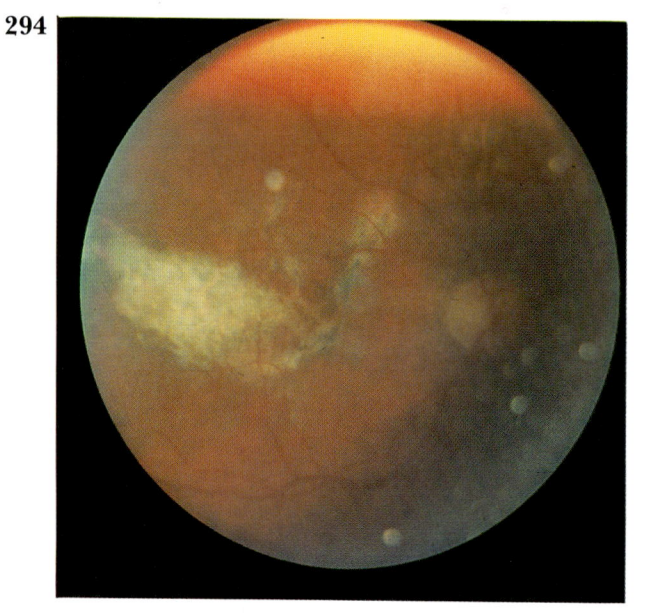

294 Profound scarring of perimacular retina and retinal pigment epithelium in patient who recovered from aspergillus endophthalmitis secondary to intravenous drug abuse.

295 Typical fungal fluff ball. Classic presentation of large vitreous fluff ball surrounded by intense vitreous inflammation in a patient suffering from candida endophthalmitis secondary to intravenous drug abuse.

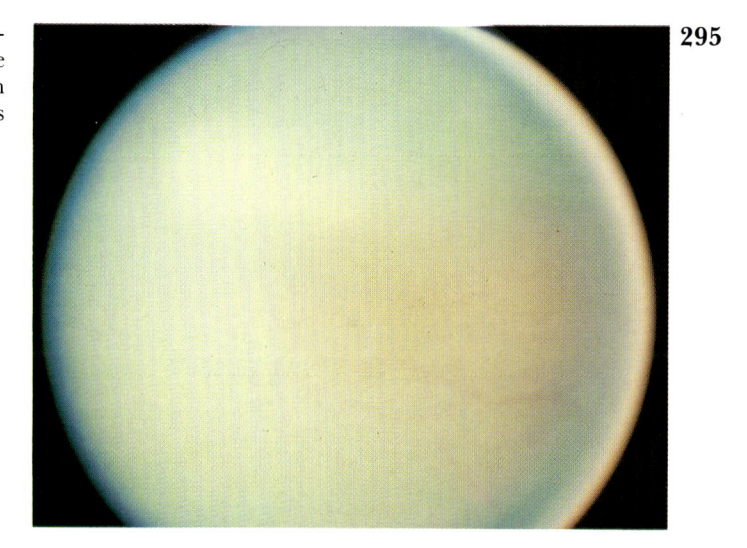

296 Resolving vitritis. The patient's vitreous is clearing and the puff ball almost totally eliminated by pars plana vitrectomy in combination with intravenous amphotericin B treatment.

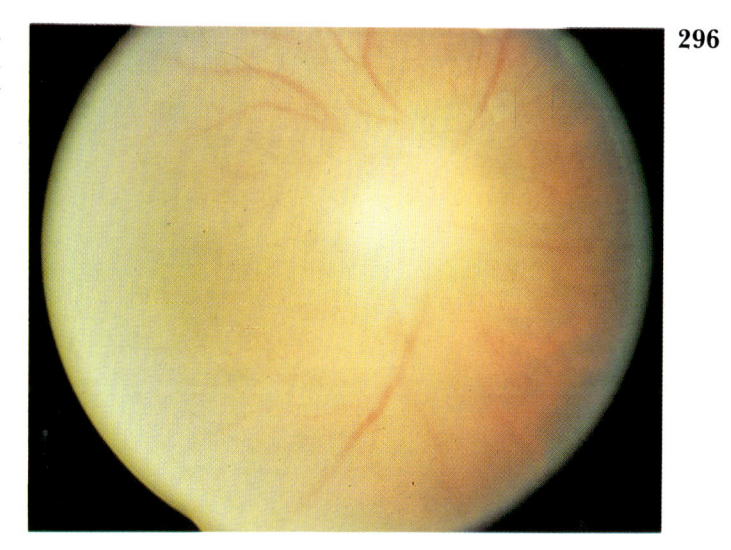

297 Resolved candida infection. Patient recovered from intraocular inflammation secondary to candida endophthalmitis from intravenous drug abuse. Note the striae in retina through the macula radiating from the optic papilla, which has resorbed all the inflammation around where the vitreous fluff ball had settled over the nerve head. A final visual acuity was reduced to 20/100 due to the retinal striae through the macula.

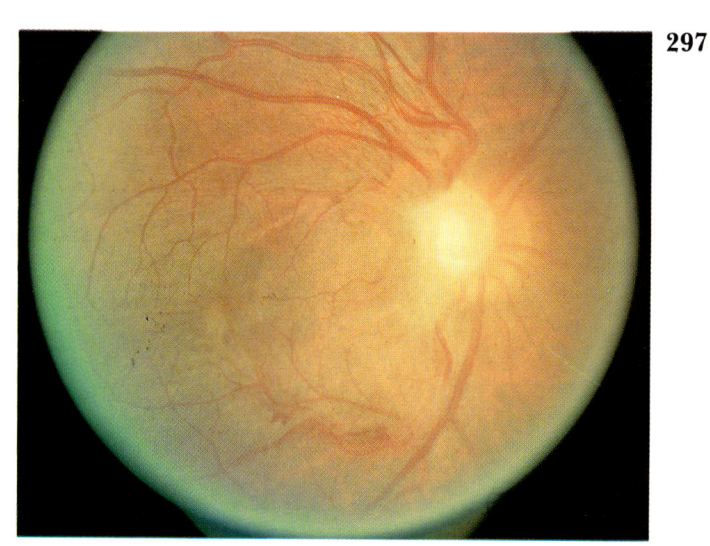

298 Shower of particulate emboli in the posterior pole of patient known to be abusing intravenous Ritalin. (*Courtesy of Howard Schatz, M.D.*)

Natural and Intraocular Lenses

Lens-Induced Uveitis (Phacoanaphylactic Endophthalmitis, Phacotoxic Uveitis)

Phacoanaphylactic uveitis is a sterile granulomatous inflammatory response to lens material which is secondary to autosensitization to the patient's own lens protein. It occurs typically after traumatic or surgical rupture of the lens capsule with escape of cortical material. In rare instances, an otherwise successful intraocular lens (IOL) implantation after extracapsular cataract extraction (ECCE or phaco) can be complicated by a non-infectious inflammatory reaction may not be a result of the IOL itself, but rather a hypersensitivity reaction to the patient's own lens protein. This protein, derived from residual lens material following ECCE, may cause a transient phacotoxic response that usually subsides rapidly on steroids, or it may induce a true phacoanaphylactic reaction.

Less commonly, actual infections with low-grade indolent organisms, have been reported to ensue long after IOL implantation, or to smolder along on steroid medication alone, masquerading as non-infectious, inflammatory reactions which necessitate removal of the capsule and its associated infection. Most studies have shown that infectious endophthalmitis occurring in intervals from 2 months to 2 years after surgery with low-grade, indolent organisms such as Propionibacterium acnes, *staph. epiderdimis*, and rhodococcus. While many of these cases were culture negative from aqueous and vitreous, these organisms were identified or cultured from the capsular bag, where they apparently smoldered along in foci of inflammation in and around the posterior capsule. In such cases, removal of the IOL and anterior vitrectomy excising the capsule cured the condition.

Intraocular Lens-Induced Uveitis

Intraocular inflammation may result as a consequence of a misplaced or displaced IOL whose structure is causing disruption of iris, iris pigment epithelium, or stroma. Older model implants, those especially with titanium clips and sharp-edged Choyce style haptics 'jammed' into the angle and trabecular meshwork, were examples of uveitis-inducing lenses. The 'UGH' syndrome, made manifest by uveitis, glaucoma, and hyphema, is a direct consequence of such ill-fitting lenses, and necessitate removal of the offending implant.

When an intraocular lens is noted to be causing an intraocular corrosion or erosion problem, the implant is best removed surgically immediately, with as little manipulation of the surrounding inflamed tissues as possible. Vitrectomy of the surrounding gel may be necessary, especially if the ongoing inflammation causes a 'wick' syndrome leading to inflammatory and traction cystoid macular edema. A posterior chamber lens, often fibrosed into position with its haptics securely in place, may require that those haptics be cut with firm scissors and left in place. If the offending structure is a haptic eroding throught the iris stroma (**299**), a portion of the iris may have to be surgically cut or teased away to free the entrapped portion.

IOL choice for Uveitis

IOLs are generally contraindicated in the uveitic syndromes when cataract development occurs. Recurrent inflammation tends to 'coat' the IOL, or to encase it in a 'cocoon' of fibrous tissue (**300**), rendering the implant as opaque or more opaque than the original cataract. It is now accepted that Fuch's heterochromic cyclitis is an acceptable risk for IOL implantation, while 'burned out' pars planitis, 'posterior' cases such as toxoplasmosis, toxocara, etc, and inactive cases are slightly less acceptable since intercurrent inflammation may 'coat' these lenses. Other uveitic syndromes are not candidates for IOLs.

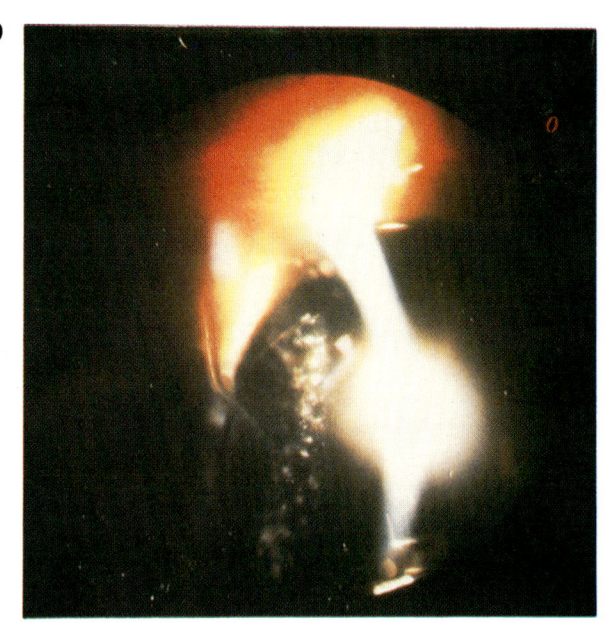

299 A 78-year-old patient, after cataract extraction with anterior chamber lens eroding iris surface and causing an unremitting iridocyclitis. This intractable IOL-induced uveitis necessitated removal of the implant as a surgical cure.

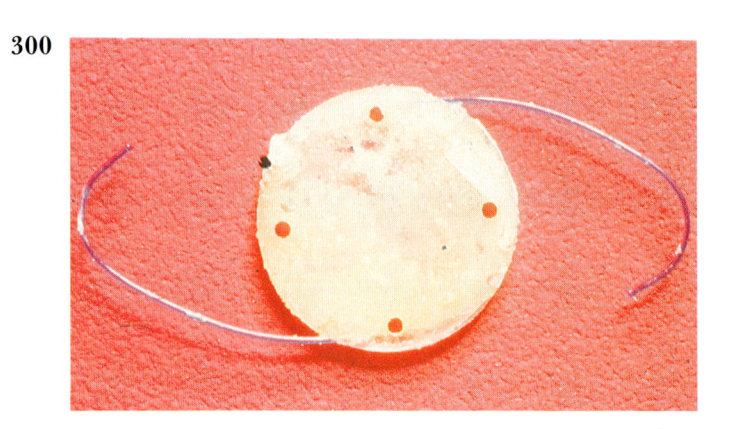

300 Posterior chamber lens removed from a patient with uveitis whose entire surface is coated with thick exudate almost completely obscuring the lens itself.

References

Aaberg T.M.: The expanding ophthalmologic spectrum of Lyme disease. *Am. J. Ophthalmol.* **107**: 77–80, 1989.
Aaberg T.M., Cesarz T.J., Flinkinger R.R.: Treatment of peripheral uveoretinitis by cryotherapy. *Am. J. Ophthalmol.* **73**: 685, 1973.
Aaberg T.M., Cesarz T.J., Rytel M.W.: Correlation of virology and clinical course of cytomegalovirus retinitis. *Am. J. Ophthalmol.* **74**: 407, 1972.
Acers T.E.: Toxoplasmic retinochoroiditis. A double-blind therapeutic study. *Arch. Ophthalmol.* **71**: 58, 1964.
Aguilar G.L., Blumenkrantz M.S., Egbert P.R., McCulley J.P.: Candida endophthalmitis after intravenous drug abuse. *Arch. Ophthalmol.* **97**: 96, 1979.
Albert D.M., Nordlund J.J., Lerner A.B.: Ocular abnormalities occurring with vitiligo. *Ophthalmology.* **86**: 1145, 1979.
Alexander A., Baer A., Fair J.R., Gochenour W.S., King J.H., Yager R.H.: Leptospiral uveitis. Report of bacteriologically verified cases. *Arch. Ophthalmol.* **62**: 150, 1966.
Allen J.C.: Sympathetic uveitis and phacoanaphylaxis. *Am. J. Ophthalmol.* **63**: 280–283, 1967.
Allen J.H.: The pathology of ocular leprosy. II. Miliary lepromas of the iris. *Am. J. Ophthalmol.* **61**: 987, 1966.
Alvarez R.G., Lopez-Villegas A.: Primary oculat sporotrichosis. *Am. J. Ophthalmol.* **62**: 150, 1966.
Anderson B.: Ocular lesions in relapsing polychondritis and other rheumatoid syndromes. The Edward Jackson Memorial Lecture. *Am. J. Ophthalmol.* **64**: 35, 1967.
Annesley W.H., Tomer T.L., Shields J.A.: Multifocal placoid pigment epitheliopathy. *Am. J. Ophthalmol.* **76**: 511, 1973.
Appen R.E.: Posterior uveitis and primary cerebral reticulum cell sarcoma. *Arch. Ophthalmol.* **93**: 123, 1975.
Aronson S., et al. (eds.): *Clinical Methods in Uveitis*, St Louis, C.V. Mosby Co., 1968.
Aronson S.B., Elliott J.H.: *Ocular Inflammation*, St. Louis, C.V. Mosby Co., 1972.
Asbury T.: The status of presumed ocular histoplasmosis: Including a report of a survey. *Trans. Am. Ophthalmol. Soc.* **64**: 371, 1966.
Ashton N.: Larval granulomatosis of the retina due to *Toxocara*. *Br. J. Ophthalmol.* **44**: 129–148, 1960.
Baldone J.A., Clark W.B., Jung R.C.: Nematode ophthalmitis. *Am. J. Ophthalmol.* **57**: 763, 1964.
Barr C.C., Green W.R., Payne J.W., et al.: Intraocular reticulum cell sarcoma. *Surv. Ophthalmol.* **19**: 224, 1975.
Baum J., Barza M., Weinstein P., et al.: Bilateral keratitis as a manifestation of Lyme Disease. *Am. J. Ophthalmol.* **105**: 75–77, 1988.
Belmont J.B., Michelson J.B.: Vitrectomy in uveitis associated with ankylosing spondylitis. *Am. J. Ophthalmol.* **94**: 300–304, 1982.
Bergaust B., Westby R.: Zoster ophthalmicus, local treatment with cortisone. *Acta. Ophthalmol.* **45**: 787, 1967.
Berger B.B., Weinberg R.S., Tessler H.H.: Bilateral cytomegalovirus panuveitis after high dose corticosteroid therapy. *Am. J. Ophthalmol.* **88**: 1020, 1979.
Bialasiewicz A.A., Ruprecht K.W., Naumann G.O.H.,
Blenk H.: Bilateral diffuse choroiditis and exudative retinal detachment with evidence of Lyme disease. *Am. J. Ophthalmol.* **105**: 419–420, 1988.
Biglan A.W., Glickman L.T., Lobes L.A.: Serum and vitreous toxocara antibody in nematode endophthalmitis. *Am. J. Ophthalmol.* **88**: 898, 1979.
Billson F.A., De Dombal F.T., Watkinson G., et al.: Ocular complications of ulcerative colitis. *Gut* **8**: 102, 1967.
Birbeck M.Q., Buckler W.S.-J., Mason R.M., et al.: Iritis as the presenting symptom in ankylosing spondylitis. *Lancet* **2**: 802, 1951.
Bird A.C., Hamilton A.M.: Placoid pigment epitheliopathy presenting with bilateral serous detachment. *Br. J. Ophthalmol.* **56**: 886, 1972.
Bird A.C., Smith J.L., Curtin V.T.: Nematode optic neuritis. *Am. J. Ophthalmol.* **69**: 72, 1970.
Blodi F.C., Hervouet F.: Syphilitic chorioretinitis. *Arch. Ophthalmol.* **79**: 294, 1968.
Blumenkranz M.S., Stevens D.A.: Endogenous coccidioidal endophthalmitis. *Ophthalmol.* **87**: 974, 1980.
Bornstein J.S., Frank M.I., Radner D.B.: Conjunctival biopsy in the diagnosis of sarcoidosis. *N. Engl. J. Med.* **267**: 60, 1962.
Boyden B.S., Yee D.S.: Bilateral coccidioidomycosis choroiditis. *Trans. Am. Acad. Ophthalmol. Otolaryngol.* **75**: 1006, 1971.
Bradley R.D., Meredith T.A., Aabert T.M., et al.: The prevalency of HLA-B-7 in presumed ocular histoplasmosis. *Am. J. Ophthalmol.* **85**: 859–861, 1978.
Braley A.E., Hamilton H.E.: Serous choroiditis associated with amebiasis. *Arch. Ophthalmol.* **58**: 1, 1957.
Brauninger G.E., Polack F.M.: Sympathetic ophthalmitis. *Am. J. Ophthalmol.* **72**: 967, 1971.
Brewerton D.A., Caffrey M., Nicholls A., et al.: Acute anterior uveitis and HL-A 27. *Lancet* **2**: 994, 1973.
Brézin A.P., Egwauagu C.E., Burnier M., Jr., Silveira C., Mahdi R.M., Gazzinelli R.T., Belfort R., Jr., Nussenblatt R.B.: Identification of *Toxoplasma gondii* in paraffin-embedded sections by the polymerase chain reaction. *Am. J. Ophthalmol.* **110**: 599–604, 1990.
Brockhurst R.J., Schepens C.L., et al.: Peripheral uveitis I. *Am. J. Ophthalmol.* **42**: 545, 1956.
Brockhurst R.J., Schepens C.L., et al.: Peripheral uveitis II. *Am. J. Ophthalmol.* **49**: 1257, 1960.
Brockhurst R.J., Schepens C.L., et al.: Peripheral uveitis III. *Am. J. Ophthalmol.* **51**: 19, 1961.
Brockhurst R.J., Schepens C.L., et al.: Peripheral uveitis IV. *Arch. Ophthalmol.* **80**: 747–753, 1968.
Broughton W.L., Cupples H.P., Parver L.: Bilateral retinal detachment following cytomegalovirus retinitis. *Arch. Ophthalmol.* **96**: 618, 1978.
Brown D.H.: Ocular Toxocara canis: II. Clinical review. *J. Pediatr. Ophthalmol.* **7**: 182, 1970.
Byers B., Kimura S.J.: Uveitis after death of larva in the vitreous cavity. *Am. J. Ophthalmol.* **77**: 63, 1974.
Campinchi R.: Uveitis of tuberculous origin. Campinchi R., Faure J.P., Bloch-Michel E., Haut J. (eds.). In: *Uveitis, Immunologic and Allergic Phenomena,* Springfield, IL, Charles

C. Thomas, 1973, p. 366.

Carlson M.R., Kerman B.M.: Hemorrhagic macular detachment in the Vogt–Koyanagi–Harada syndrome. *Am. J. Ophthalmol.* **84**: 632, 1977.

Carney M.D., Peyman G.A., Goldberg M.F., *et al.*: Acute retinal necrosis. *Retina* **6**: 85–94, 1986.

Cassidy J.T., Brody G.L., Martel W.: Monoarticular juvenile rheumatoid arthritis. *J. Pediatr.* **70**: 867, 1967.

Catterall R.D., Perkins E.S.: Uveitis and urogenital disease in the male. *Br. J. Ophthalmol.* **45**: 109, 1961.

Char D.H., Margolis L., Newman A.B.: Ocular reticulum cell sarcoma. *Am. J. Ophthalmol.* **91**: 480, 1981.

Chumbley L.C., Kearns T.P.: Retinopathy of sarcoidosis. *Am. J. Ophthalmol.* **80**: 807, 1975.

Clarkson J.G., Blumenkranz M.S., Culbertson W.W., *et al.*: Retinal detachment following the acute retinal necrosis syndrome. *Ophthalmology* **91**: 1665–1668, 1984.

Cogan D.G.: Immunosuppression and eye disease. *Am. J. Ophthalmol.* **83**: 777–788, 1977.

Cogan D.G., Kuwabara T., Young G.F., Knox D.L.: Herpes simplex retinopathy in an infant. *Arch. Ophthalmol.* **72**: 641, 1964.

Coleman S.L., Brull S., Green W.R.: Sarcoid of the lacrimal sac and surrounding area. *Arch. Ophthalmol.* **88**: 645, 1972.

Colvard D.M., Robertoson D.M., O'Duffy J.D.: The ocular manifestations of Behçet's disease. *Arch. Ophthalmol.* **95**: 1813, 1977.

Cowper A.R.: Harada's disease and Vogt–Koyanagi syndrome: Uveoencephalitis. *Arch. Ophthalmol.* **45**: 367, 1951.

Crohn, B.B.: Ocular lesions complicating ulcerative colitis. *Am. J. Med. Soc.* **160**: 260, 1925.

Culbertson W.W., Blumenkranz M.S., Haines H., *et al.*: The acute retinal necrosis syndrome. Part 2: Histopathology and etiology. *Ophthalmology* **89**: 1317–1325, 1982.

Culbertson W.W., Blumenkranz M.S., Pepose J.S., *et al.*: Varicella zoster virus is a cause of the acute retinal necrosis syndrome. *Ophthalmology* **93**: 559–569, 1986.

Cutler J.E., Binder P.S., Paul T.O., *et al.*: Metastatic coccidioidal endophthalmitis. *Arch. Ophthalmol.* **96**: 689, 1978.

Darrell R.W.: Acute tuberculous panophthalmitis. *Arch. Ophthalmol.* **78**: 51, 1967.

Darrell R.W.: Endogenous aspergillus uveitis following heart surgery. *Arch. Ophthalmol.* **78**: 354, 1967.

Desmonts G.: Definitive serologic diagnosis of ocular toxoplasmosis. *Arch. Ophthalmol.* **76**: 839, 1966.

Deutman A.F., Grizzard W.S.: Rubella retinopathy and subretinal neovascularization. *Am. J. Ophthalmol.* **85**: 82, 1978.

Deutman A.F., Oosterhuis J.A., Boen-Tan T.N., Aan de Kerk A.L.: Acute posterior multifocal placoid pigment epitheliopathy. *Br. J. Ophthalmol.* **56**: 863, 1972.

de Veer J.A.: Bilateral endophthalmitis phacoanaphylactica. *Arch. Ophthalmol.* **49**: 607, 1953.

de Venecia G., Zu Rhein G.M., Pratt V.V., *et al.*: Cytomegalic inclusion retinitis in an adult. *Arch. Ophthalmol.* **86**: 44, 1971.

Dobbie J.G.: Cryotherapy in the management of toxoplasma retinochoroiditis. *Trans. Am. Acad. Ophthalmol. Otolaryngol.* **72**: 364, 1968.

Dobbie J.G.: Toxoplasma retinochoroiditis. *Ann. Ophthalmol.* **2**: 509, 1970.

Duker J.S., Nielsen J.C., Eagle R.C., Jr., Bosley T.M., Granadier R., Benson W.E.: Rapidly progressive acute retinal necrosis secondary to herpes simplex virus, type 1. *Ophthalmology* **97**: 1638–1643, 1990.

Duker, J.S., Blumenkranz, M.S.: Diagnosis and Management of the Acute Retinal Necrosis (ARN) Syndrome. *Surv. Ophthalmol.* **35**: 327–343, 1991.

Easom H.A., Zimmerman L.E.: Sympathetic ophthalmia and bilateral phacoanaphylaxis. *Arch. Ophthalmol.* **72**: 9, 1964.

Edwards T.F.: Ophthalmic complications from varicella. *J. Pediatr. Ophthalmol.* **2**: 37, 1965.

Elis P.P., Gentry J.H.: Ocular complications of ulcerative colitis. *Am. J. Ophthalmol.* **58**: 779, 1964.

Elliott J.H., Jackson D.J.: Presumed histoplasmic maculopathy. Clinical course and prognosis in nonphotocoagulated eyes. *Int. Ophthalmol. Clin.* **15**: 29, 1975.

Elliott J.H., O'Day D.M., Gutow G.S.: Mycotic endophthalmitis in drug abusers. *Am. J. Ophthalmol.* **88**: 66, 1979.

Epstein D.L., Jedzuniak J.A., Grant W.M.: Identification of Heavy-molecular-weight soluble lens protein in aqueous humor in human phacolytic glaucoma. *Invest. Ophthalmol.* **17**: 398, 1978.

Felberg N.T., Shields J.A., Federman J.L.: Antibody to *Toxocara canis* in aqueous humor. *Arch. Ophthalmol.* **99**: 1563–1564, 1981.

Fisher J.P., Lewis M.L., Blumenkranz M.S., *et al.*: The acute retinal necrosis syndrome. Part 1: Clinical manifestations. *Ophthalmology* **89**: 1309–1316, 1982.

Fishman L.S., Griffin J.R., Sapico F.L., *et al.*: Hematogenous Candida endophthalmitis – complication of candidema. *N. Engl. J. Med.* **286**: 675, 1972.

Fitzgerald C.R.: Pars plana vitrectomy for vitreous opacity secondary to presumed toxoplasmosis. *Arch. Ophthalmol.* **98**: 321, 1980.

Fitzpatrick P.J., Robertson D.M.: Acute posterior multifocal placoid pigment epitheliopathy. *Arch. Ophthalmol.* **89**: 373, 1973.

Flocks M., Littwin C.S., Zimmerman L.E.: Phacolytic glaucoma. *Arch. Ophthalmol.* **54**: 37, 1955.

Font R.L., Rao N.A., Issarescu S.: Ocular involvement in Whipple's disease. *Arch. Ophthalmol.* **96**: 1431, 1978.

Foster C.S., Fong L.P., Singh G.: Cataract surgery and intraocular lens implantation in patients with uveitis. *Ophthalmology* **96**: 281–288, 1989.

Franceschetti A.: Heterochromic cyclitis (Fuchs' syndrome). *Am. J. Ophthalmol.* **39**: 50, 1955.

Freeman W.R., Thomas E.L., Rao N.A., *et al.*: Demonstration of herpes group virus in acute retinal necrosis syndrome. *Am. J. Ophthalmol.* **102**: 701–709, 1986.

Frenkel J.K.: Pathogenesis of toxoplasmosis with a consideration of cyst rupture in Besnoitia infection. *Surv. Ophthalmol.* **6**: 799, 1961.

Frenkel J.K., Jacobs L.: Ocular toxoplasmosis. Pathogenesis, diagnosis, and treatment. *Arch. Ophthalmol.* **59**: 260, 1958.

Friedlander M.: *Allergy and Immunology of the Eye*, Hagerstown, MD, Harper & Row, 1979.

Friedman A.H., Deutsch-Sokol R.H.: Sugiuras sign: Perilimbal vitiligo in the Vogt–Koyanagi–Harada Syndrome. *Ophthalmology* **88**: 1159, 1981.

Friedmann C.T., Knox D.L.: Variations in active toxoplasmic retinochoroiditis. *Arch. Ophthalmol.* **81**: 481, 1969.

Fujikawa L.S.: Advances in immunology and uveitis. *Ophthalmology* **96**: 1115–1120, 1989.

Fujikawa L.S., Haugen J.-P.: Immunopathology of vitreous and retinochoroidal biopsy in posterior uveitis. *Ophthalmology* **97**: 1644–1653, 1990.

Gass J.D.M.: Pathogenesis of disciform detachment of the neuroepithelium. V. Disciform macular degeneration secondary to focal choroiditis. *Am. J. Ophthalmol.* **63**: 661, 1967.

Gass J.D.M.: Acute posterior multifocal placoid pigment epitheliopathy. *Arch. Ophthalmol.* **80**: 177, 1968.

Gass J.D.M.: Vitiliginous chorioretinitis. *Arch. Ophthalmol.* **99**: 1778–1787, 1981.

Gass J.D.M.: Uveal effusion syndrome. *Retina* **3**: 159–163, 1983.

Gass J.D.M., Olson C.L.: Sarcoidosis with optic nerve and retinal involvement: A clinicopathologic case report. *Trans. Am. Acad. Ophthalmol. Otolaryngol.* **77**: 739, 1973.

Gass J.D.M., Wilkinson C.P.: Follow-up study of presumed ocular histoplasmosis. *Trans. Am. Acad. Ophthalmol. Otolaryngol.* **76**: 672, 1972.

Gass J.D.M., Jallow S.: Idiopathic serous detachment of the choroid, ciliary body, and retina (uveal effusion) syndrome. *Ophthalmology* **89**: 1018–1032, 1982.

Gee S.S., Khalid F.T.: Extracapsular cataract extraction in Fuchs' heterochromic iridocyclitis. *Am. J. Ophthalmol.* **108**: 310–314, 1989.

Ghartey K.N., Brockhurst R.J.: Photocoagulation of active toxoplasmic retinochoroiditis. *Am. J. Ophthalmol.* **89**: 854, 1980.

Giles C.L.: The treatment of Toxoplasma uveitis with pyrimethamine and folonic acid. *Am. J. Ophthalmol.* **58**: 611, 1964.

Giles C.L.: Peripheral uveitis in patients with multiple sclerosis. *Am. J. Ophthalmol.* **70**: 17, 1970.

Giles C.L.: Pyrimethamine (Daraprim) and the treatment of toxoplasmic uveitis. *Surv. Ophthalmol.* **16**: 88, 1971.

Girard L.J., Rodriguez J., Mailman M.L., Romano T.J.: Cataract and uveitis management by pars plana lensectomy and vitrectomy by ultrasonic fragmentation. *Retina* **5**: 107–114, 1985.

Godfrey W.A., Sabates R., Cross D.D.: Association of presumed ocular histoplasmosis with HLA-B7. *Am. J. Ophthalmol.* **85**: 845, 1978.

Goldberg M.F.: Cytological diagnosis of phacolytic glaucoma utilizing millipore filtration of the aqueous. *Br. J. Ophthalmol.* **51**: 847, 1967.

Goldberg M.F., Croxan Y., Duke J.R., et al.: Cytopathologic and histopathologic aspect of Fuchs' heterochromic iridocyclitis. *Arch. Ophthalmol.* **74**: 604, 1965.

Gorman B.D., Nadel A.J., Coles R.S.: Acute retinal necrosis. *Ophthalmology* **89**: 809–814, 1982.

Gravina R.F., Nakanishi A.S., Faden A.: Subacute sclerosing panencephalitis. *Am. J. Ophthalmol.* **86**: 106, 1978.

Green W.R., Bennett J.E.: Coccidiomycosis. *Arch. Ophthalmol.* **77**: 337, 1967.

Grieco M.H., Freilich D.B.: Diagnosis of cryptococcal uveitis with hypertonic media. *Am. J. Ophthalmol.* **72**: 171, 1971.

Griffin J.R., Pettit T.H., Fishman L.S., et al.: Bloodborne Candida endophthalmitis. *Arch. Ophthalmol.* **89**: 450, 1973.

Haarr M.: Rheumatic iridocyclitis. *Acta. Ophthalmol.* **38**: 37, 1960.

Hamilton A.M., Bird A.C.: Geographical choroidopathy. *Br. J. Ophthalmol.* **58**: 777, 1974.

Hanscom T.A., Diddie K.R.: Early surgical drainage of macular subretinal hemorrhage. *Arch. Ophthalmol.* **105**: 1722, 1987.

Harada Y.: Beitrag zur klinischen Kenntnis von nichteitriger choroiditis. (Choroiditis diffusa acuta.) *Acta. Soc. Ophthalmol. Jpn.* **30**: 356, 1926.

Harris D., Birch C.L.: Bilateral uveitis associated with gastrointestinal *Entamoeba histolytica* infection: Case report. *Am. J. Ophthalmol.* **50**: 496, 1960.

Hart W.M., Reed C.A., Freedman H.L., et al.: Cytomegalovirus in juvenile iridocyclitis. *Am. J. Ophthalmol.* **86**: 329, 1978.

Hinzpeter E.N., Naumann G., Bartelheimer H.K.: Ocular histopathology in Still's disease. *Ophthalmol. Res.* **2**: 16, 1971.

Hodes B.L., Stern G.: Phacoanaphylactic endophthalmitis: Echographic diagnosis of phacoanaphylactic endophthalmitis. *Ophthalmic Surg.* **7**: 60, 1976.

Hogan M.J.: Ocular toxoplasmosis. *Am. J. Ophthalmol.* **46**: 467, 1958.

Hogan M.J., Kimura S.J., Spencer W.H.: Visceral larva migrans and peripheral retinitis. *J. Am. Med. Assoc.* **194**: 1345, 1965.

Holland G.N., Engstrom R.E., Jr., Glasgow B.J., et al.: Ocular toxoplasmosis in patients with acquired immunodeficiency syndrome. *Am. J. Ophthalmol.* **106**: 653, 1988.

Hyvarinen L., Lerer R.J., Knox D.L.: Fluorescent angiographic findings in presumed ocular histoplasmosis. *Am. J. Ophthalmol.* **71**: 449, 1971.

Intraocular Inflammation, Uveitis and Ocular Tumors, Ophthalmology Basic and Clinical Science Course (Section 3). *Am. Acad. Ophthalmol.*, San Francisco, 1981–1982.

Irvine A.R., Jr.: Nematodiosis: Clinical description and pathology. In: Kimura S., Caygill W. (eds.), *Retinal Diseases*. Philadelphia, Lea and Febiger, 1979, pp. 348–251.

Irvine A.R., Spencer W.H., Hogan M.J., et al.: Presumed chronic ocular histoplasmosis syndrome: A clinical-pathologic case report. *Trans. Am. Ophthalmol. Soc.* **74**: 91, 1976.

Irvine S.R., Irvine A.R., Jr.: Lens induced uveitis and glaucoma. Part II. The 'phacotoxic' reaction. *Am. J. Ophthalmol.* **35**: 370, 1952.

Irvine W.C., Irvine A.R., Jr.: Nematode endophthalmitis, *Toxocara canis*. *Am. J. Ophthalmol.* **47**: 185–191, 1959.

James D.G.: Ocular lesions in sarcoidosis. *Am. J. Med.* **26**: 331, 1959.

James D.J., Anderson R., Langley D., et al.: Ocular sarcoidosis. *Br. J. Ophthalmol.* **48**: 461, 1964.

Jampel H.D., Jabs D.A., Quigely H.A.: Trabeculectomy with 5-fluorouracil for adult inflammatory glaucoma. *Am. J. Ophthalmol.* **109**: 168–173, 1990.

Jensen E.: Retino-choroiditis juxtapapillaris. *Arch. Ophthalmol.* **69**: 41, 1909.

Kalina P.H., Pach J.M., Buettner H., Robertson D.M.: Neovascularization of the disc in pars planitis. *Retina* **10**: 269–273, 1990.

Kaplan H.J.: Discussion of cataract surgery and intraocular lens implantation in patients with uveitis. *Ophthalmology* **96**: 287–288, 1989.

Kaplan H.J., Aaberg T.M.: Birdshot retinochoroidopathy.

Am. J. Ophthalmol. **90**: 773, 1980.

Kaufman H.E., Kanai A., Ellison W.E.D.: Herpetic iritis: Demonstration of virus in the anterior chamber by fluorescent antibody techniques and electron microscopy. *Am. J. Ophthalmol.* **71**: 465, 1971.

Kelley J.S., Green W.R.: Sarcoidosis involving the optic nervehead. *Arch. Ophthalmol.* **89**: 486, 1973.

Kelly P.J., Weiter J.J.: Resolution of optic disk neovascularization associated with intraocular inflammation. *Am. J. Ophthalmol.* **90**: 545–548, 1980.

Kimura S.J., Hogan M.J., Tjhygeson P.: Fuchs' syndrome of heterochromic cyclitis. *Arch. Ophthalmol.* **54**: 186, 1955.

Kimura S., Hogan L.: Chronic cyclitis. *Arch. Ophthalmol.* **71**: 183, 1964.

Kimura S.J., Hogan J.J., O'Connor G.R., et al.: Uveitis and joint diseases. *Arch. Ophthalmol.* **77**: 309, 1967.

Klingele T.G., Hogan M.J.: Ocular reticulum cell sarcoma. *Am. J. Ophthalmol.* **79**: 39, 1975.

Landers M.B., Klintworth G.K.: Subacute sclerosing panencephalitis (SSPE). *Arch. Ophthalmol.* **86**: 156, 1971.

Lewis M.L., Van Newkirk M.R., Gass J.D.M.: Follow-up study of presumed ocular histoplasmosis syndrome. *Ophthalmology* **87**: 390, 1980.

Lichter P.R.: Intraocular lenses in uveitis patients. *Ophthalmology* **96**: 279–280, 1989.

Liesegang T.J.: Clinical features and prognosis in Fuchs' uveitis syndrome. *Arch. Ophthalmol.* **100**: 1622, 1982.

Lowenfeld I.E., Thompson H.S.: Fuchs' heterochromic cyclitis: A critical review of the literature. I. Clinical characteristic of the syndrome. *Surv. Ophthalmol.* **17**: 394, 1973.

Lowenfeld I.E., Thompson H.S.: Fuchs' heterochromic cyclitis: A critical review of the literature. II. Etiology and mechanisms. *Surv. Ophthalmol.* **18**: 2, 1973.

Lubin J.R., Albery D.M., Weinstein M.: 65 years of sympathetic ophthalmia: A clinicopathologic review of 105 cases (1913–1978). *Ophthalmology* **87**: 109, 1980.

Macular Photocoagulation Study Group: Argon laser for ocular histoplasmosis. Results of a randomized clinical trial. *Arch. Ophthalmol.* **101**: 1347, 1983.

Makley T.A., Jr.: Heterochromic cyclitis in identical twins. *Am. J. Ophthalmol.* **41**: 768, 1956.

Makley T.A., Azar A.: Sympathetic ophthalmia. *Arch. Ophthalmol.* **96**: 257, 1978.

Mamo J.G., Azzam S.A.: Treatment of Behçet's disease with chlorambucil. *Arch. Ophthalmol.* **84**: 446, 1970.

Margolis L., Fraser R., Lichter A., et al.: The role of radiation therapy and the management of ocular reticulum cell sarcoma. *Cancer* **45**: 688, 1980.

Matsuda H.: Electron microscopic studies on Vogt–Koyanagi–Harada syndrome and sympathetic ophthalmia with special reference to the melanocyte. *Acta. Soc. Ophthalmol. Jpn.* **74**: 1107, 1970.

Maumenee A.E.: Clinical entities in uveitis. *Trans. Am. Acad. Ophthalmol. Otolaryngol.* **74**: 473, 1970.

Meredith T.A., Green W.R., Key S.N., et al.: Ocular histoplasmosis. Clinicopathologic correlation of 3 cases. *Surv. Ophthalmol.* **22**: 189, 1977.

Michels R.G., Know D.L., Eronsan N.S.: Intraocular reticulum cell sarcoma. *Arch. Ophthalmol.* **93**: 1331, 1975.

Michelson J.B.: Infectious clinical uveitis. *Current Opinion in Ophthalmology* **1**: 373–384, 1990.

Michelson J.B., Friedlaender M.H.: Behçet's disease. *Int. Ophthalmol. Clin.* **30**: 271–278, 1990.

Michelson J.B., Friedlaender M.H.: Endophthalmitis of drug abuse. *Int. Ophthalmol. Clin.* **27**: 120–126, 1987.

Michelson J.B., Friedlaender M.H., Nozik R.A.: Lens implant surgery in pars planitis. *Ophthalmology* **97**: 1023–1026, 1990.

Michelson J.B., Friedlaender M.H., O'Connor G.R.: Keratocentesis and vitreous biopsy. In: Duane T.D., Jaeger E.A. (eds.) *Clinical Ophthalmology*, Philadelphia, J.B. Lippincott, 1988.

Michelson J.B., Shields J.A., McDonald P.R., et al.: Retinitis secondary to acquired systemic toxoplasmosis with isolation of the parasite. *Am. J. Ophthalmol.* **86**: 548, 1978.

Michelson J.B., Roth A.M., Waring G.O.: Lepromatous iridocyclitis diagnosed by anterior chamber paracentesis. *Am. J. Ophthalmol.* **88**: 674, 1979.

Michelson J.B., et al.: Foreign body granuloma of the retina associated with intravenous cocaine addiction. *Am. J. Ophthalmol.* **87**: 278, 1979.

Michelson J.B., et al.: Subretinal neovascular membrane and disciform scar in Behçet's disease. *Am. J. Ophthalmol.* **90**: 182, 1980.

Michelson J.B., et al.: Ocular reticulum cell sarcoma: Presentation as retinal detachment with demonstration of monoclonal immunoglobulins light chains on the vitreous cells. *Arch. Ophthalmol.* **99**: 1409, 1981.

Michelson J.B., Freedman S.D., Boyden D.G.: Aspergillus endophthalmitis in a drug abuser. *Ann. Ophthalmol.* **14**: 1051–1057, 1982.

Michelson J.B., Chisari F.V.: Behçet's disease, a review. *Surv. Ophthalmol.* **26**: 190–203, 1982.

Michelson J.B., Belmont J.B., Higginbottom, P.: Juxtapapillary choroiditis associated with chronic meningitis due to *Coccidiodes immitis*. *Ann. Ophthamol.* **15**: 666–668, 1983.

Michelson J.B.: 'Melting Corneas and Collapsing Nose' Relapsing Polychondritis-C.P.C.—clinical challenges. *Surv. Ophthalmol.* (in press).

Michelson P., Stark W., Reeser F., Green W.R.: Endogenous Candida Endophthalmitis: Report of Thirteen Cases and a Review of the Literature. *International Ophthalmol Clinics, Ocular Pathology*, Vol. II, No. 3, pp. 125–147, Fall, 1971. Excerpts in Audio Digest, Volume 8, No. 11, 1970.

Michelson P, Knox D., Green W.R.: Ischemic ocular inflammation: A clinicopathologic case report. *Arch. Ophthalmol.* **86**: 274, 1971.

Mieler W.F., Will B.R., Lewis H., Aaberg T.M.: Vitrectomy in the management of peripheral uveitis. *Ophthalmology* **95**: 859–864, 1988.

Mills K.B., Rosen E.S.: Intraocular lens implantation following cataract extraction in Fuchs' heterochromic uveitis. *Ophthalmic Surg.* **13**: 467–469, 1982.

Minckler D.S., Font R.L., Zimmerman L.E.: Uveitis and reticulum cell sarcoma of brain with bilateral neoplastic seeding of the vitreous without retinal or uveal involvement. *Am. J. Ophthalmol.* **80**: 433, 1975.

Murray H.W., Knox D.L., Green W.R., et al.: Cytomegalovirus retinitis in adults: A manifestation of disseminated virus infection. *Am. J. Med.* **63**: 574, 1977.

Neumann E., Gunders A.E.: Pathogenesis of the posterior segment lesions of ocular onchocerciasis. *Am. J. Ophthalmol.* **75**: 82, 1973.

Nichols C.W., Eagle R.C., Yanoff M.: Conjunctival biopsy as an aid in the evaluation of the patient with suspected sarcoidosis. *Ophthalmology* **87**, 1980.

Nicholson D.H.: Cytomegalovirus infection of the retina.

Int. Ophthalmol. Clin. **15**: 37, 1975.
Nobe J.R., Kokoris N., Diddie K.R., et al.: Lensectomy–vitrectomy in chronic uveitis. *Retina* **3**: 71–76, 1983.
Nozik R.A., Vignette: The tailored laboratory investigation of urveitis ophthalmology: Basic and Clinical Science Course, Section III, Intraocular inflammation uveitis and ocular tumors. *Am. Acad. Ophthalmol.* 1981–1982, pp. 142–150.
Nozik R.A., Smith R.E., Michelson J.B., Weinberg R.S.: Practical uveitis A.A.O. course. Ophthalmology Annual Meeting Supplement, 1983.
Obenauf C.D., Shaw H.E., Sydnor C.F., et al.: Sarcoidosis and its ocular manifestations. *Am. J. Ophthalmol.* **86**, 1978.
O'Connor G.R.: The influence of hypersensitivity on the pathogenesis of ocular toxoplasmosis. *Trans. Am. Ophthalmol. Soc.* **68**: 501, 1970.
O'Connor G.R.: Manifestations and management of ocular toxoplasmosis. *Bull. N.Y. Acad. Med.* **50**: 192, 1974.
O'Connor G.R., Frenkel J.K.: Dangers of steroid treatment in toxoplasmosis: Periocular injections and systemic therapy. *Arch. Ophthalmol.* **94**: 213, 1976.
O'Connor G.R.: Uveitis and the immunologically compromised host. *N. Engl. J. Med.* **299**: 130–132, 1978.
O'Connor P.R.: Visceral larva migrans of the eye: Subretinal tube formation. *Arch. Ophthalmol.* **88**: 526, 1972.
Ohno S., Char D.H., Kimura S.J., et al.: Vogt–Koyanagi–Harada syndrome *Am. J. Ophthalmol.* **83**: 735, 1977.
Ohno S., Kimura S.J., O'Connor G.R., et al.: HLA antigens and uveitis. *Br. J. Ophthalmol.* **61**: 62, 1977.
Ophir A., Ticho U.: Remission of anterior uveitis by subconjunctival fluorouracil. *Arch. Ophthalmol.* **109**: 12–13, 1991.
Ostler H.B., Dawson C.R., Schacter J., et al.: Reiter's syndrome. *Am. J. Ophthalmol.* **71**: 986, 1971.
Palmer E.A.: Endogenous Candida endophthalmitis in infants. *Am. J. Ophthalmol.* **89**: 388, 1980.
Parver L.M., Font R.L.: Malignant lymphoma of the retina and brain: Initial diagnosis by cytologic examination of vitreous aspirate. *Arch. Ophthalmol.* **97**: 1505, 1979.
Pederson J.E., Kenyon K.R., Green W.R., et al.: Pathology of pars planitis. *Am. J. Ophthalmol.* **86**: 762–774, 1978.
Perkins E.S.: Patterns of uveitis in children. *Br. J. Ophthalmol.* **50**: 169, 1966.
Perkins, E.S.: Ocular toxoplasmosis. *Br. J. Ophthalmol.* **57**: 1, 1973.
Perry H.D., Font R.L.: Clinical and histopathologic observations in severe Vogt–Koyanagi–Harada syndrome. *Am. J. Ophthalmol.* **83**: 242, 1977.
Pettit T.H., Learn R., Foos R.Y.: Intraocular coccidioidomycosis. *Arch. Ophthalmol.* **77**: 655, 1967.
Petrilli A.M., Belfort R., Jr., Abreu M.T., et al.: Ultrasonic fragmentation of cataract in uveitis. *Retina* **6**: 61–65, 1986.
Phillips C.A., Fanning W.L., Gump D.W., et al.: Cytomegalovirus encephalitis in immunologically normal adults: Successful treatment with vidarabine. *J. Am. Med. Assoc.* **238**: 2299, 1977.
Pollard Z.F., Jarrett W.H., Hagler W.S., et al.: ELISA for diagnosis of ocular toxocariasis. *Ophthalmology* **86**: 743, 1979.
Pollard Z.F.: Ocular Toxocara in siblings of two families. *Arch. Ophthalmol.* **97**: 2319, 1979.
Price F.W., Schlaegel T.F., Jr.: Bilateral acute retinal necrosis. *Am. J. Ophthalmol.* **89**: 419–424, 1980.
Pruett R.C., Brockhurst R.J., Letts N.F.: Fluorescein angiography of peripheral uveitis. *Am. J. Ophthalmol.* **77**: 448, 1974.
Rainen E.A., Little H.L.: Ocular coccidioidomycosis: A clinicopathologic case report. *Trans. Am. Acad. Ophthalmol. Otolaryngol.* **76**: 645, 1972.
Ramsey M.S., Willis N.R.: Endogenous Candida endophthalmitis. *Can. J. Ophthalmol.* **7**: 126, 1972.
Richards W.W., Arrington J.M.: Unsuspected ocular leprosy. *Am. J. Ophthalmol.* **68**: 491, 1969.
Riise P.: Endophthalmitis phacoanaphylactica. *Am. J. Ophthalmol.* **69**: 911, 1965.
Robb R.M., Waters G.V.: Ophthalmic manifestations of subacute sclerosing panencephalitis. *Arch. Ophthalmol.* **83**: 426, 1970.
Robertson D.M., Riley F.C., Hermans P.E.: Endogenous Candida oculomycosis. *Arch. Ophthalmol.* **91**: 33, 1974.
Rockey J.H., Donnelly J.J., Stromberg B.E., et al.: Immunopathology of *Toxocara canis* and *Ascaris suum* infections of the eye: The role of the eosinophil. *Invest. Ophthalmol. Vis. Sci.* **18**: 1172, 1979.
Rodenbiker H.T., Ganley J.P.: Ocular coccidioidomycosis. *Surv. Ophthalmol.* **24**: 263, 1980.
Rose L.: Filarial worm in anterior chamber of eye of man. *Arch. Ophthalmol.* **75**: 13, 1965.
Ross W.H., Sutton H.F.S.: Acquired syphilitic uveitis. *Arch. Ophthalmol.* **98**: 496, 1980.
Ryan S.J.: De novo subretinal neovascularization is histoplasmosis syndrome. *Arch. Ophthalmol.* **94**: 321, 1976.
Ryan S.J., Maumenee A.E.: Acute posterior multifocal placoid epitheliopathy. *Am. J. Ophthalmol.* **74**: 1066, 1972.
Ryan S.J., Maumenee A.E.: Birdshot retinochoroidopathy. *Am. J. Ophthalmol.* **89**: 31, 1980.
Saari M., Vuorre I., Kaila J., et al.: Family studies of ocular manifestations in arthritis. *Can. J. Ophthamol.* **13**: 144, 1978.
Saari M., Vuorre I., Neiminen H., et al.: Acquired toxoplasmic chorioretinitis. *Arch. Ophthalmol.* **94**: 1485, 1976.
Sabates R., Pruett R.C., Brockhurst R.J.: Fulminant ocular toxoplasmosis. *Am. J. Ophthalmol.* **92**: 497, 1981.
Sawelson H., Goldberg R.E., Annesley W.H., Jr., et al.: Presumed ocular histoplasmosis syndrome. *Arch. Ophthalmol.* **94**: 221, 1976.
Schaller J.S., Johnson G.D., Holborow E.J., et al.: The association of ANA with chronic iridocyclitis of JRA. *Arthritis Rheum.* **17**: 409, 1974.
Schaller J., Kupfer C., Wedgwood R.J.: Iridocyclitis in juvenile rheumatoid arthritis. *Pediatrics* **44**: 92, 1969.
Schantz P.M., Glickman L.T.: Toxocaral visceral larva migrans. *N. Engl. J. Med.* **298**: 436, 1978.
Scharf J., Miller B., et al.: HL-A 27 antigen associated with uveitis and ankylosing spondylitis in a family. *Am. J. Ophthalmol.* **82**: 139, 1976.
Scheie H.G., McLellan T.G.: Treatment of herpes zoster ophthalmicus with corticotropin and corticosteroids. *Arch. Ophthalmol.* **62**: 579, 1959.
Scheie H.G., Morse P.H.: Rubeola retinopathy. *Arch. Ophthalmol.* **88**: 341, 1972.
Schepens C.L., Brockhurst R.J.: Uveal effusion. I. Clinical picture. *Arch. Ophthalmol.* **70**: 189, 1963.
Schlaegel T.F., O'Connor G.R.: Tuberculosis and syphilis. *Arch. Ophthalmol.* **99**: 2206, 1981.
Schlaegel T.F.: The natural history of histo spots in the disc-macular area. *Int. Ophthalmol. Clin.* **15**: 19, 1975.
Schlaegel T.F., Jr.: *Essentials of Uveitis*, Boston, Little,

Brown & Co., 1969, Ch. 4–12.

Schlaegel T.F., Jr.: Granulomatous uveitis: An etiologic survey of 100 cases. *Trans. Am. Acad. Ophthalmol. Otolaryngol.* **62**: 813, 1958.

Schlaegel T.F., Jr., Knox D.L.: Toxocariasis. In: *Duane's Clinical Ophthalmology*, T.D. Duane (ed.), Vol. 4, Ch. 52, Hagerstown, MD, Harper & Row, 1976.

Schlaegel T.F., Jr., Weber J.C.: Double-blind therapeutic trial of isoniazid in 344 patients with uveitis. *Br. J. Ophthalmol.* **53**: 42, 1968.

Schofield P.B.: Phacolytic glaucoma. *Trans. Ophthalmol. Soc. UK* **77**: 193, 1977.

Schwartz L.K., O'Connor G.R.: Secondary syphilis with iris papules. *Am. J. Ophthalmol.* **90**: 380, 1980.

Sheffer A., Green W.R., Fine S.L., *et al.*: Presumed ocular histoplasmosis syndrome. A clinicopathologic correlation of a treated case. *Arch Ophthalmol.* **98**: 335, 1980.

Shields J.A.: Ocular toxocariasis: Review. *Surv. Ophthalmol.* **28**: 361–381, 1984.

Shimada K., O'Connor G.R., Yoneda C.: Cyst formation by *Toxoplasma gondii* (RH strain) *in vitro*. *Arch. Ophthalmol.* **92**: 496, 1974.

Siltzbach L.E., James D.G., Neville E.: Course and prognosis of sarcoidosis around the world. *Am. J. Med.* **57**: 847, 1974.

Silveira C., Belfort R., Jr., Burnier J., Jr., Nussenblatt R.B.: Acquired toxoplasmic infection as the cause of toxoplasmic retinochoroiditis in families. *Am. J. Ophthalmol.* **106**: 362, 1988.

Silverman M.S., Hughes S.E.: Transplantation of photoreceptors to light-damaged retina. *Invest. Ophthalmol. Vis. Sci.* **30**: 1684, 1989.

Silverstein A.M., O'Connor G.R. (eds.): *Immunology and Immunopathology of the Eye*, New York, Masson, 1979.

Simpson G.V.: Diagnosis and treatment of uveitis in association with sarcoidosis. *Trans. Am. Ophthalmol. Soc.* **66**: 117, 1968.

Slem G.: Clinical studies of ocular leprosy. *Am. J. Ophthalmol.* **71**: 431, 1971.

Smiley A.E.: The eye in juvenile rheumatoid arthritis. *Trans. Ophthalmol. Soc. UK* **94**: 817, 1974.

Smith J.L.: Recent observations on the treatment of late ocular syphilis and neurosyphilis. *Trans. Am. Acad. Ophthalmol. Otolaryngol.* **73**: 1113, 1969.

Smith M.E.: Retinal involvement in adult cytomegalic inclusion disease. *Arch. Ophthalmol.* **72**: 44, 1964.

Smith P.H., Greer C.H.: Unusual presentation of ocular *Toxocara* infestation. *Br. J. Ophthalmol.* **55**: 317, 1971.

Smith R.E., Nozik R.A.: *Uveitis. A Clinical Approach to Diagnosis and Management*, Baltimore, Williams & Wilkins, 1983, pp. 185–187.

Smith R.E.: Ocular histoplasmosis. In: S.J. Ryan, R.E. Smith (eds.), *Selected Topics on the Eye in Systemic Disease*, New York, Grune and Stratton, 1974, p. 135.

Smith R.E., Ganley J.P.: Presumed ocular histoplasmosis. I. Histoplasmin skin test sensitivity in cases identified during a community survey. *Arch. Ophthalmol.* **87**: 245, 1972.

Smith R.E., Nozik R.A.: *Uveitis, a Clinical Approach to Diagnosis and Management*, Baltimore, Williams & Wilkins, 1983.

Smith R.E., Godfrey S.A., Kimura S.J.: Chronic cyclitis. I. Course and visual prognosis. *Trans. Am. Acad. Ophthalmol. Otolaryngol.* **77**: 760, 1973.

Smith R.E., Godfrey S.A., Kimura S.J.: Complications of chronic cyclitis. *Am. J. Ophthalmol.* **82**: 277–282, 1976.

Smith R.E., O'Connor G.R.: Cataract extraction in Fuchs' syndrome. *Arch. Ophthalmol.* **91**: 39, 1974.

Snyder D.A., Tessler H.H.: Vogt–Koyanagi–Harada syndrome. *Am. J. Ophthalmol.* **90**: 69, 1980.

Sullivan S.F., Dallow R.L.: Intraocular reticulum cell sarcoma – its dramatic response to systemic chemotherapy and its angiogenic potential. *Ann. Ophthalmol.* **9**: 401, 1977.

Tabbara K.F., O'Connor G.R.: Treatment of ocular toxoplasmosis with clindomycin and sulfadiazine. *Ophthalmology* **87**: 129, 1980.

Thomas M.A., Kaplan H.J.: Surgical removal of subfoveal neovascularization in the presumed ocular histoplasmosis syndrome. *Am. J. Ophthalmol.* **111**: 1–7, 1991.

Tjhygeson P., Ostler H.B.: Zoster and herpes simplex virus uveitis: A comparison. In: *Immunology and Immunopathology of the Eye*, New York, Masson, 1979, p.230.

Toussaint D., Danis P.: Retinopathy in generalized Loa-Loa filariasis. *Arch. Ophthalmol.* **74**: 470, 1965.

Uchida Y., Kakehashi Y., Kameyama K.: Juxtapapillary retinochoroiditis with a psychiatric disorder possibly caused by *Toxoplasma*. *Am. J. Ophthalmol.* **86**: 791, 1978.

VanMetre T.E., Jr., Maumenee A.E.: Specific ocular uveal lesions in patients with evidence of histoplasmosis. *Arch. Ophthalmol.* **71**: 314, 1964.

von Noorden G.K., Guck A.A.: Ocular onchocerciasis. *Arch. Ophthalmol.* **80**: 26, 1978.

Wade E.C., Flynn H.W., Jr., Olsen K.R., Blumenkranz M.S., Nicholson D.H.: Subretinal hemorrhage management by pars plana vitrectomy and internal drainage. *Arch. Ophthalmol.* **108**: 973, 1990.

Wagoner M.D., Goner J.R., Albert D.M., *et al.*: Intraocular reticulum cell sarcoma. *Ophthalmology* **87**: 724, 1980.

Wan W.L., Cano M.R., Pince K.J., Green R.L.: Echographic characteristics of ocular toxocariasis. *Ophthalmology* **98**: 28–32, 1991.

Weinberg R., Tessler H.: Serum lysozyme in sarcoid uveitis. *Am. J. Ophthalmol.* **82**: 105, 1976.

Weinreb R.N., Barth R., Kimura S.J.: Limited Gallium scans and angiotensin converting enzyme in granulomatous uveitis. *Ophthalmology* **87**: 207, 1980.

Weinreb R.N., Kimura S.J.: Uveitis associated with sarcoidosis and angiotensin converting enzyme. *Am. J. Ophthalmol.* **89**: 180, 1980.

Weiss M.J., Velazquez N., Hofeldt A.J.: Serologic tests in the diagnosis of presumed toxoplasmic retinochoroiditis. *Am. J. Ophthalmol.* **109**: 407, 1990.

Wilder H.C.: Nematode endophthalmitis. *Trans. Am. Acad. Ophthalmol. Otolaryngol.* **55**: 99, 1950.

Wilder H.C.: Nematode endophthalmitis. *Trans. Am. Acad. Ophthalmol. Otolaryngol.* **42**: 129, 1960.

Wilkinson C.P., Welch R.B.: Intraocular Toxocara. *Am. J. Ophthalmol.* **71**: 921, 1971.

Winterkorn J.M.S.: Lyme Disease: Neurologic and ophthalmic manifestations. *Surv. Ophthalmol.* **35**: 191–204, 1990.

Wirostko E., Spalter H.F.: Lens induced uveitis. *Arch. Ophthalmol.* **78**: 1, 1967.

Wolff S.M.: The ocular manifestations of congenital rubella. *Trans. Am. Ophthalmol. Soc.* **70**: 577, 1972.

Woods A.C., Guyton, J.S.: Role of a sarcoidosis and of brucellosis in uveitis. *Arch. Ophthalmol.* **31**: 469, 1944.

Woods A.C.: *Endogenous Inflammation of the Uveal Tract*, Baltimore, Williams and Wilkins Co., 1961, p.357.

Index

Index

All numerals refer to page numbers

A

Acquired immune deficiency syndrome (AIDS), 55–7
   cytomegalovirus, 119
   toxoplasmosis, 92
Acquired syphilis, 63
Acute hemorrhaging subretinal neovascular membrane, 29
Acute multifocal placoid pigment epitheliopathy (AMPPE), 127
Acute multifocal posterior plaquoid epitheliopathy, 27
Acute necrotizing herpes zoster retinitis, 55
Acute ocular histoplasmosis syndrome, 28
Acute syphilitic infection, 58
AIDS-related complex, 55
Amphoterocin B, 83, 143
Anesthetic nodules, 110, 111
Angioid streaks, 35, 81
Ankylosing spondylitis, 5, 45–6
   Koeppe nodule, 16
   steroid treatment, 21
Anterior segment ischemia, 9
Anterior uveitis in Behçet's disease, 97
Aphthous ulcer, 97, 98
   on tongue, 9
ARN syndrome *see* bilateral acute retinal necrosis
Arthritic uveitides, 5
Aspergillus endophthalmitis, 141
Astrocytic hamartoma, 31
Azathioprine (AZT), 119, 121

B

Bamboo spine, 46
Band keratopathy, 12, 42, 125
   with sarcoidosis, 49, 50
BARN syndrome *see* bilateral acute retinal necrosis
Behçet's disease, 8, 9, 15, 97–101
   ciliary circulation vasculitis, 30
   hypopyon, 15
   inactive vasculitis, 23
   Molteno implantation, 36
   necrotizing vasculitis, 23
   ocular symptoms, 97
   profound retinal infarction, 23
   traction retinal detachment, 36
Berlin's nodules, 22
   with sarcoidosis, 49
Bilateral acute retinal necrosis, 131–2
Birdshot choroidopathy, 133–4
Borrelia burgdorferi, 59
Bot fly larva, 89
Brain
   multiple small foci, 61
   reticulum cell sarcoma, 104, 106
Busacca nodules, 17
   with sarcoidosis, 49
Butterfly eruptions on lids and maxilla, 65

C

Candida endophthalmitis, 143
Candidiasis, 55
Candle wax drippings, 49, 53
Cataract
   in Fuch's heterochromic iridocyclitis, 135, 136
   in pars planitis, 125
   surgery, 43
   with monarticular rheumatoid arthritis, 43
   with sarcoidosis, 49
Chlorambucil, 97
Chorioretinitis in MEWDS, 130
Chorioretinopathy in relapsing polychondritis, 137
Choroidal infiltration, focal, 113
Choroiditis
   in Vogt–Koyanagi–Harada syndrome, 69
   multifocal, 133
   Mycobacterium tuberculosis, 113
   with coccidioidomycosis, 84
   with sarcoidosis, 49
Chronic atrophic polychondritis *see* relapsing polychondritis
Chronic bilateral diffuse granulomatous uveitis, 5
Chronic cyclitis, 125–6
Chronic iridocyclitis, 5
   steroid treatment, 21
Chronic relapsing polychondritis, 12, 65
Ciliary circulation vasculitis, 30
Classification of uveitis, 5
Clindamycin, 92
CMV *see* cytomegalovirus
Coats' disease, 25, 34
   serous retinal detachment, 34
Coccidioidomycosis, 83–4
   choroiditis, 27
Colchicine, 97
Collagen vascular diseases, 65–8
Congenital syphilis, 63
Conjunctiva biopsy, 7
Connective tissue inflammation *see* collagen vascular diseases
Corneal inflammation, 137
Corneal melt with rheumatoid arthritis, 39
Cotton wool
   exudation, 57
   spots, 65, 68
Cryptococcus neoformans, 55

Cyclitic membrane, 11, 43
Cyclosporin, 97, 121
Cysts of iris pigment epithelium, 14
Cytoid bodies, 65, 66
Cytomegalic inclusion
 disease, 58
 retinitis, 119, 120
Cytomegalic occlusion disease, 115
Cytomegalovirus, 115
 inclusion disease (CID), 119–120
 retinitis, 55–6

D
Dermal vesicles from acute herpetic skin infection, 118
Desert fever *see* San Joaquin Valley Fever
Diagnosis of uveitis, 5
Diffuse focal choroidal infiltrates, 28
Diffuse vasculitis, 67
Disorganized retinal architecture, 25
Drug abuse, 139–144
 aspergillus endophthalmitis, 141, 142
 particulate emboli, 139, 140, 144
Dry eye syndrome, 38
 secondary, 21
 with rheumatoid arthritis, 37

E
Eale's disease, 27
Embolism, particulate matter, 139, 140, 144
Endophthalmitis, 15
 in toxocariasis, 87, 88
 metastatic, 139
 with drug abuse, 139, 141, 142, 143
Episcleritis, 39, 137, 138
Epstein–Barr virus, 115, 116
Erythema
 migrans, 61
 nodosum with maculopapular eruption, 99
Exanthematous eruption, 91
 in toxoplasmosis, 93
Exudative retinopathy, 67

F
Facial nerve dermitome, 120
Fibrous bands in toxoplasmosis, 95
Filamentary keratitis, 21, 38
Focal hemorrhage in retina, 23
Foscarnet, 119
FTA–ABS for syphilis, 63
Fuch's heterochromic cyclitis, 5, 13, 145
Fuch's heterochromic iridocyclitis, 135–6
Fungal fluff ball, 143

G
Gancyclovir, 119
Geographic choroiditis, 35, 121
Geographic ulcer with herpes simplex keratitis, 118

Giant iris stromal nodule, 52
Glaucoma, 5
 in Fuch's heterochromic iridocyclitis, 135
 with herpes virus, 115
 with sarcoidosis, 49
Granuloma in toxocariasis, 87
Granulomatous iridocyclitis, 9
 mutton-fat KP, 14
Granulomatous uveitis, 7
 toxoplasmosis, 91–2

H
Hansen's disease *see* leprosy
Harada syndrome, 29, 30, 69, 71
Helicoid choroidopathy, 121
Hemophthalmitis, 20
Hemorrhagic papillitis, 61
Herpes
 dendrite, 10, 116
 virus, 115–8
Herpes simplex
 disease, 117, 118
 hominis (HSH) disease, 116
 infection, 7
 keratouveitis, 10
 retinitis, 55
 virus, 115
Herpes zoster, 56
 ophthalmicus, 115, 120
 uveitis, 117
 virus, 115
Herpetic iridocyclitis with iris trophy, 10
Herpetic keratitis, 117, 118
Herpetic ulceration of the cornea, 15
Heterochromia, 5
HLA b27 antigen, 45
HLA b8, 49
Human immunodeficiency virus (HIV), 55
Hypertensive retinopathy, 67
Hypopyon, 18
 herpes simplex disease, 118
 in Behçet's disease, 97, 99

I
Immunoglobulin molecules, 105
Immunosuppression, 119, 120
Immunosuppressives, 97
Interstitial keratitis, 21
Intraocular lens choice, 145
Intraocular lens-induced uveitis, 145, 146
Intraocular lenses, 145
Iridocyclitis, 5
 acute plastic, 111, 112
 and juvenile rheumatoid arthritis, 41, 42, 43
 in Behçet's disease, 97
 in birdshot choroidopathy, 133
 in coccidioidomycosis, 83
 in syphilis, 63

recurrent flare-up, 43
with ankylosing spondylitis, 45
with herpes virus, 115
with Reiter's disease, 47
with rheumatoid arthritis, 37
with sarcoidosis, 49
Iris
  atrophy, 117, 118
  heterochromia, 9
  infiltrate in reticulum cell sarcoma, 107
  nodules with sarcoidosis, 49
  pigment epithelium cysts, 14
Ixodes dammini, 62

J
Juvenile rheumatoid arthritis, 5, 15, 41–3
  band keratopathy, 12
  cataract surgery, 43
  cyclitic membrane, 11, 16

K
Kaposi's sarcoma, 55, 57
Keratic precipitates (KP)
  granulomatous, 13
  in Fuch's heterochromic iridocyclitis, 135
  masquerade mutton fat, 106
  mutton fat, 14, 92, 96
  mutton fat granulomatous, 49, 52
  pigmented, 11
  pigmented mutton fat, 107
  with juvenile rheumatoid arthritis, 42
Keratitis, disciform, 117
Keratitis sicca
  filamentary keratitis, 38
  in collagen vascular diseases, 65
  with rheumatoid arthritis, 37
  with sarcoidosis, 50
Keratoconjunctivitis sicca, 137
Keratomalacia, 37
Koeppe nodules, 16
  with sarcoidosis, 49

L
Lens-induced uveitis, 145
Leonine facies of lepromatous leprosy, 110
Lepromatous iridocyclitis, 8, 17
  hypopyon, 18
Lepromatous leprosy, 16, 109, 110, 111
Lepromatous uveitis, 8
Leprosy, 16, 109
Leutic choroiditis and vasculitis, 64
Loa loa worm, 89
Lupus erythematosus, 65, 68
Lyme disease, 59–62
  brain scan, 61
  diagnosis, 60
  stages, 60
Lymphadenopathic infection, 91, 94

Lymphocytic leukemia, 108

M
Macroaneurysm, 31
Macular abscess in toxocariasis, 86
Macular hemorrhage, acute, 80
Macular scar, 81
  atrophic, 80
  in toxoplasmosis, 92
Maculopapular eruption, 99
Malignant melanoma
  infiltrating conjunctival, 20
  serous retinal detachment, 33
Marie–Strümpel spine, 45
Masquerade syndrome of iritis, 14
Measles virus infection, 124
Meningoencephalitic syndrome, 91
Metastatic bronchogenic carcinoma, 32
Minocycline, 92
Molteno implantation, 36, 70
Monarticular rheumatoid arthritis, 41, 42, 43
Multiple evanescent white dot syndrome (MEWDS), 129–130
Mycobacteria, 109–114
Mycobacterium leprae, 109
Mycobacterium tuberculosis, 113
Myelinated nerve fibers, 30

N
Nasal cartilage, resorbed, 8
Natural and intraocular lenses, 145
Necrotic vasculitis, 67
Necrotizing vasculitis, 23
  in Behçet's disease, 100
Nodular lepromata, 16, 17, 112
  anesthetic, 110
Nodular scleritis, 38
Noncaseating granuloma, 49
  with sarcoidosis, 51
Nongranulomatous iritis, 37

O
Occlusive vasculitis, 66
  in Behçet's disease, 98
Ocular histoplasmosis syndrome, 28
Ocular toxocariasis, 85–9
Optic nerve
  fluffy white enlargement, 53
  in sarcoidosis, 49, 53
Optic neuritis, 137
Osseous choristoma, 33

P
Panophthalmitis cataract, 36
Panuveitis, 113
Papillary conjunctivitis, 47
Papilledema, 65
Papillitis

in toxoplasmosis, 95
with Lyme disease, 61
with sarcoidosis, 53
Parinaud's ocular glandular syndrome, 113
Pars plana
    dense exudation, 125, 126
    infiltrate, 18
    vitrectomy, 143
Pars planitis, 5, 18, 125–6
    and juvenile rheumatoid arthritis, 41
Penicillamine, 63
Penicillin, 63
Peripapillary inflammation, 123
Peripheral anterior synechiae, 52
Peripheral uveitis, 125–6
Periphlebitis, 22
    with sarcoidosis, 49
Perivascular sheathing, 68
Phacoanaphylactic endophthalmitis, 145
Phacotoxic uveitis, 145
Phakomatosis, 31
Phlebitis, candle wax drippings, 53
Pinna swelling, 137, 138
Pizza pie retinopathy, 119
Pneumocystis carinii, 55
    choroiditis, 56
Poliosis in Vogt–Koyanagi–Harada syndrome, 69, 70
Polyarteritis nodosum, 65, 67
Polyarticular juvenile rheumatoid arthritis, 41
Polychondritis, chronic relapsing, 12
Posterior chamber lens, 146
Posterior subcapsular cataract, 21
Prednisone, 121
Prepapillary depigmentation, 78
Presumed ocular histoplasmosis (POHS), 77–81
Pseudanthoma elasticum syndrome, angioid streaks, 35
Pseudo-reticulum cell sarcoma, 108
Pyrimethamine, 92, 94

R

Radiation therapy, 103
Recurrent inflammation in toxoplasmosis, 96
Reiter's disease, 5, 12, 47–48
Relapsing polychondritis, 137–8
Reticulum cell sarcoma, 5, 19, 103–8
Retina
    abscess in toxocariasis, 86, 87
    hemorrhage in Behçet's disease, 99
    inflammation in toxoplasmosis, 93, 95
    physiology in MEWDS, 129
    scar in toxoplasmosis, 94
    serous detachment, 72, 73
    tear, 24
Retinal angioma, 32
Retinal detachment
    in bilateral acute retinal necrosis, 131
    obscured, 24
    serous, 33, 34
Retinal infarction, 23
    in Behçet's disease, 100, 101
Retinal necrosis
    acute, 116
    in bilateral acute retinal necrosis, 131, 132
Retinal pigment epithelium
    after uveal effusion, 76
    changes in Behçet's disease, 101
    hyperpigmentation, 72
    hypertrophy, 92
    in acute multifocal placoid pigment epitheliopathy (AMPPE), 127, 128
    in bilateral acute retinal necrosis, 132
    in birdshot choroidopathy, 133, 134
    in multiple evanescent white dot syndrome (MEWDS), 129
    in serpiginous choroidopathy, 121, 122
    in toxoplasmosis, 95
    inflammation, 73
    pinpoint leakages, 71
    scarring, 72
Retinal vascular sheathing, with Lyme disease, 60
Retinal vasculitis with sarcoidosis, 49
Retinal-choroidal scar in toxocariasis, 86
Retinitis
    cytomegalovirus inclusion disease (CID), 119
    in subacute sclerosing panencephalitis (SSPE), 124
    toxoplasmosis, 91, 93
Retinoblastoma, 31
Retinochoroiditis in toxoplasmosis, 91–2
Retinopathy of AIDS, 55
Rheumatoid arthritis, 37–40
Rheumatoid scleral uveitis, 39
Richter syndrome, 107
Roth spot, 96
Rubeola infection, 124
Rubeosis iridis, 9

S

Sabin tetrad, 91
Sacroiliac sclerosis, 46
Saddle nose, 138
Salt and pepper fundus inflammation of retinal pigment epithelium, 63
San Joaquin Valley Fever, 83
Sarcoid, 7
    granuloma, 51
    iridocyclitis, 52
    nodules, 22, 49, 51
    uveitis, 10
Sarcoidosis, 5, 7, 49–53
    filamentary keratitis, 21
    hilar adenopathy, 50
    lachrymal and salivary glands, 50
    nasal and pharyngeal mucosa, 50

pulmonary, 22
Satellite lesion in toxoplasmosis, 96
Scleral nodules, 111
Scleritis, 39
  with rheumatoid arthritis, 37
Sclero-keratitis with rheumatoid arthritis, 37
Secondary uveitis, 7
Serous retinal detachment, 33
  Coats' disease, 34
Serpiginous choroiditis *see* geographic choroiditis
Serpiginous choroidopathy, 121–3
  see also geographic choroiditis
Sickle salmon patch, 32
Sickle-cell disease, retinopathy, 32
Signs of uveitis, 6
Snowball opacities in vitreous, 125, 126
Steroids, 21, 97
  for serpiginous choroidopathy, 121
Still's disease, 42
Sturge–Weber telangiectasia, 11
Subacute sclerosing panencephalitis (SSPE), 124
Subconjunctival hemorrhage, 9
Subconjunctival lymphoma, 7
Subretinal neovascular membrane, 28
  old scarred-up macular disciform lesion, 29
    with presumed ocular histoplasmosis (POHS), 77, 78, 79, 80
Sulfadiazine, 92
Synechiaed pupil, 48
Syphilis, 63–4
Syphilitic infection, 58
Systemic sarcoidosis, 49

T
T-cell helper inducer cells, 55
Talc granuloma, 140
Thalasia californiensis, 88
Tick-borne disease, 59
Toxocara canis, 25, 26, 85
Toxocariasis, 25
  acute infestation, 26
  ocular, 85–9
Toxoplasma gondii, 55, 91
Toxoplasmic papillitis, 20
Toxoplasmic retinochoroiditis, 5
Toxoplasmosis, 19, 91–6
  focal hemorrhage in retina, 23
  inactive scar, 24
  reactivation, 19
  recurrent, 25
  trophozoites, 94
Traction retinal detachment, 36
Tuberculoid leprosy, 109

Tuberculous nodules, 113

U
Uveal effusion, 75–6
  with rheumatoid arthritis, 40

V
Varicella-zoster chorioretinitis, 56
Vasculitis
  acquired ocular tuberculosis, 113, 114
  central nervous system, 69
  in Behçet's disease, 97, 99, 100, 101
  in bilateral acute retinal necrosis, 131
  in collagen vascular diseases, 65, 66, 67, 68
  in drug abuse, 141
  in pars planitis, 125
  inactive, 23
  mycobacterial, 113, 114
  Mycobacterium tuberculosis, 113
  with Lyme disease, 60
Vitiligo
  facial, 69, 70
  in Vogt–Koyanagi–Harada syndrome, 69, 70, 71
Vitreitis, 19, 20
Vitreous
  B-cell infiltrate, 105
  hemorrhage, 24
  inflammation, 143
  with reticulum cell sarcoma, 104, 105, 108
Vitritis
  herpes zoster, 115
  in drug abuse, 143
  in toxoplasmosis, 93, 95
  in Vogt–Koyanagi–Harada syndrome, 73
  reticulum cell sarcoma, 103, 105, 106, 107
Vogt–Koyanagi iridocyclitis, 17
Vogt–Koyanagi–Harada syndrome, 5, 13, 69–74
  Busacca nodules, 17
  Molteno implantation, 36
  pigment migration, 29
  recurrent serous detachment of retina, 30
  serous retinal detachment, 33
  uveitis, 69, 70
Voissus' ring, 13
Von Hippel–Lindau syndrome, 32

W
Wallerian degeneration of neurons, 65, 66
Wegener's disease, 65

Z
Zoster vesicle, 120